A Public Health Guide to Ending the Opioid Epidemic

A Public Health Guide to Ending the Opioid Epidemic

**MICHAEL R. FRASER, PHD, MS
AND JAY C. BUTLER, MD**
Editors

with

PHILICIA TUCKER, MPH
Managing Editor

OXFORD
UNIVERSITY PRESS

Oxford University Press is a department of the University of Oxford. It furthers
the University's objective of excellence in research, scholarship, and education
by publishing worldwide. Oxford is a registered trade mark of Oxford University
Press in the UK and certain other countries.

Published in the United States of America by Oxford University Press
198 Madison Avenue, New York, NY 10016, United States of America.

Library of Congress Cataloging-in-Publication Data
Names: Fraser, Michael R., editor. | Butler, Jay C., editor.
Title: A public health guide to ending the opioid epidemic / Michael R. Fraser,
Jay C. Butler, editors; with Philicia Tucker, managing editor.
Description: New York, NY : Oxford University Press, 2019. |
Includes index.
Identifiers: LCCN 2019019523 | ISBN 9780190056810 (pbk.) |
ISBN 9780190056827 (updf) | ISBN 9780190056834 (epub) | ISBN 9780190056841 (online)
Subjects: | MESH: Opioid-Related Disorders—prevention & control |
Drug Overdose—prevention & control | Epidemics—prevention & control |
Models, Organizational | United States
Classification: LCC RC568.O45 | NLM WM 284 | DDC 362.29/3—dc23
LC record available at https://lccn.loc.gov/2019019523

9 8 7 6 5 4 3 2 1

Printed by LSC Communications, United States of America

CONTENTS

ACKNOWLEDGMENTS

Just like the work of public health, editing a book is a "team sport." We would like to thank our team, all of whom had instrumental roles in moving this idea across the finish line as the complete volume you are reading. First, we acknowledge all of the authors who were core members of the team. Our authors and contributors willingly shared their expertise with us and graciously accepted edits and additions to their chapters. Philicia Tucker provided excellent administrative oversight of the development of this book and admirably served as our Chief Author Wrangler and liaison with our colleagues at Oxford University Press. The Oxford University Press team was instrumental, vital, and ever encouraging: Thanks to Chad Zimmerman, Chloe Layman, and Niveda. The staff at the Association of County and City Health Officials (ASTHO), including Christi Mackie and Andy Baker-White, were important to supporting several pieces in this book and provided expert advice and feedback. Finally, we thank our "home team"—those who supported and sustained us during long hours and late nights of editing and organizing this book's content despite amazingly busy "real jobs."

For everyone's efforts, we are truly grateful.

Jay C. Butler
Michael R. Fraser
Editors

ACKNOWLEDGMENTS

FOREWORD: A RECOVERY JOURNEY

GREG WILLIAMS

M *y name is Greg Williams and I am a person in long-term recovery from addiction.* There are many deeply important layers to those 15 short words. My journey through addiction culminated in heavy use of opioids as an adolescent. It was not a journey I sought out; in many ways it "just happened." For reasons I could not explain then, but have more clarity around now, in three short years my seemingly innocent use of marijuana and alcohol as I was just becoming a teenager manifested into an opioid dependency beyond my control.

It was 1999, I was 15 years old, and the early signs of the opioid crisis were just beginning in Appalachia—but I was in Stamford, Connecticut, just 40 minutes from the other "ground zero." Doctors were being shamed for not treating pain patients appropriately and pain pills had begun to show up en masse in medicine cabinets across the country. Peers introduced me to diverted opioids and benzodiazepines. We would promptly look up the imprint codes on the pills using the internet to ensure they had "good" side effects. It started innocently enough, but what transpired next—addiction—was not something I signed up for or chose.

In *The Anonymous People*, a feature-length documentary film I produced on this topic (Figures I.1 and I.2), I chose to visualize the lack of choice I felt by slowly zooming in tight on an image of my high school yearbook photo while narrating: "Public perception of addiction to alcohol and other drugs continues to be something very different than the science. What that perception does is look at this 15-year-old kid, with a genetic predisposition and still-developing brain, and suggest I made an independent, rational choice to become addicted."[1]

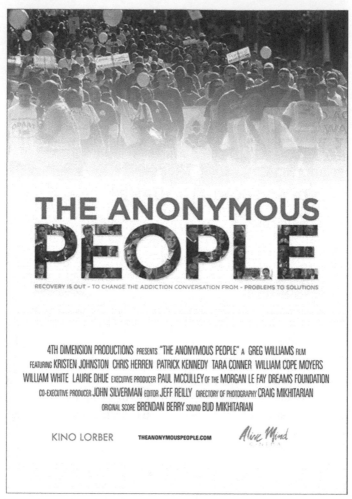

FIGURE I.1. *The Anonymous People* movie poster.

What is important now is that we use a science-based understanding of addiction to end the crisis. Addiction is *not* a choice. Addiction is a chronic disease of the brain and, as with any chronic disease, it requires quality, evidence-based treatment and active public health education and health promotion campaigns to prevent it.

My recovery was established in 2001, after a near-fatal car accident at age 17 landed me in the hospital, and then an adolescent psychiatric unit, then a quality adolescent addiction treatment program, then a recovery house for 90 days. Recovery was not my idea. I was a reluctant participant and thought of myself as "too young to be an addict." Today, I realize my belief that I was too young to struggle with addiction came from the media messages surrounding the topic. I was born in 1983, and my childhood included the fear-driven era

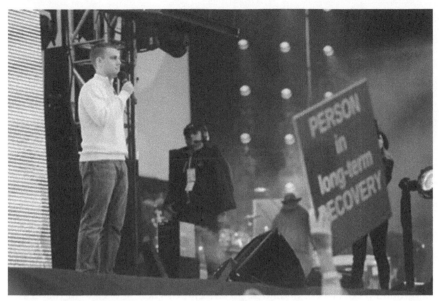

FIGURE I.2. Greg Williams at the UNITE to Face Addiction Rally, Washington, DC, October 4, 2015. (Photo credit: National Council on Alcoholism and Drug Dependence and Kate Meyer.)

where people who used drugs were viewed as "public enemy number one." The images and messages transmitted to me were not of young high school kids smoking marijuana, drinking alcohol, or taking pills. They were of older people most often using crack cocaine or injecting heroin. I could not relate to those images at the time and therefore thought, "I must not be an addict."

It took a lot of time, a lot of education, a lot of therapy, and a lot of self-acceptance to overcome those deeply entrenched beliefs about what addiction is and that it actually impacts young people. Today, I am grateful to be alive and not incarcerated, given the volume of substances ingested and the risky and illegal behavior I engaged in as an adolescent suffering from a substance use disorder. As a result of my personal freedom from active addiction, not only have I survived one of the deadliest health problems facing young people in America today, but I have thrived. I have been blessed with incredible opportunities to learn, chase dreams, and live a life full of purpose. I am not alone: There are 23 million other Americans living in recovery. That is more than those who are currently struggling with all substance use disorders combined, including opioids.[2] But historically we have been a silent and marginalized group of people. I was actually taught in recovery to stay *anonymous* out of the fear of future discrimination I might face if I told my story.

Individuals in recovery and their families are a heterogeneous group and have never collectively mobilized and organized to affect policy, change our culture, and attract others to life in recovery. There are deep parallels to what we face and what is possible to overcome when looking at the HIV/AIDS movement in the late 1980s and early 1990s, led in large part by the LGBT community. However, a revolution in cultural perception requires a united message of the reality of recovery to shift public discourse, change stigma, and ultimately improve policy responses. Desperately needed are robust local, state, and national advocacy efforts aimed at informing the transition from a criminal justice–centered approach toward a health-centered approach that will improve prevention, treatment, and recovery policies across all systems.

In his book *Let's Go Make Some History: Chronicles of the New Addiction Recovery Advocacy Movement*, William White argues that existing "underground" recovery communities hold the answers for the future grounded in a new public recovery movement.[3] Understandably, some people in recovery are reluctant to go public with their addiction status. But when someone does tell his or her story and put a face and a voice on recovery, the public can finally access the powerful message of hope that has resonated for years in these underground recovery communities. At the end of each interview of the nearly 100 recovery community leaders for my *The Anonymous People* documentary, I would ask interviewees about their vision for the future. Almost all of them said they wanted to "one day see thousands of people like me, our families, and those who have lost loved ones gather on the National Mall to create a moment just like other civil rights movements in our country's history have done" (Figure I.3).

In 2015, as the death toll from opioids was rising to unfathomable levels, it became apparent that this was our moment. And in the face of incredible odds, we did it: we gathered on the National Mall in Washington, DC, and marked a turning point in American history. The start of the chapter "Recovery" in the first-ever *Surgeon General's Report on Alcohol, Drugs, and Health: Facing Addiction in America* begins with this passage:

> On October 4, 2015, tens of thousands of people attended the UNITE to Face Addiction rally in Washington, D.C. The event was one of many signs that a new movement is emerging in America: People in recovery, their family members, and other supporters are banding together to decrease the discrimination associated with substance use disorders and spread the message that people do recover.[4(p. 5)]

On that dreary cold day on the National Mall we launched the "Facing Addiction" movement, which in just over two short years has merged with the oldest national advocacy organization battling alcohol and other drug problems, the National Council on Alcoholism and Drug Dependence (NCADD). Our visionary founder, Marty Mann, understood that addiction was an illness that must be treated as a public health problem. Her vision, forged in 1944, is based on two significant focal points:

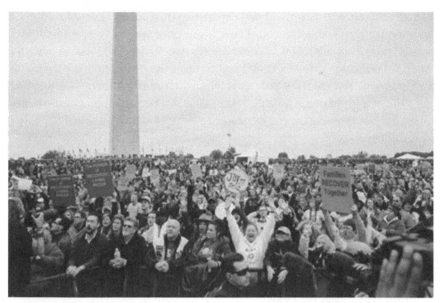

FIGURE I.3. Crowd at the UNITE to Face Addiction Rally, Washington, DC, October 4, 2015. (Photo credit: National Council on Alcoholism and Drug Dependence and Kate Meyer.)

- People with the illness of addiction can be helped and are worth helping.
- Addiction is a public health problem and, therefore, a public responsibility to address.

Facing Addiction with NCADD, the merger of Facing Addiction and the National Council on Alcoholism and Drug Dependence, now provides a national platform for a coalition with over 850 Action Network Partners, 80 affiliate organizations, and a national voice of grassroots advocacy for individuals and families impacted by addiction. People in recovery from addiction, our families, and our allies have a duty to respond to the ignorance, prejudice, and injustice that continue to pervade our culture. Lives depend on it. In spite of a broken system and failed community response, many of us have been given the gift of recovery, and that can have profound cultural, political, health care, criminal justice, and economic implications.

Few people are aware that through recovery, more than 25 million of us have gotten well, families have been reunited, and our communities have been the ultimate beneficiary. Congress does not believe we exist in such significant numbers (yet) and the media continue to ignore this major facet of the addiction story. It is our duty to share our stories with a unified message to a new audience so that future generations can live free from the greatest barriers to recovery: stigma, shame, and discrimination. Like many health professionals, public health practitioners are important allies in this work, including those who have the lived experience of recovery, know loved ones who are battling with addiction, know loved ones who have recovered, and see the ravages of addiction in communities nationwide and what is possible when we dedicate ourselves to and invest adequately in addiction prevention and treatment and recovery programs. No matter how addiction has touched your life or a loved one's, I invite you to consider becoming one of the many emerging faces sharing the recovery stories in harmony with a growing chorus of revolutionaries.

References

1. *The Anonymous People*. [DVD] Directed by G. Williams. Van Nuys, CA: Dimension Productions; 2013.
2. Recovery Research Institute. 1 in 10 Americans report having resolved a significant substance use problem. https://www.recoveryanswers.org/research-post/1-in-10-americans-report-having-resolved-a-significant-substance-use-problem/ [no date]. Accessed December 19, 2018.
3. White WL. *Let's Go Make Some History: Chronicles of the New Addiction Recovery Advocacy Movement*. Washington, DC: Johnson Institute Foundation; 2006.
4. US Department of Health and Human Services (HHS), Office of the Surgeon General. *Facing Addiction in America: The Surgeon General's Report on Alcohol, Drugs, and Health*. Washington, DC: HHS; 2016.

FOREWORD: COUNTERING THE OPIOID EPIDEMIC

MEENA VYTHILINGAM, KUMIKO LIPPOLD,
AND BRETT P. GIROIR

The ongoing epidemic of opioid addiction and opioid-related deaths is devastating communities, families, and individuals across our nation. In 2017 alone, the US Centers for Disease Control and Prevention (CDC) estimated that 70,237 Americans died from drug overdoses[1] and the majority (47,600) of these deaths involved opioids.[2] More than 130 Americans die every day from an opioid-related overdose and an estimated 2.1 million Americans aged 12 and older meet the criteria for opioid use disorder (OUD).[3] The economic cost of our nation's opioid crisis in 2015 alone was a staggering $504 billion, equating to approximately 2.8% of the US gross domestic product (GDP).[4] The opioid crisis is the most important public health crisis of our time and combating it remains a top priority across our agency, the US Department of Health and Human Services (HHS), and for the Trump administration as a whole.

The far-reaching devastation caused by the opioid epidemic has necessitated the design and rapid implementation of a strategic plan that incorporates the latest research findings and evidence-based practices.[5] Partnerships and collaborations across public, private, nonprofit, and academic health systems are critical in defeating the opioid scourge. The HHS Office of Assistant Secretary for Health (OASH) plays a key role in coordinating the numerous federal initiatives related to opioids and pain and has prioritized a five-pronged public health strategy to address this public health emergency (Figure II.1). The strategies are described below.

HHS 5-POINT STRATEGY TO COMBAT THE OPIOIDS CRISIS

| **Better** addiction prevention, treatment, and recovery services | **Better** data | **Better** pain management | **Better** targeting of overdose reversing drugs | **Better** research |

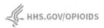

FIGURE II.1. HHS 5-point strategy to combat the opioids crisis.
Source: HHS.GOV/Opioids.

Access: Better Prevention, Treatment, and Recovery Services

In 2018, HHS invested more than $4.4 billion to combat opioid abuse, misuse, and overdose deaths by funding treatment, prevention, and recovery efforts. States, tribes, and communities across America can apply for these newly appropriated funds to address the opioid crisis. In addition, the US Centers for Medicare and Medicaid Services (CMS) launched two innovative programs, the Maternal Opioid Misuse (MOM) model and the Integrated Care for Kids (InCK) initiative, to address gaps in coordinated care for pregnant and post-partum women with OUD and their children. Recent improvements in access to evidence-based treatments are supported by the fact that the number of unique patients with OUD receiving buprenorphine, a medication-assisted treatment (MAT) option, has increased by 31% per month between January 2017 and May 2019.[6]

Data: Better Data on the Epidemic

The ever-changing landscape of the opioid epidemic requires constant vigilance and situational awareness. The CDC leads a robust surveillance program to monitor the opioid crisis. CDC publishes monthly updates on drug and opioid mortality at the national and state levels, including longitudinal trends, and the reported and predicted number of overdose deaths. In addition to fatal overdose deaths, data on nonfatal overdoses and syndromic surveillance data from 32 states and the District of Columbia are analyzed by CDC's Enhanced State Opioid Overdose Surveillance (ESOOS) program, which serves as an

FIGURE II.2. Surgeon General's advisory on naloxone and opioid overdose.
Source: US Department of Health and Human Services, Office of the Surgeon General.
https://www.surgeongeneral.gov/priorities/opioid-overdose-prevention/naloxone-advisory.html

early warning system to help identify opioid overdose outbreaks. Together, these CDC programs provide critical surveillance data that can inform national, state, and local opioid prevention efforts and assist with targeted resource allocation.

Pain: Better Pain Management

Since overprescription of opioids by clinicians initially contributed to this epidemic, undoing this crisis will involve educating clinicians about the risks of opioids and the importance of adhering to evidence-based prescribing guidelines. Providing evidence-based pain management is also a critical step in preventing inappropriate exposure to prescription opioids. The publication of the CDC's Guideline for Prescribing Opioids for Chronic Pain and the Pain Management Best Practices Inter-Agency Task Force recommendations represent two examples of collaborative efforts to translate the latest science into clinical practice.[7,8] Federally funded prescription drug monitoring programs (PDMPs) allow for state- and territorial-level interventions to monitor appropriate prescribing of opioids, influence clinical practice, and protect at-risk patients.

Overdoses: Better Targeting of Naloxone

Improving access to naloxone, the lifesaving opioid overdose-reversing medication, is an effective approach to prevent opioid related deaths. In April 2018, the Surgeon General's Advisory on Naloxone and Opioid Overdose emphasized the importance of increasing naloxone access to at-risk patients, their friends, family, and the local community (Figure II.2).[9,10] The number of monthly naloxone prescriptions has increased by more than 504% from

January 2017 to May 2019,[6] in addition to millions of doses being distributed directly to states, municipalities, first responders, and nonprofit organizations. Clinicians are advised to co-prescribe naloxone for patients who are also receiving opioids at doses greater than 50 morphine milligram equivalents (MME) or other risk factors such as sleep apnea and OUD.

Research: Better Research on Pain and Addiction

HHS, through the National Institutes of Health (NIH), supports cutting-edge research to elucidate the neurobiology of pain and addiction in order to develop novel treatments. This is exemplified through Helping to End Addiction Long Term (HEAL), an NIH-led, multi-agency effort to advance recent research and translation of scientific solutions into clinical practice by facilitating public–private partnerships.

Preliminary data suggest that these upstream and downstream efforts across the continuum of care are beginning to make inroads into the opioid crisis. The total number of opioid prescriptions dispensed monthly by pharmacies has declined by approximately 21% from January 2017 to May 2019,[6] the number of patients receiving medication-assisted treatment (MAT) has increased, and the extent of opioid pain reliever misuse and first-time heroin use has also decreased substantially according to the 2017 National Survey on Drug Use and Health.[3] According to provisional data from the CDC, the seemingly relentless trend of rising overdose deaths seems to be slowing and the curve is finally bending in the right direction. However, plateauing at a still high opioid-related mortality rate is hardly an opportunity to declare victory. It is critical to maintain a sense of urgency and continue an "all hands on deck" approach in order to win this war against opioids.

To reiterate, the opioid epidemic will only be curbed by a "whole society" approach, for which the role of state and territorial health officials and other public health practitioners is both central and essential. As key leaders of the public health response in their respective jurisdictions, public health officials can provide strategic direction and technical guidance to stakeholders at all levels of the government, including city, county, and tribal agencies, to ensure that we win the opioid war. Public health practitioners are critical to implementing evidence-based treatment, recovery, and prevention programs. There are multiple opportunities for all health care professionals, legislators, law enforcement officials, and the general public to help curb the tide of opioid overdose.

Communities can implement CDC's 10 evidence-based strategies for preventing opioid overdose (Text Box II.1), including establishing syringe services programs, and the public should provide input into the activities of HHS through advocacy and submitting public comments on opioid policies and

---

**TEXT BOX II.1 TEN EVIDENCE-BASED STRATEGIES
FOR PREVENTING OPIOID OVERDOSE**

1. Targeted naloxone distribution
2. Medication-assisted treatment (MAT)
3. Academic detailing
4. Eliminating prior-authorization requirements for medications for opioid use disorder
5. Screening for fentanyl in routine clinical toxicology testing
6. 911 Good Samaritan laws
7. Naloxone distribution in treatment centers and criminal justice settings
8. MAT in criminal justice settings and on release
9. Initiating buprenorphine-based MAT in emergency departments
10. Syringe services programs

For more information on these strategies, visit:
https://www.cdc.gov/drugoverdose/pdf/pubs/2018-evidence-based-strategies.pdf

---

programs.[11] Finally, health professionals, friends, families, and the judicial and law enforcement communities can help reduce stigma by recognizing OUD as a brain illness and encouraging individuals to seek treatment. Only then can we bring our brothers, mothers, daughters, and friends back to their loved ones.

References

1. Ahmad FB, Rossen LM, Spencer MR, et al. Provisional drug overdose death counts. CDC website. https://www.cdc.gov/nchs/nvss/vsrr/drug-overdose-data.htm. Accessed February 5, 2019.
2. Hedegaard H, Miniño AM, Warner M. Drug overdose deaths in the United States, 1999–2017. NCHS Data Brief, no. 329. Hyattsville, MD: National Center for Health Statistics; 2018. https://www.cdc.gov/nchs/data/databriefs/db329-h.pdf. Accessed February 5, 2019.
3. US Substance Abuse and Mental Health Services Administration (SAMHSA). Key substance use and mental health indicators in the United States: Results from the 2017 national survey on drug use and health. https://www.samhsa.gov/data/sites/default/files/cbhsq-reports/NSDUHFFR2017/NSDUHFFR2017.pdf. Accessed February 5, 2019.
4. Council of Economic Advisers. The underestimated cost of the opioid crisis. https://www.whitehouse.gov/briefings-statements/cea-report-underestimated-cost-opioid-crisis. 2017. Accessed February 5, 2019.
5. US Department of Health and Human Services. Strategy to combat opioid abuse, misuse, and overdose: A framework based on the five-point strategy. 2019. https://www.hhs.gov/opioids/sites/default/files/2018-09/opioid-fivepoint-strategy-20180917-508compliant.pdf. Accessed February 5, 2019.

6. IQVIA National Prescription Audit. Data retrieved on November 9, 2018. *Note: Data presented for the retail and mail channels only.*

7. Dowell D, Haegerich TM, Chou R. CDC guideline for prescribing opioids for chronic pain—United States, 2016. *MMWR Morb Mortal Wklyl Rep.* 2016; 65(No. RR-1):1–49.

8. U.S. Department of Health and Human Services (2019, May). Pain Management Best Practices Inter-Agency Task Force Report: Updates, Gaps, Inconsistencies, and Recommendations. Retrieved from U. S. Department of Health and Human Services website: https://www.hhs.gov/ash/advisory-committees/pain/reports/index.html

9. Adams JM. Surgeon General's advisory on naloxone and opioid overdose. U.S. Department of Health and Human Services. https://www.surgeongeneral.gov/priorities/opioid-overdose-prevention/naloxone-advisory.html. Accessed February 5, 2019.

10. Adams JM. Increasing naloxone awareness and use: The role of health care practitioners. *JAMA.* 2018; 319(20):2073–2074.

11. Caroll JJ, Green TC, Noonan RK. Evidence-based strategies for preventing opioid overdose: What's working in the United States. National Center for Injury Prevention and Control, Centers for Disease Control and Prevention, US Department of Health and Human Services. 2018. http://www.cdc.gov/drugoverdose/pdf/pubs/2018-evidence-based-strategies.pdf. Accessed February 5, 2019.

I | Fundamentals and Frameworks

1. Fundamentals and Frameworks

1 | Introduction

WHY A PUBLIC HEALTH GUIDE TO ENDING THE OPIOID CRISIS?

MICHAEL R. FRASER AND JAY C. BUTLER

F EW CONTRIBUTIONS TO THE field concerning the current opioid crisis in
the United States focus sufficient attention on the public health aspects
of the epidemic and share actual examples that practitioners can use to
learn how to successfully integrate primary, secondary, and tertiary prevention strategies across multiple sectors to prevent opioid use disorder and the
broader issues of substance misuse and addiction. Justifiably, a great deal of
prior work has concentrated on health care and clinical perspectives related to
the crisis due to the exponential rise in opioid-related overdose deaths and the
urgent demand for access to evidence-based treatment and recovery programs.
This work includes developing prescribing guidelines, enhancing prescription
drug monitoring programs, scaling up access to overdose reversal medication,
and making medication-assisted treatment (MAT) more widely available nationwide. However, in our review of many of the efforts to end the epidemic,
comparable attention has not been paid to the central tenets of the public health
approach. These tenets include (1) how to best support community-based, primary prevention of substance misuse and addiction in various settings with
diverse populations, (2) how to prevent addiction across the life course using a
public health approach, and (3) how to effectively address the cultural, social,
and environmental aspects of health that are driving the current epidemic.

The paucity of research on and practical guidance for how local, state, and
federal governmental public health agencies and their partners can move "upstream" to respond to the crisis, and lead community partnerships to end it,
drove us to propose this *Guide* and engage so many talented colleagues to
produce it. All of the authors who contributed to this work are personally and/
or professionally engaged in responding to the crisis from different vantage
points inside and outside of government, from the center and periphery of

public health practice, and from their lived experience of recovering from substance use disorder and addiction or supporting individual recovery journeys as family members and friends, and as practitioners working with and managing individual patients and entire communities facing addiction.

The contributions in this volume describe how public health has played a significant role in responding to the epidemic, in public health's traditional approach to disease surveillance and control but also in contemporary approaches to health promotion that include building community resilience, addressing the impact of adverse childhood events (ACEs), and mitigating the root causes of addiction community-wide. This *Guide* also describes the multiple partnerships public health agencies need to develop with many different stakeholders, including substance abuse and drug and alcohol program directors, primary and specialty health care providers, law enforcement and corrections officials, health care insurers and payers, medical societies, community development organizations, and myriad others.

While we intended the *Guide* to be comprehensive, there are many facets of the crisis that are not included in this volume due to the sheer number and variety of ways public health is responding to the crisis and the many different approaches being taken to end it. The contributions herein emphasize the role of public health practice in the prevention of substance misuse and addiction or represent the work of a sector with which public health needs to become much more closely engaged. The chapters in Part I highlight fundamental frameworks and approaches to understanding the crisis from the vantage point of public health and share information that public health practitioners should consider as they develop contemporary opioid response programs and policies. Part II examines the ways that public health and health care partners, including providers and payers, have worked together to address the epidemic from the nexus of clinical medicine and community health practice. This focus on clinical practice is important given the existing focus on secondary and tertiary prevention, the urgent need to expand screening and treatment for substance misuse and addiction, and the tremendous opportunities for improving health that come from integrated public health and health care partnerships. In Part III, contributions illustrate the need for comprehensive, systems-level approaches that address the drivers of the crisis and the multiple leverage points at which public health can intervene to end it. Part III also includes an exploration of what it really means to address primary prevention of addiction, ways that public health agencies have used their traditional surveillance and epidemiology roles to better understand the epidemic, and how public health practitioners can develop new models to support "opioid stewardship" at the local, state, and federal levels.

As the Assistant Secretary of Health Dr. Brett Giroir and his team at the US Department of Health and Human Services (HHS) describe in the foreword to this volume, federal health officials have laid out five key strategies to address the opioid crisis. National leadership to end the crisis has been galvanized through state and federal emergency declarations and by high-level strategy development meetings between cities, states, and federal officials at the White House and HHS. Congress has prioritized treatment, recovery, and prevention and appropriated billions of new dollars to develop new and expand current programs.

The new political will and increase in fiscal resources are vital to reaching a goal we all share: ending the current epidemic of overdose deaths, as we also address the broader and longstanding problems of substance misuse and addiction of which opioid misuse is but one part. But these new resources did not come with a step-by-step protocol or instruction manual that could be applied to all communities in the same way. For example, expanding access to MAT will look different in a rural or frontier state, or a state that has expanded Medicaid versus a state that has not. Another reason is that sharing what is working and describing the public health role takes time that most public health practitioners do not have: They are busy responding to the crisis and doing the work urgently needed to address overdose deaths in their jurisdictions. Many of the contributors to this volume agreed to write their chapters knowing that it would be done on nights and weekends, or another "duty as assigned," but also knowing that sharing their contribution could have significant impact on the lives of others through describing their experience or sharing their knowledge. As Greg Williams aptly reminds us in his foreword to the *Guide*, recovery is possible and sustainable, and success is achievable, but more needs to be done to support the community of those in recovery and to prevent substance misuse and addiction in the first place.

While titled a "guide," this volume may more aptly be described as a collection of stories about how talented, dedicated, and inspiring leaders have taken a variety of efforts to prevent opioid misuse and addiction. It is not a cookbook with a list of ingredients to be assembled and prepared or a Google map with all the steps clearly laid for the journey. Instead, this *Guide* shares the diverse experience and insight of seasoned researchers and practitioners about the current crisis and efforts to end it. The application and implementation of the lessons and insights they share in each chapter then become the purview of readers, who, we hope, will be inspired and informed by its contents. If our readers feel a little overwhelmed by all that needs to be done to achieve a lasting and sustainable impact, our goal of painting an accurate picture of the situation will be met. But working together across sectors, we are confident that a lasting and sustainable impact can be achieved.

Public health practitioners know that there is no way to end the current crisis without addressing the broad social, economic, and environmental factors that have created and sustained its growth, factors that go well beyond changing the prescribing behavior of health care providers and interrupting the supply of illicit opioids. Naloxone dispensing, monitoring prescribing behavior, expanding access to MAT, increasing the use of alternative treatments for pain, and researching new cures for addiction all need to be complemented by approaches that address the demand for opioids in the first place. This involves working in what Fraser and Plescia refer to as the public health "sweet spot":[1] the primary prevention of substance misuse and addiction and working to expand evidence-based programs and policies that promote healthy communities and build individual, family, and community resilience. We understand that until we truly address the root causes of addiction, it will be difficult to end the crisis once and for all. To put it another way, we are not going to arrest or treat our way out of the opioid crisis; instead, we have to focus on preventing it. This *Guide* is intended to help show where we have been in these prevention efforts, where we are today, and where we are headed in the future.

Reference

1. Fraser M, Plescia M. The opioid epidemic's prevention problem. *Am J Public Health.* 2019; 109(2):215–217.

2 | The Emergence of an Epidemic

ELIZABETH M. FINKELMAN AND J. MICHAEL MCGINNIS

THE OPIOID EPIDEMIC STEMS from roots that course deeply throughout human history but whose alarming recent spread has positioned it as the most rapidly increasing killer of Americans. Derived from the extract of seeds of a poppy plant that has been growing on the planet for thousands of years, the use of opium poppy by humans may reach back more than 5,000 years to Mesopotamia, when the Sumerians began systematically using it for both medicinal and recreational purposes. With the advent of broad ocean travel and trade, opium became a focus of commerce, and, as often occurs in matters of trade, a prominent object of competition and conflict.

Today, the United States finds itself in the throes of a devastating opioid use epidemic, the deadliest addiction crisis of our time. Between 1999 and 2016, the US opioid epidemic claimed the lives of over 350,000 Americans.[1] Driven by the epidemic, drug overdose is now the leading cause of unintentional death in the United States, taking the lives of over 170 Americans every day. Overdose has become the leading cause of death for Americans under the age of 50, and its toll continues to worsen. In 2016, over 64,000 Americans died from drug overdose, a 21% increase from 2015, and of those deaths approximately 42,000 were linked to opioids. While the crisis does not discriminate in terms of who or where it touches, opioid overdose deaths are most common among non-Hispanic whites, among individuals aged 25 to 54 years old, and in the Northeast, Midwest, and Southern US Census Bureau regions. Beyond the devastating human toll, the epidemic has inflicted a tremendous economic burden. A 2018 report estimated that the epidemic cost the nation about $1 trillion between 2001 and 2017, and it is projected that it will cost the economy an additional $500 billion between now and 2020.[2]

With consequences that are tragic and unprecedented, the opioid epidemic will leave an impact that spans generations of Americans. As various sectors seek to mobilize cooperatively to identify solutions, this chapter explores the origins of the epidemic. With root causes that are multiple and complex, a confluence of drivers that cuts across the health system and societal, legal, and socioeconomic domains has been integral to its progression.

The Evolution of Opioid Use in the United States

Use of opiates (opium and opium derivatives) as a sanctioned intervention for pain relief in the United States dates back to the nation's founding, when opium was used to treat wounded soldiers of the British and Continental armies during the Revolutionary War. But it was the 1805 isolation of morphine, the active ingredient in the opium poppy, by German pharmacist Friedrich Serturner that truly transformed and expanded its medical use, eventually igniting the beginnings of America's first opioid epidemic around the time of the Civil War. Initially, morphine was administered in tablet form or applied topically, and then through hypodermic syringes when they were introduced in the 1850s. With few alternatives, and limited understanding of or education on its addictive properties, physicians used morphine extensively to treat a broad spectrum of conditions ranging from asthma to headaches to menstrual cramps.[3] In 1874, the British chemist C. R. Alder Wright developed heroin by boiling morphine with acetic anhydride, but it was not until 1897 that Felix Hoffmann, the German chemist who had created aspirin for the Bayer Corporation, developed heroin for introduction for medical use to commercial markets (Figure 2.1). At the time, Bayer marketed heroin as an effective alternative to morphine, particularly for the treatment of children's colds and coughs. Clinical use of opiates, including morphine and heroin, led many to medical addiction to these drugs and the occurrence of an earlier version of a national opioid addiction epidemic in the United States.

By the turn of the century, clinical use began to slow. Between advances in public health and medicine (including the introduction of aspirin in 1899 and the passage of the federal Pure Food and Drug Act of 1906) and a growing understanding of the addictive properties of morphine and heroin, doctors began to taper their prescription of opiates. In tandem, recreational or "street" use of heroin and opium smoking was growing. In an effort to address both the rise in medically induced dependence and recreational use of opiates, Congress passed the Harrison Narcotic Act of 1914,[4] which imposed taxes and regulations on the production, importation, and distribution of opiates and coca-derived products.

By 1924, Congress expanded the Act to ban the importation, sale, or manufacture of heroin, prompting an era of "opiophobia" in the treatment of chronic pain that would persist until late in the 20th century, marked by an inherent tension between a physician's "desire to relieve the patient's pain and fear of inducing addiction."[5] Even in the treatment of cancer pain, physicians were extremely wary of administering narcotics, often adhering to the notion that

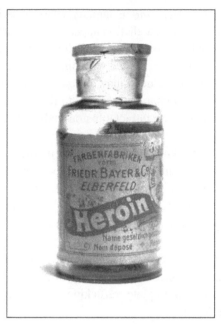

FIGURE 2.1. Bayer Corporation—Opium Bottle, c. 1924.
Source: This work has been released into the public domain by its author, Mpv_51. This applies worldwide.

"every effort should be made to put off [their] use until all other measures have been exhausted . . . and the patient's life can be measured in weeks."[6]

Substantially unrelated to the treatment of pain, use and abuse of opiates for the mood-altering effects that had also long promoted their attractiveness took a dramatic jump in the United States during the late 1960s. The combination of new supply sources, soldiers accessing heroin in Vietnam, estranged inner-city populations, and counterculture influences all fueled trafficking and use. Because many of the products used in this period were from illicit sources, and the victims of opiate addiction tended to be concentrated in marginalized social strata, the medical treatment system was substantially uninvolved in the response to the patients and public health effects of the problem, and much of the responsibility for managing the challenge fell to law enforcement and social services. As a result, the health care training, treatment, insurance coverage, and supportive services required to address the needs of addicted persons were not developed as a skill and capacity set essential to address the core health needs of millions of Americans.

Then came a shifting focus on pain management. During the 1980s, a number of articles published in prominent medical journals called into question the risk of opioid addiction when opioids were used in the treatment of long-term, non-cancer pain. Most notable is a brief letter published in the

New England Journal of Medicine in January 1980, observing that from the authors' assessment of records, addiction appeared to be rare among inpatients treated with narcotics with no history of addiction.[7] A few years later, in 1986, in a paper evaluating 38 patients treated with opioid analgesics for non-cancer pain, Portenoy and Foley concluded that "opioid maintenance therapy can be a safe, salutary and more humane alternative to the options of surgery or no treatment in those patients with intractable non-malignant pain and no history of drug abuse."[8]

Although researchers acknowledged the limits on their rigor and generalizability, the reports of these and selected other papers provided the foundation for a substantial reversal of the accepted narrative for medical treatment of pain, and aggressive commercial marketing of opioids. Treating patients' pain became the central priority and opioids offered an expeditious, affordable, and seemingly "safe" means for doing so. The tragic casualty of this premature, ill-informed, and unmeasured therapeutic doctrine was a dramatic increase in opioid prescribing and intensive marketing to prescribers, which, in concert with new tactics in illicit opiate trafficking, resulted in an unprecedented opioid addiction epidemic.

Drivers of the Epidemic

Increased opioid use and addiction rates have been driven by multiple factors. Biology is a fundamental driving factor (i.e., the physiologic response systems triggered by exposure to certain substances). As with variation in immune response systems on exposure to allergens, there are myriad variations among individuals in their susceptibilities to the addictive properties of opioids. For a given individual, therefore, the basic starting point driving addictive predisposition is biologic. From that baseline, personal social circumstances and interactions serve to potentiate or buffer against susceptibility to addiction, again with substantial variation from person to person.

The determinants of whether or when a problem progresses from an individual challenge to a society-wide epidemic are systems-based and include the prevalence of the exposure source, knowledge about the agent and the susceptibility profile, the capability of the response system, and societal understanding and will to engage. In the case of opioids, supply was not only unchecked but actively promoted. The health system was unprepared qualitatively and quantitatively, and culturally society's instinct was to marginalize and moralize the threat, underestimate its reach, underappreciate the science of addiction, and stigmatize individuals experiencing opioid use disorder. Several of these drivers of the epidemic are described in more detail below.

Supply Drivers

Three interacting factors shape the role of supply as a driver in the use of opioids: supply, demand, and proximity of the demand to supply. When heroin use and deaths rose sharply during the Vietnam War, it was driven directly by the size of the Southeast Asian growth of the opium poppy, the 1968 peak presence of 550,000 US troops in Vietnam, and policies that some have said provided shadow support to the drug trade. When soldiers returned home, some brought their newly acquired heroin use with them, which contributed, along with other domestic factors, to the rapid increase in heroin deaths experienced during the 1960s. Although heroin deaths were disproportionately experienced in poor and marginalized communities in this period, the association of heroin use with crime and disease led to a more general reaction and public concern about addiction that also brought about uneasiness in the medical community and the public about the use of prescription opioids, and restraints on their use. Both demand and supply decreased.

Coincident and countervailing forces then emerged. The growth in chronic diseases accompanied both an aging population (a natural outcome of increasing life expectancy) and the development of treatments that prolonged, albeit sometimes marginally, survival rates and therefore increased the prevalence of often painful conditions. Demand for pain management increased. Contributing to the demand was the rapid response of commercial marketing practices to the published reflections that prescribed opioids might not be as addictive as previously thought. Although these observations were very early and quite limited—and were later shown to be premature and erroneous—certain pharmaceutical manufacturers based substantial and well-funded marketing efforts on the notion. Three characteristics of these efforts were especially notable: (1) the support for efforts to position pain as the "fifth vital sign," (2) increased product detailing to clinicians, and (3) the growth of direct-to-consumer advertising.

In the mid-1990s, the American Pain Society began a campaign marketing pain as the "fifth vital sign," responding to, in part, a heightened sense across the medical community that chronic pain patients were not receiving adequate care. By the late 1990s, many health care organizations had adopted the mandate that pain must be assessed and treated, and the effectiveness of pain treatment became an important determinant of patient satisfaction scores. A major unintended consequence of this was the overutilization of opioids as the first-line treatment of chronic, non-cancer pain. In conjunction, pharmaceutical companies saw clear opportunities to develop and market new opioid drugs for this purpose, with OxyContin (extended-release oxycodone) being among the most prominent examples.

Released by Purdue Pharma in 1996, OxyContin was aggressively promoted with labeling approved by the US Food and Drug Administration (FDA) indicating that the drug could not be easily abused and that iatrogenic addiction was "very rare"[9] (Figure 2.2). Cornerstones of the company's marketing plan included pharmaceutical detailing practices (using prescriber profiling data to augment prescribing), direct-to-consumer marketing (through the distribution of pamphlets, TV ads, and videos), and professional education programming. Between 1996 and 2000, Purdue Pharma sponsored over 20,000 educational and continuing medical education programs promoting the long-term use of opioids for the treatment of non-cancer pain.[10] During that same time period, sales figures for OxyContin increased from $48 million to over $1 billion.[11] In 2001, responding to growing reports of diversion and misuse of OxyContin, the FDA amended the drug label to warn of the drug's potential to be misused and abused. Despite the new warnings, however, OxyContin sales

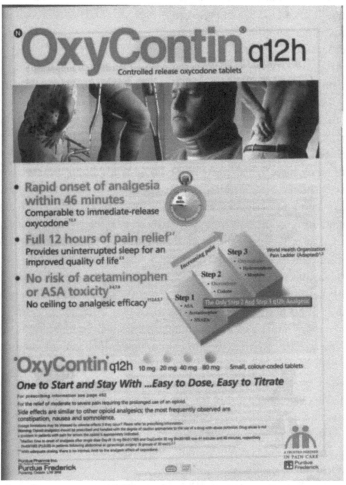

FIGURE 2.2. Example of OxyContin advertisement from Purdue Pharma.
Source: *Canadian Family Physician*, 2000.

continued to rise. As the supply of OxyContin and other opioid analgesics increased, so too did rates of diversion, misuse, abuse, and addiction. Between 1999 and 2011, oxycodone consumption (including OxyContin) increased by 500% and hydrocodone consumption doubled.[12] During approximately the same time period the number of people seeking treatment for opioid addiction increased over 900%[12] and the number of deaths from opioid analgesics nearly quadrupled.[13]

Rates of prescription opioid abuse began to level off in 2010, attributable to a range of efforts, including the introduction of abuse-deterrent formulations of opioid analgesics, the implementation of prescription drug monitoring programs and other efforts to reduce "doctor shopping," the crackdown on and closure of "pill mills" (clinics that prescribed large volumes of opioids with little or no medical justification), as well as the introduction of local, state, and federal government programs to improve opioid prescribing practices more broadly.[14] As the supply of prescription opioids was curtailed, prices of the drugs rose and overall access became more difficult. In turn, those who had become addicted to prescription opioids turned to cheaper, more accessible, and more potent drugs, such as heroin. Between 2003 and 2013, an estimated three out of four new heroin users reported previous misuse of prescription opioids prior to using heroin.[15] The supply of illicit sources and products expanded to usher in another wave of opioid-related deaths, beginning in 2013 and continuing (Figure 2.3). In 2016, synthetic and illicitly manufactured opioids, such

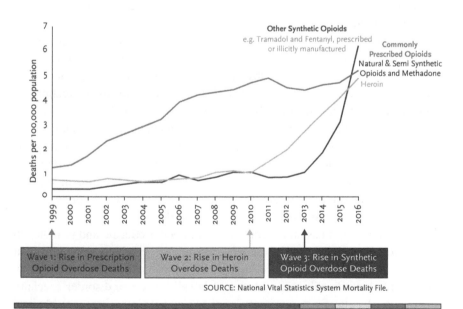

SOURCE: National Vital Statistics System Mortality File.

FIGURE 2.3. Three waves of the rise in opioid overdose deaths.
Source: CDC, 2017.[1]

as fentanyl and other synthetic opioids, were involved in nearly 50% of all opioid-related deaths, well surpassing the number of overdose deaths associated with prescription opioids.[16]

Societal Myopia

Beyond the addictive properties and supply drivers of opiates themselves, perhaps the most determining factor in the emergence of the epidemic has been the strong stigma resident in the societal view of addiction. Instead of treating substance use disorders like other chronic brain conditions, historically addiction has been stigmatized as a moral failing and categorized as a social problem best handled by individuals themselves, their families, or the social infrastructure of their communities. More often than not, substance use disorders have been addressed through punitive measures, such as "tough on crime" laws and incarceration for illicit drug possession and use. This has not only prevented individuals from getting the care they need but has also diverted resources from prevention, treatment, and recovery services where they are most needed. Further, society's stigmatization of addiction is reflected in the structure and financing of mainstream medicine, which has in many ways placed unintended and enduring barriers on treating substance use disorders.

Health System Drivers

As the use and abuse of opiates was rapidly increasing, the consequences were confronted by a health system both unprepared to handle the challenge and slow, if not unwilling, to change to accommodate it. Despite the fact that addiction treatment requires a blend of management by sustained counseling, testing, and pharmaceutical intervention (like most other chronic diseases), the millions of Americans who currently suffer from addiction to drugs, both prescribed and illicit, or other substances, such as alcohol, often go untreated. For those suffering from opioid use disorder, 80% are not receiving treatment.[17] They face formidable treatment barriers not as much from the complexities of addiction treatment as from the reality that the financial, professional, social, and cultural influences at work in our health care system are structured to discourage engagement. The 2016 Surgeon General's report *Facing Addiction in America* put it aptly: "[D]espite a compelling national need for treatment, [historically] the health care system was neither trained to care for nor especially eager to accept patients with substance use disorders."[18]

The opioid crisis has underscored a need to better educate and train health professionals to screen for, recognize, and treat addiction, as well as to treat and manage pain. Reports have highlighted the skill shortage that exists in both the broader health care system and in substance use disorder specialty programs. Results from a survey by the Liaison Committee on Medical Education found that of the 125 accredited US medical schools, 95% provided training in substance use treatment as part of a larger required course, only 8% had a separate required course, and 36% offered an elective course.[19,20] Regarding pain management education, a 2011 study found that US medical schools allocate a median of nine classroom hours to pain and its management, amounting to roughly 0.3% of total curriculum hours.[21] In addition to insufficient education and training, stigma and misconceptions about treatment for opioid use disorders also pose major barriers. Most notably, there still exists a strong belief among some providers that medication-assisted treatment (MAT), which is now widely accepted as the gold standard of care for treatment of opioid use disorders, amounts to no more than substituting one drug or addiction for another.

Beyond deficiencies in health professionals' competencies, and at times their willingness to recognize, treat, and manage substance use disorders, the administration, financing, and regulation of treatment for substance use disorders and addiction have long stood outside of "mainstream" health care. In addition to being structurally and culturally removed, historically treatment for substance use disorders was focused solely on addiction. This focus overlooks the more widely prevalent cases of mild or moderate substance use disorders and in effect eliminates opportunities to prevent what would become more severe cases. In recent years, there has been marked progress toward integrating addiction and mental health with primary care, most notably the passage of the Wellstone-Domenici Mental Health Parity and Addiction Equity Act in 2008, the Patient Protection and Affordable Care Act (ACA) in 2010, and an overall movement in health care toward greater care integration. Even so, critical barriers remain to realizing more coordinated and integrated care for substance use disorders. These challenges span several factors but most notably include infrastructure issues, such as (1) electronic health information exchange, (2) confidentiality regulations and privacy laws, (3) the capacity and composition of the healthcare workforce, and (4) financing.

Incomplete electronic health information exchange across providers, due in large part to limited technical assistance and funding support for electronic health record implementation, has made care coordination for substance use disorders cumbersome and challenging. Confidentiality regulations, most notably federal law 42 CFR Part 2 and state privacy laws, have also made exchanging treatment-related information difficult, in some cases threatening the safety of patients. While ensuring the confidentiality of sensitive patient information is essential, it can be deleterious to the patient when a care provider is not aware of a patient's history with substance misuse or concurrent medication-assisted treatment and prescribes treatment that is inappropriate.

Of course, for effective care coordination and integration to take place, a diverse and robust health care workforce is needed to deliver it across the care continuum. For mental health and substance use disorder treatment, the capacity of the workforce has been inadequate and is only being strained further by the opioid epidemic. Building the workforce capacity needed will necessitate that health professionals broadly have the core competencies, supports, and incentives to prevent and treat substance use disorders. Diversity in skill and expertise is essential from primary care providers to substance use disorder specialists, behavioral health providers, nurses, nurse practitioners, physician assistants, pharmacists, and social workers, among others.

Finally, financing disincentives have posed major challenges for the coordination and integration of substance use disorder treatment with mainstream health care. These disincentives cut across a range of issues, including the low pay and salary structure of the substance use disorder treatment workforce,[22] as well as the varied coverage that exists for substance use disorder treatment, and related, non-health-care supportive services that are essential for long-term recovery and success. To varying degrees, substance use disorder treatment is financed by private insurance; Medicaid; Medicare; other federal, state, or local government financing; or out-of-pocket payment by patients themselves and their families and friends. In 2014, 45% of substance use disorder treatment was financed through private insurance, Medicaid, or Medicare.[18] Notably, coverage for essential social and community-based services that are needed for long-term recovery are rarely covered by insurance, and most often are supported by a combination of federal, state, and local government funding, along with support from nonprofit organizations.

Implications for Controlling the Epidemic

Given the numerous and complex origins of the opioid epidemic, many diverse but coordinated strategies will be needed across sectors to control and overcome the crisis. In several cases, the solutions are well known or understood but structural barriers, policies, regulations, or, in some instances, lack of national will remain impediments to implementation and progress.

Particularly challenging will be overcoming the social and cultural stigma that has historically not only permeated how the public views substance misuse and addiction but how the health care system has developed to treat (or not treat) these chronic illnesses of the brain. While notable progress has been made in this respect, more is needed. Further, progress depends on the ability to address the many structural barriers to integrated and coordinated care services. In particular, the importance of bridging medical and social interventions is not unique to addiction, but priming the health care system to deal more effectively across medical-social service boundaries will also ready it for better engaging the challenges posed by other high-need patients, including the 5% of patients who drive 50% of health care costs.

Notably, addressing these overarching systemic and cultural factors will help foster the strong public health and prevention framework that is needed to avoid worsening the crisis or repeating it in the years and decades ahead. As the nation witnesses an increasing number of "deaths of despair" (deaths from suicide, alcoholism, or drug overdose), ensuring that the health care system can deliver robust and comprehensive mental health and substance use disorder prevention and treatment services is essential to its long-term success. Though the task is formidable, overcoming the opioid epidemic as a unified health care ecosystem and as a nation offers a tremendous opportunity to realize better health futures for us all.

Authors' Note

While the authors are both with the National Academy of Medicine, the responsibility for the content of this piece is that of the authors alone and not the National Academy of Medicine.

References

1. US Centers for Disease Control and Prevention. Understanding the epidemic. https://www.cdc.gov/drugoverdose/epidemic/index.html. Accessed January 2, 2019.
2. Altarum. Economic toll of opioid crisis in U.S. exceeded $1 trillion since 2001. https://altarum.org/news/economic-toll-opioid-crisis-us-exceeded-1-trillion-2001. Accessed January 8, 2019.
3. Trickey E. Inside the story of America's 19th century opiate addiction. *Smithsonian*. https://www.smithsonianmag.com/history/inside-story-americas-19th-century-opiate-addiction-180967673/#G2QqRK2rD4Pt1ryc.99. Accessed January 2, 2019.
4. Jones MR, Viswanath O, Peck J, et al. A brief history of the opioid epidemic and strategies for pain medicine. *Pain Ther*. 2018; 7(1):13–21.
5. Meldrum ML. A capsule of history of pain management. *JAMA*. 2003; 290(18):2470–2475.
6. Schiffrin MJ. *The Management of Pain in Cancer*. St. Louis, MO: Year Book; 1956:7–8.
7. Porter J, Jick H. Addiction rare in patients treated with narcotics. *N Engl J Med*. 1980; 302(2):123.
8. Portenoy RK, Foley KM. Chronic use of opioid analgesics in non-malignant pain: Report of 38 cases. *Pain*. 1986; 25(2):171–186.
9. Tompkins DA, Hobelmann JG, Compton P. Providing chronic pain management in the "Fifth Vital Sign" era: Historical and treatment perspectives on a modern-day medical dilemma. *Drug Alcohol Depend*. 2017; 173(1):s11–s21.
10. U.S. General Accounting Office. Prescription drugs: OxyContin abuse and diversion and efforts to address the problem. 2003. http://www.gao.gov/new.items/d04110.pdf. Accessed January 2, 2019.

11. VanZee A. The promotion and marketing of OxyContin: Commercial triumph, public health tragedy. *Am J Public Health*. 2009; 99(2):221–227.

12 Andrew K, Courtwright DT, Hwang CS, et al. The prescription opioid and heroin crisis: A public health approach to an epidemic of addiction. *Annu Rev Public Health*. 2015; 36(1): 559–574.

13. Chen LH, Hedegaard HM. Drug-poisoning deaths involving opioid analgesics: United States, 1999–2011. NCHS Data Brief No. 166. 2014. Hyattsville, MD: National Center for Health Statistics.

14. Dart RC, Surratt HL, Cicero TJ, et al. Trends in opioid analgesic abuse and mortality in the United States. *N Engl J Med*. 2015; 372(3):241–248.

15. Cicero TJ, Ellis MS, Surratt, HL. The changing face of heroin use in the United States: A retrospective analysis of the past 50 years. *JAMA Psychiatry*. 2014; 71(7):821–826.

16. U.S. National Institutes of Health. Fentanyl and other synthetic opioids: drug overdose deaths. 2016. https://www.drugabuse.gov/related-topics/trends-statistics/infographics/fentanyl-other-synthetic-opioids-drug-overdose-deaths. Accessed January 2, 2019.

17. Saloner B, Karthikeyan S. Changes in substance abuse treatment use among individuals with opioid use disorders in the United States, 2004–2013. *JAMA*. 2015; 314:1515–1517.

18. U.S. Department of Health and Human Services (HHS), Office of the Surgeon General. *Facing Addiction in America: The Surgeon General's Report on Alcohol, Drugs, and Health*. 2016. Washington, DC: HHS.

19. Haack MR, Adger H, eds. *Strategic Plan for Interdisciplinary Faculty Development: Arming the Nation's Health Professional Workforce for a New Approach to Substance Use Disorders*. Dordrecht, the Netherlands: Kluwer Academic/Plenum Publishers; 2002.

20. Institute of Medicine. *Improving the Quality of Health Care for Mental and Substance-Use Conditions*. 2006. Washington, DC: National Academies Press.

21. Mezei L, Hogans B. Pain education in North American medical schools. *J Pain*. 2011; 2:1199–1208.

22. Mark TL, Yee T, Levit KR, et al. Insurance financing increased for mental health conditions but not for substance use disorders, 1984–2014. *Health Aff*. 2016; 35(6):958–965.

3 | Public Health Approaches to Preventing Substance Misuse and Addiction

JAY C. BUTLER

T HE THREE-TIERED FRAMEWORK DEVELOPED for the 2017 Association of State and Territorial Health Officials (ASTHO) President's Challenge (see p. 141) provides a paradigm for how public health agencies can address the health effects of substance misuse and addiction, especially for the current epidemic of opioid-related adverse health events. Over the past two years, public health agencies have implemented many of these concepts, and preliminary data for 2017 and 2018 indicate progress in reducing misuse of opioids and the number of overdose deaths. As of the publication of this *Guide*, there are many areas where the emerging science of addiction is being translated into evidence-based policy as we also work to address ongoing challenges at each of the three levels of prevention.

Tertiary prevention has been an area of significant activity. Syringe and needle service programs have expanded in many jurisdictions. Further analysis of the HIV outbreak in southern Indiana has shown that in the absence of syringe and needle service programs, transmission can be explosive but unrecognized until many are infected.[1] Waiting until an outbreak occurs before increasing access to clean injection equipment is a costly delay. Consideration of safe-injection facilities in a few US communities continues, informed by a growing body of evidence from other countries suggesting that these programs may facilitate not only decreased risk of overdose and needle-borne infection, but also entry into addiction treatment programs, countering claims that these services merely enable illicit drug use.[2] The majority of states have taken steps to increase access to naloxone, and in April 2018, US Surgeon General Jerome Adams issued a public health advisory to increase awareness of naloxone as an life-saving intervention and, when accompanied by secondary and primary prevention strategies, a foundational part of the public health response to the opioid crisis.[3]

Secondary prevention requires increasing access and removing barriers to treatment. Recent encouraging trends include an increasing number of providers receiving Drug Addiction Treatment Act of 2000 (DATA 2000) waivers in order to prescribe buprenorphine for opioid addiction, and there has been increased recognition among clinicians that addiction treatment is within the purview and responsibility of primary care providers and non-addiction specialists.[4–6] There has been increased recognition that providing treatment to persons with addiction during incarceration represents an underutilized public health invention to address the epidemic as well as a critical part of breaking the cycle of addiction-related crime and repeated incarceration. A recent court ruling in Massachusetts deemed that discontinuing opioid addiction treatment, with the attendant risk of precipitating withdrawal during incarceration, violates the prohibition against cruel and unusual punishment in the Eighth Amendment to the US Constitution and protections provided under the Americans with Disabilities Act.[7] Increased use of medication-assisted treatments in the Rhode Island prison system was associated with a 60% reduction in overdose deaths among the recently incarcerated.[8]

Primary prevention addresses both the supply of and demand for opioids. Improved pain management strategies, including dispensing an appropriate number of opioid doses for a single episode of acute pain, is limiting the number of prescription opioids available in the community for diversion and misuse. Public health, social service, and criminal justice agencies, as well as medical professional organizations, are increasingly promoting trauma-informed care as an evidence-informed method to address adverse childhood experiences and to build personal resilience.

Although the progress to date is encouraging, there is much left to do and many new challenges. As the flood of prescription opioids in our communities has been reduced, some chronic pain patients who have been stable on opioid pain relievers find that they can no longer access their medications. Additionally, more data are needed to determine the optimal methods for implementing dispensing limits for episodes of acute pain.[9] Gains in prevention of overdoses from prescription opioids and heroin have been tempered, and in some areas obliterated, by the introduction of fentanyl and related illicit synthetic opioids, such as U-47700, into the illicit drug supply. Risk of overdose is enhanced by inadvertent exposures that can occur when opioids such as heroin or other drugs, including cocaine and methamphetamine, are contaminated with fentanyl.[10]

The 2017 ASTHO President's Challenge remains a relevant and important framework for organizing current efforts to end the opioid crisis. The multitiered and multisector response to the opioid crisis must continue. To paraphrase Robert Frost, we in public health "have promises to keep, and miles to go before we sleep" in addressing the opioid crisis.

Editor's Note

The material that follows was originally published as "2017 ASTHO President's Challenge: Public Health Approaches to Preventing Substance Misuse and Addiction," *Journal of Public Health Management and Practice*, September/October 2017; 23(5):531–536.
[insert Butler, 2017 reprint here]

References

1. Campbell EM, Jia H, Shankar A, et al. Detailed transmission network analysis of a large opiate-driven outbreak of HIV infection in the United States. *J Infect Dis.* 2017; 216(9):1053–1062.
2. Gostin LO, Hodge JG, Gulinson CL. Supervised injection facilities: Legal and policy reforms. *JAMA.* 2019; 321(8):745–746.
3. Adams JM. Increasing naloxone awareness and use: The role of health care practitioners. *JAMA.* 2018; 319(20):2073–2074.
4. Wakeman SE, Barnett ML. Primary care and the opioid-overdose crisis—Buprenorphine myths and realities. *N Engl J Med.* 2018; 379(1):1–4.
5. Rapoport AB, Christopher CF. Stretching the scope—Becoming frontline addiction-medicine providers. *N Engl J Med.* 2017; 377(8):705–707.
6. D'Onofrio G, McCormick RP, Hawk K. Emergency departments—A 24/7/365 option for combating the opioid crisis. *N Engl J Med.* 2018; 379(26):2487–2490.
7. Binswanger IA. Opioid use disorder and incarceration—Hope of ensuring the continuity of treatment. *N Engl J Med.* 2019; 380:1193–1195.
8. Green TC, Clarke J, Brinkley-Rubinstein L, et al. Postincarceration fatal overdoses after implementing medications for addiction treatment in a statewide correctional system. *JAMA Psychiatry.* 2018; 75(4):405–407.
9. Chua K-P, Brummett CM, Walijee JF. Opioid prescribing limits for acute pain: Potential problems with design and implementation. *JAMA.* 2019; 321(7):643–644.
10. Khatri UG, Viner K, Perrone J. Lethal fentanyl and cocaine intoxication. *N Engl J Med.* 2018; 379(18):1782.

4 | Public Health Approaches to Overdose Prevention and Harm Reduction

MARK LYSYSHYN AND MARK TYNDALL

HARM REDUCTION AIMS TO reduce the negative consequences of drug use in people unable or unwilling to stop.[1] Harm reduction policies, programs, and practices aim to meet people where they are at and are focused on preventing harms such as overdose rather than preventing drug use itself. Harm reduction approaches are meant to be complementary to prevention and treatment approaches, acknowledging that it is not currently possible to prevent or treat all cases of problematic substance use and also that addiction is a relapsing chronic condition.

Home to North America's first and only legal supervised injection site for over a decade, Vancouver and the province of British Columbia (BC) have been considered leaders in the field of harm reduction.[2] Harm reduction interventions were adopted in response to increasing overdose deaths and an HIV epidemic in the late 1990s. Harm reduction was officially endorsed in 2005 as an essential component of Vancouver's "four pillar" drug prevention policy for preventing harm from psychoactive substance use, along with prevention, treatment, and enforcement.[3]

Recently, increasing contamination of the illicit drug supply with fentanyl and other highly potent synthetic opioids has led to rapid increases in overdose deaths in BC, like it has in much of North America. BC has been considered the epicenter of this crisis in Canada, leading to the declaration of a public health emergency by the Provincial Health Officer in April 2016. In response to the crisis, BC has had to scale up and expand its harm reduction response, focusing on supervised consumption, overdose prevention and drug checking services, naloxone and peer programs, as well as harm reducing treatment approaches such as injectable opioid agonist therapy.[4,5]

Supervised Consumption and Overdose Prevention Sites

Supervised consumption sites or supervised injections sites are facilities where people who use drugs can legally consume pre-obtained drugs under the supervision of health professionals who can respond should an overdose occur. They typically also provide other harm reduction services such as naloxone and harm reduction supply distribution as well as referral to addiction treatment and health and social services. There are currently more than 100 facilities offering supervised consumption services worldwide. The majority of these facilities are located in Europe; however, facilities also exist in Australia and Canada. Most operate under a legal exemption to local drug laws.

Insite, North America's first supervised consumption site, opened in Vancouver in 2003 and has arguably been subjected to the most rigorous scientific evaluation. The evaluation showed that Insite reduces overdose risk and prevents overdose deaths; indeed, nobody has ever died of an overdose at Insite.[6] Insite also decreases the risk of HIV and hepatitis C transmission, increases uptake of addiction treatment services, offers medical care for injection-related infections, provides greater safety for women who use drugs, and improves public order by reducing public injection and injection-related litter. The evaluation also found that Insite did not lead to increased drug use or increased crime.[7] A recent evidence review of drug consumption rooms by the European Monitoring Centre for Drugs and Drug Addiction came to similar conclusions.[8]

When BC's public health emergency was declared in April 2016, Insite and one other small site in Vancouver were the only facilities providing legal supervised consumption services in BC and also in Canada. Now, two years later, legal supervised injection services are being offered at 25 sites across Canada, including three sites in Vancouver and six sites in the rest of BC. Although most services operate out of fixed sites, innovative mobile services are being offered in a number of locations.[9] And although the majority of clients consume drugs by injection at these sites, most now offer supervised injection, oral, and intranasal consumption.[4,10] A site in Lethbridge, Alberta, is the first and only site in Canada currently offering legal supervised inhalation.

Even so, the process for establishing supervised consumption sites has not kept pace with community need. Following the lead of activists that set up "pop-up" supervised injection sites, BC's government issued an emergency order allowing health authorities to establish Canada's first overdose prevention sites in December 2016.[11] These are low-barrier services, typically operated in partnership with community agencies and peers, where clients are monitored while using drugs without authorization from the Canadian government. As of March 31, 2018, 25 overdose prevention sites in BC had received

826,064 visits and reversed 5,386 overdoses with no deaths.[12] The unprecedented rise in overdose deaths and the consistent public health messaging that people should not be using drugs on their own have made these sites a central component of the overdose response. The flexible model has led to innovative practices such as peer supervision and supervision of inhalation via an outdoor tent.[13] It has also allowed smaller, more rural communities to offer overdose prevention services and for agencies to create specialized services targeting vulnerable populations such as women and people living in high-risk housing complexes.[14–16] Overdose prevention sites have since been established in other provinces, and the Canadian government has created a streamlined process to authorize them.[17,18]

Drug Checking and Alerting

Drug checking is a harm reduction intervention that offers testing of street drugs to assess their composition in order to allow for more informed decision making by people who use drugs. Drug checking services can vary in a number of ways, including the testing technique (e.g., reagents, test strips, spectrometry), type of results provided (e.g., presence vs. absence, quantitative), service setting (e.g., at home, mobile, fixed site), and use of results (e.g., individual harm reduction, public health action, market monitoring). While drug checking services are available in Europe, they are considered illegal in North America, although sometimes they are available in music festival settings on an ad hoc basis.

Faced with a contaminated drug supply, Vancouver implemented Canada's first legal drug checking service. A one-year pilot at Insite showed that drug checking using test strips designed to test urine for fentanyl could prevent overdose by encouraging clients to reduce their dose.[19] Since then, fentanyl drug checking using fentanyl test strips has been expanded to other supervised consumption sites and overdose prevention sites across BC, with calls for further expansion. More advanced drug checking combining fentanyl test strips and infrared spectrometry is currently being evaluated at several sites throughout BC.[20]

This approach has been supported by the Fentanyl Overdose Reduction Checking Analysis Study (FORECAST) conducted by the Bloomberg School of Public Health at Johns Hopkins University, which recommended that public health agencies implement drug checking programs using fentanyl test strips and/or infrared spectrometry. Fentanyl test strips are also being distributed across the United States and a number of groups are trying to evaluate their effectiveness when used in this way.[21] While the optimal technology and setting for drug checking remains to be determined, the current options remain limited for people who find that they have purchased contaminated drugs but still want or need to use them.

To extend the benefits of drug checking services and to share information about potential drug contamination events, overdose alerting systems can be set up. These systems connect stakeholders with information about overdose events such as first responders, health authorities, police, coroners, community service providers, laboratories, and poison information centers so that information can be shared and disseminated. This information can be shared with people who use drugs via the media, social media, or posters placed at harm reduction supply distribution points. Typical alerts contain information and/or photos of the drug, the contaminant of concern, overdose features to look out for, and information about how to reduce harm. Information about drugs is being shared directly with the drug-using community in the Vancouver region through a novel anonymous text-based, two-way messaging service called the RADAR network.[22] Members of the network can report unusual overdoses or suspected drug contamination events and receive overdose alerts.

"Take Home Naloxone"

The BC Centre for Disease Control established a provincial Take Home Naloxone program in 2012 in response to persistently high rates of opioid overdose deaths.[23] The program, which provides training and kits containing naloxone (an antidote to opioid overdose), has been massively scaled up due to the overdose epidemic. In 2017, 56,000 kits were distributed, with at least 14,000 kits used to reverse overdoses that year.[24,25] A recent study estimated that 226 deaths were averted by the administration of naloxone in 2016 during the early stages of the provincial naloxone expansion.[26]

The primary recipients of naloxone kits and overdose response training are those who are at risk of an opioid overdose themselves or those who may witness one. It is now common to see people in the community carrying small black cases that contain three vials of naloxone, a syringe, and other equipment. Peer engagement has been excellent, and lives have been saved by the rapid response. The kits have also been used by community-based overdose responders to create innovative programs such as "Spikes on Bikes," a mobile overdose prevention and response service.[27]

The toll on the community overdose responders has been significant and is often underappreciated. These are often people dealing with serious health and social challenges themselves, and reversing an overdose can be a very traumatic experience. Supports need to be in place to debrief and provide counseling to those involved in naloxone programs. The Take Home Naloxone program is a critical addition to the naloxone now carried by all first responders in BC. However, the biggest limitation with such a program is that overdose deaths occur mostly when people overdose alone and there is no opportunity to intervene.

Injectable Therapies

Opioid agonist therapy (OAT) or medication-assisted treatment is an evidence-based approach for treating opioid use disorder. OAT improves retention in treatment, decreases illicit opioid use, and improves morbidity and mortality, but it does not work for everybody. Around half of patients treated with OAT will discontinue treatment within a year and relapse to opioid use. As such, jurisdictions such as BC now offer injectable opioid agonist therapies (iOAT) using synthetic heroin (diacetylmorphine) and hydromorphone.

Prescribed heroin is available in Switzerland, Germany, the Netherlands, Denmark, and Canada. Research has shown that it improves treatment retention, reduces illicit opioid use, reduces criminal activity and incarceration, and improves mortality.[28] A Cochrane review concluded that treatment with heroin was superior to methadone in people who had previously failed treatment with methadone.[29] Injectable therapies have been well evaluated in the North American context. The North American Opiate Medication Initiative (NAOMI) enrolled participants in Montreal and Vancouver and demonstrated that prescribed heroin was more effective than optimized methadone maintenance therapy for people who had not benefited from other treatments.[30] Following NAOMI, the Study to Assess Long-term Opioid Medication Effectiveness (SALOME) enrolled participants in Vancouver and demonstrated that injectable hydromorphone worked as well as heroin and that participants could not tell the difference between the two medication, meaning that injectable hydromorphone could be used in jurisdictions where heroin is not available.[31]

Although iOAT is an effective treatment strategy for people who have not benefited from OAT in the past, it can also be used as a harm reduction strategy for people not willing to try OAT or not ready to stop using injection drugs. It is a bridging intervention that can help move people from a harm reduction paradigm into a treatment paradigm. In addition to having significant health and social benefits to the individual, iOAT is cost-effective and benefits the community by reducing criminal activity and health care costs.[32]

In almost all countries where iOAT is available, it is provided within supervised settings to ensure compliance, to monitor for safety, and to prevent diversion. Although effective, the model used at the Crosstown Clinic in Vancouver for the NAOMI and SALOME trials is expensive and other models have started to emerge in BC, including iOAT supervised at community health centers, community pharmacies, overdose prevention sites, and social housing settings. But given the scale of the overdose crisis and the demand for iOAT, other more innovative models may also be needed.

Hydromorphone Distribution

Increasingly, the public health response to the opioid overdose epidemic in BC has focused on providing a regulated supply of pharmaceutical-grade opioids.[33] The concept has been proven with OAT and iOAT, which is provided under clinical supervision. However, there are limitations to these programs due to cost, infrastructure requirements, inclusion criteria, and uptake.

A more scalable model may involve the use of hydromorphone pills, which are easier to distribute, already widely used, and inexpensive. Devising a program that provides a regulated source of hydromorphone pills to registered participants would directly address current poisonings due to the unregulated and toxic illicit opioid market. While most participants would likely crush the pills for injection, oral ingestion would also be possible. Protocols have been developed that would allow supervised use of hydromorphone in settings like supervised injection sites and use of hydromorphone in other settings without supervision. The programs would provide access to other supports and services to reduce the risk of diversion and to optimize safe use. Dispensing could take place in supportive housing environments, supervised injection sites, or standalone locations. A potential way to distribute the pills would be through secure dispensing machines that could provide individualized dosing, scheduling, and monitoring. Such technology might allow implementation in communities that lack adequate harm reduction or treatment services. A pilot program is currently being planned for 2018 in Vancouver.

Engaging Peers

Peers have been instrumental in the design, implementation, and operation of successful harm reduction programs and peer-led organizations such as the Vancouver Network of Drug Users (VANDU), and other frontline community and advocacy groups have been critical in bringing attention to the issue of illegal drug use and the need for harm reduction programs in communities across Canada.[34]

Increasingly, efforts to build up the capacity of peers and peer-based groups has been supported through ensuring inclusion at stakeholder meetings, providing training and employment opportunities, and giving a venue to directly influence the design of harm reduction interventions.[35] Best practices for peer engagement and use of respectful language have been developed, and peers in Vancouver can now obtain a "street degree" in overdose prevention at the Molson Learning Lab.[36,37] While some success has been achieved, the overall approach to engagement is challenging, especially for individuals who remain actively engaged in illegal drug use. In many communities the severe repression and stigma have driven people using drugs to the margins of society, and most do not feel safe identifying as a "drug user." It is imperative that safe places are established where drug users can gather, organize, and have a voice.

Summary

The introduction of fentanyl and other synthetic opioids to the illegal drug market in many communities throughout North America is largely responsible for the rapid rise in overdose and overdose death. If nothing else, the opioid overdose epidemic has exposed the precarious situation facing people who use illegal drugs. Harm reduction interventions provide a critical first line of defense by creating environments that can bring people out of the shadows and the isolation that currently makes using illegal drugs so dangerous. The same public health approach has been critical to reducing the transmission of infectious diseases, connecting people with social services and addiction treatment, and making communities safer.

The overdose epidemic has also exposed the limitations of harm reduction approaches in the face of a highly contaminated drug supply. From a public health perspective, it is not acceptable to ignore the damage caused by structural factors such as poverty, homelessness, prohibition, and the use of the criminal justice system to enforce laws that directly contribute to the suffering and death of people who use drugs. It is clear that making drugs illegal does little to stop people from using them, especially those who are already dependent on them.

Harm reduction is really the only approach that attempts to take drug use out of the criminal justice sphere and approaches addiction for what it really is, a health and social issue. A harm reduction approach is in no way at odds with the critical need to improve access to health and social services, increase access to addiction treatment, and provide opportunities for abstinence-based recovery programs. Unfortunately, ignoring evidence-based harm reduction interventions means that many people may never get the opportunity.

References

1. Harm Reduction International. What is harm reduction? https://www.hri.global/what-is-harm-reduction. Accessed February 12, 2019.
2. Hyshka E, Bubela T, Wild TC. Prospects for scaling up supervised injection facilities in Canada: The role of evidence in legal and political decision-making. *Addiction.* 2013; 108(3):468–476.
3. City of Vancouver, British Columbia. Four pillars drug strategy. https://vancouver.ca/people-programs/four-pillars-drug-strategy.aspx. Accessed February 12, 2019.
4. Office of the Chief Coroner, Ministry of Public Safety & Solicitor General. Illicit Drug Overdose Deaths in B.C. 2018. https://www2.gov.bc.ca/assets/gov/public-safety-and-emergency-services/death-investigation/statistical/illicit-drug.pdf. Accessed February 12, 2019.

5. Government of British Columbia. Provincial health officer declares public health emergency. https://news.gov.bc.ca/releases/2016HLTH0026-000568. Accessed February 12, 2019.
6. Milloy MJ, Kerr T, Tyndall M, et al. Estimated drug overdose deaths averted by North America's first medically-supervised safer injection facility. *PLoS One*. 2008; 3(10):e3351.
7. Urban Health Research Initiative, Vancouver, B.C., Center for Excellence in HIV/AIDS. Insight into Insite. 2010. http://www.bccsu.ca/wp-content/uploads/2016/10/insight_into_insite.pdf. Accessed February 12, 2019.
8. European Monitoring Center for Drugs and Drug Addiction. Drug consumption room: An overview of provision and evidence (perspectives on drugs). http://www.emcdda.europa.eu/publications/pods/drug-consumption-rooms_en. Accessed February 12, 2019.
9. Government of Canada. Supervised consumption sites: Status of applications. https://www.canada.ca/en/health-canada/services/substance-abuse/supervised-consumption-sites/status-application.html. Accessed February 12, 2019.
10. Fraser Health. Fraser Health receives exemption to supervise consumption of oral and intra-nasal substances. http://news.fraserhealth.ca/News/June-2017/Exemption-supervised-consumption-oral-intra-nasal.aspx. Accessed February 12, 2019.
11. Government of British Columbia. Ministerial order support urgent overdose response action. https://news.gov.bc.ca/releases/2016HLTH0094-002737. Accessed February 12, 2019.
12. British Columbia Centre for Disease Control. Overdose data and reports: Overdose services. http://www.bccdc.ca/health-professionals/clinical-resources/harm-reduction/overdose-data-reports. Accessed February 12, 2019.
13. PHS Community Services Society. Vancouver: Overdose prevention sites. https://www.phs.ca/index.php/project/overdose-prevention-sites/. Accessed February 12, 2019.
14. Vancouver Island Health Authority. Overdose prevention. http://www.viha.ca/mho/overdose.htm. Accessed February 12, 2019.
15. Atira Women's Resource Society. Vancouver: SisterSpace, shared using room for women. http://www.atira.bc.ca/sisterspace-shared-using-room-women. Accessed February 12, 2019.
16. Bardwell G, Collins AB, McNeil R, Boyd J. Housing and overdose: An opportunity for scale-up of overdose prevention interventions? *Harm Reduct J*. 2017; 14(1):77.
17. Government of Ontario, Ministry of Health and Long-Term Care. Applications now open for overdose prevention sites. http://www.health.gov.on.ca/en/news/bulletin/2018/hb_20180111.aspx. Accessed February 12, 2018.
18. Government of Canada. Statement from the Minister of Health regarding the opioid crisis. https://www.canada.ca/en/health-canada/news/2017/12/statement_from_theministerofhealthregardingtheopioidcrisis.html. Accessed February 12, 2019.
19. Karamouzian M, Dohoo C, Forsting S, et al. Evaluation of a fentanyl drug checking service for clients of a supervised injection facility, Vancouver, Canada. *Harm Reduct J*. 2018. 15:46.
20. Province expands fentanyl testing and launches drug checking pilot in Vancouver. Vancouver Coastal Health. http://www.vch.ca/about-us/news/province-expands-fentanyl-testing-and-launches-drug-checking-pilot-in-vancouver. Accessed February 12, 2019.

21. Johns Hopkins Bloomberg School of Public Health. Fentanyl Overdose Reduction Checking Analysis Study. 2018. https://americanhealth.jhu.edu/sites/default/files/inline-files/Fentanyl_Executive_Summary_032018.pdf. Accessed February 12, 2019.

22. Vancouver Coastal Health, New alert system starts for bad dope [Internet]. Vancouver: Vancouver Coastal Health; 2017. Available from: http://www.vch.ca/about-us/news/new-alert-system-starts-for-bad-dope. Accessed July 3, 2019.

23. Oluwajenyo Banjo, Tzemis D, Al-Qutub D, et al. A quantitative and qualitative evaluation of the British Columbia Take Home Naloxone program. *CMAJ Open.* 2014; 2(3): E153–E161.

24. British Columbia Centre for Disease Control. Take Home Naloxone Program in B.C. http://towardtheheart.com/thn-in-bc-infograph. Accessed February 12, 2019.

25. Buxton JA, Gilbert M, Wilson M, Ogborne-Hill E. Patient and physician resources for naloxone use in B.C. *BC Med J.* 2018; 60(2):84–85.

26. Irvine MA, Buxton JA, Otterstatter M, et al. Distribution of take-home opioid antagonist kits during a synthetic opioid epidemic in British Columbia, Canada: A modelling study. *Lancet Public Health.* 2018; 3(5):e218–e225.

27. PHS Community Services Society. Vancouver: Spikes on bikes. https://www.phs.ca/index.php/project/spikes-on-bikes/. Accessed February 12, 2019.

28. Strang J, Groshkova T, Uchtenhagen A, et al. Heroin on trial: Systematic review and meta-analysis of randomised trials of diamorphine-prescribing as treatment for refractory heroin addiction. *Br J Psychiatry.* 2015; 207(1):5–14.

29. Ferri M, Davoli M, Perucci CA. Heroin maintenance for chronic heroin-dependent individuals. *Cochrane Database Syst Rev.* 2010; 9:CD003410.

30. Oviedo-Joekes E, Brissette S, Marsh DC, et al. Diacetylmorphine versus methadone for the treatment of opioid addiction. *N Engl J Med.* 2009; 361:777–786.

31. Oviedo-Joekes E, Guh D, Brissette S, et al. Hydromorphone compared with diacetylmorphine for long-term opioid dependence. *JAMA Psychiatry.* 2016; 73(5):447–455.

32. Bansback N, Guh D, Oviedo-Joekes E, et al. Cost-effectiveness of hydromorphone for severe opioid use disorder: findings from the SALOME randomized clinical trial. *Addiction.* 2018; 113(7):1264–1273.

33. Tyndall M. An emergency response to the opioid overdose crisis in Canada: A regulated opioid distribution program. *CMAJ.* 2018; 190(2):E35–E36.

34. Jozaghi E, Greer AM, Lampkin H, Buxton JA. Activism and scientific research: 20 years of community action by the Vancouver Area Network of Drug Users. *Subst Abuse Treat Prev Policy.* 2018; 13(1):18.

35. Greer AM, Luchenski SA, Amlani AA, et al. Peer engagement in harm reduction strategies and services: A critical case study and evaluation framework from British Columbia, Canada. *BMC Public Health.* 2016; 16:452.

36. British Columbia Centre for Disease Control. Peer engagement and evaluation. http://www.bccdc.ca/health-professionals/clinical-resources/harm-reduction/peer-engagement-evaluation#Resources. Accessed February 12, 2019.

37. Vancouver Coastal Health. First overdose prevention learning lab opens. http://vchnews.ca/news/2017/09/21/first-overdose-prevention-learning-lab-opens/#.WrAAHVrwaUk. Accessed February 12, 2019.

5 | Stigma and the Language of Addiction

MICHAEL BOTTICELLI AND COLLEEN L. BARRY

WHILE IT IS WIDELY agreed that the opioid epidemic gained its foothold in the early 2000s as opioid prescribing grew dramatically, this epidemic has also laid bare many of the historical contributors that made conditions ripe for the current crisis. A lack of parity in health insurance for substance use disorder (SUD) treatment, the absence of addiction medicine training in general medical education curricula, an overemphasis on criminal justice responses focused on drug supply reduction, and many other critical factors predate the opioid epidemic and primed the country to experience its worst health and social crisis since the height of the AIDS epidemic.

There is perhaps no more pernicious contributor to this epidemic than stigma and its role in tainting how we perceive and make value judgments about people with SUD. Stigma influences attitudes toward individuals and groups, and these attitudes are expressed in how we as a nation have dealt with addiction in general and the opioid crisis in particular. Stigma is defined as a strong lack of respect for a person or a group of people or a bad opinion of them because they have done something or have traits of which society disapproves.[1] The process of assigning stigma (stigmatization) involves (1) labeling the difference that defines the stigmatized group, (2) stereotyping and connecting that labeled difference with other negative attributes, (3) distinguishing the people who are stigmatized from mainstream society and assigning them reduced social status, and (4) discriminating against this group. Stigma can be a major cause of societal exclusion, social isolation, and discrimination that devalues both the person and condition.[2]

Numerous studies have shown that SUDs are among the most highly stigmatized diseases compared to other health conditions.[3] The manifestations of stigma at the individual, familial, clinical, community/societal, and public policy levels are important contributors to the low numbers of people who seek and receive treatment; the overuse of incarceration for drug possession or use, particularly among people of color; the use of highly stigmatized language;

and the general public's attitude toward addiction as a moral failing and a matter of personal choice. Any serious strategic effort to reduce the morbidity and mortality of the current opioid crisis and of SUDs more generally must focus on reducing stigma and all its expressions.

In this chapter we address how stigma pervades public attitudes about addiction, clinical manifestations of stigma, and individual or self-stigma; how changing the language we use to discuss SUDs can reduce stigma; and how communication strategies that do not stigmatize individuals and groups can promote their receptivity to treatment and recovery and ultimately improve the public's health.

Public Attitudes About Addiction

For decades, the public at large has viewed, and continues to view, addiction as simply a matter of individual choice. This view is largely driven by a lack of scientific understanding of the genetic, environmental, and neurobiologic aspects of SUDs and addiction. Those who cannot seem to "control" their behavior (which can often be distressing and highly upsetting to others) continue to be seen as weak-willed or morally flawed. A 2018 Blue Cross Blue Shield survey of Massachusetts residents found that only 39% of those surveyed said that addiction was a disease; 28% believed it was a choice.[4] In the same survey, 82% of respondents believed that those with an addiction are all, mostly, or somewhat to blame, and 66% felt that not wanting to give up their addiction was the biggest barrier for recovery.[4] We posit that studies in other states would find similar results and lack of understanding around the biology and neuroscience of addiction.

In a national, web-based public opinion survey, Barry et al.[5] found that respondents held significantly more negative views toward people with drug addiction compared to those with mental illness (Figure 5.1). More respondents were unwilling to have a person with an SUD marry into their family or work closely with them on the job and were more willing to accept discriminatory practices such as denying housing or employment to individuals with SUDs relative to those with mental illness. Furthermore, respondents were skeptical about the effectiveness of treatment and more likely to oppose public policies aimed at helping people with SUDs, such as ensuring insurance parity and supporting government funding for addiction treatment.[5]

These attitudes permeate public policy and have shaped our overall approach to reducing drug use and its consequences in the United States. In 1988, Congress authorized the formation of the White House Office of National Drug Control Policy (ONDCP) by passage of the Anti-Drug Abuse Act. The ONDCP is charged with two main functions: to annually develop the administration's National Drug Control Strategy and to lead the development

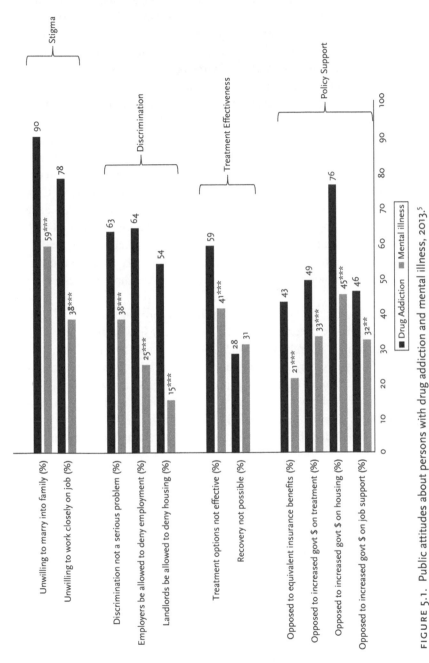

FIGURE 5.1. Public attitudes about persons with drug addiction and mental illness, 2013.[5]

Notes: 7-point Likert scales were collapsed to dichotomous stigma, discrimination, treatment effectiveness, and policy support measures. Pearson chi-square used to test whether attitudes differed based whether respondents viewed the drug addiction or mental illness version of each survey item. *$p < .05$; **$p < .01$; ***$p < .001$

of the consolidated federal drug control budget to align with its strategic priorities. Comprising actions and funding from the US Department of Health and Human Services, US Department of Justice, US Department of State, and their relevant operating divisions and agencies, the ONDCP has historically played a critical role in shaping drug policy in the United States. Not only does it set policy and fund programs, but, through its considerable bully pulpit, it can also shape public attitudes on how we view people with SUDs.

An analysis of federal government spending (Figure 5.2) indicates that since the ONDCP was established and began tracking overall federal funding, there has been far greater federal investment in law enforcement-centric approaches (supply reduction) compared to public health and prevention approaches (demand reduction). In fact, it was not until the end of the Obama administration that there was near parity in spending between supply and demand reduction, largely a result of the Patient Protection and Affordable Care Act (ACA) and increased spending for prevention. The historical overreliance on law enforcement approaches to address substance misuse, combined with discriminatory racial attitudes, led not only to incarceration of drug dealers and the pursuit of cartel leaders, but more consequentially to a large incarceration of low-level, nonviolent offenders arrested for simple possession or drug use.

Most studies indicate that 60% to 80% of those incarcerated in US jails and prisons meet diagnostic criteria for an SUD, with very few of those receiving any sort of treatment or rehabilitation.[6] Most of these low-level offenses were more a function of trying to support their own addiction than a criminogenic life.[6] The framing of addiction predominately as a law enforcement issue rather than a public health issue is reflected in news media coverage of the topic, and this framing reinforces stigma. For example, a 2015 study by McGinty et al. found that the news media more often frame the problem as a

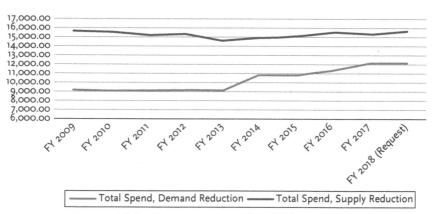

FIGURE 5.2. Historical federal drug control spending (budget authority in millions).
Source: White House Office of National Drug Control Policy[31]

criminal justice issue.[7] The most frequently mentioned cause of the problem was illegal drug dealing, and the most frequently mentioned actions were law enforcement solutions designed to arrest and prosecute the individuals responsible for diverting opioid analgesics onto the illegal market.[7]

Another major manifestation of public misperceptions and stigma toward addiction is in public policy. For example, stigma is reflected in the long history of discriminatory insurance coverage practices for public and commercial plans.[8] Lack of parity in insurance coverage for mental health and SUD treatment benefits relative to benefits for other health conditions goes back decades, with many insurers not offering a benefit or applying substantially different coverage limitations (minimal covered services, lifetime and annual limits, higher co-payments and deductibles) as well as nonquantitative practices (differing prior authorization and utilization review practices) than those provided for other similar health conditions.[9,10]

While efforts to address and increase coverage parity date back to the 1960s, it was not until the passage of the Paul Wellstone and Pete Domenici Mental Health Parity and Addiction Equity Act of 2008 that substantial progress was made.[11] Former Representative Patrick Kennedy of Rhode Island, one of the chief architects of the law, made the case for its passage on the grounds that "access to mental health services is one of the most important and most neglected civil rights issues facing the Nation. For too long, persons living with mental disorders have suffered from discriminatory treatment at all levels of society."[12] Additionally, the ACA, passed in 2010, required SUD treatment as one of the 10 essential health benefits and required both marketplace and Medicaid expansion plans to afford that coverage in accordance with federal parity.[8]

Clinical Manifestations of Stigma

It has been well documented that negative and stigmatizing attitudes of clinicians result in the undertreatment of patients with SUDs, a lack of empathy, and a reticence among patients to share important information about their substance use for fear of judgment and retribution.[13,14] Certainly, the attitudes of the general public contribute to these opinions among medical professionals, but they are also compounded by a lack of dedicated and specific training for clinical staff as part of routine medical education and clinical preparation. For example, only a very small percentage of primary care physicians have opted to take the training sponsored by the US Drug Enforcement Agency that is necessary to prescribe the addiction medication buprenorphine.[14] The Drug Abuse Treatment Act of 2000 (DATA 2000) allows physicians to treat patients with addiction medications in a variety of medical setting rather than just in specialty addiction treatment programs. Since the passage of DATA

2000 and the approval by the US Food and Drug Administration of variety of buprenorphine-based medications, only 4% of primary care physicians have gone through the training, and of these, not all actually prescribe the medications.[15] While there are many reasons that contribute to these low numbers, one cannot discount the role that stigma plays in a lack of desire to treat people with opioid addiction and other SUDs despite their prevalence in these same care settings.[16]

Encouragingly, some health care training institutions have begun to integrate core competencies into medical education. A joint effort by governmental and academic leadership in Massachusetts led to the development and implementation of a standard set of core clinical competencies among the state's four medical and three dental schools. As providers address stigma in the clinical setting, great strides can be made to reduce stigma and better treat patients with SUDs.

Self-Stigma

As is often the case with stigmatized diseases, those affected internalize those beliefs.[17] This self-stigma becomes a major determinant in why those with an SUD delay seeking care or avoid care altogether. Self-stigma also substantially contributes to a profound sense of isolation and loneliness, which can further exacerbate the disease, leading to potentially fatal consequences. Based on the results from the 2016 National Survey on Drug Use and Health, an annual telephonic survey administered by the US Substance Abuse and Mental Health Services Administration (SAMHSA), an estimated 19.9 million adults in the United States met diagnostic criteria for an SUD; this represents approximately 8.1% of all adults.[18] An estimated 2.1 million (10.8%) of these adults actually received treatment at a facility. The vast majority of remaining adults in the survey (95.5%, or 16.9 million adults) did not feel that they needed treatment and did not seek it. Only 4.5% (806,000 people) felt they needed treatment but did not seek it, or made an effort to find treatment but did not get it. The survey also asked respondents to cite the various reasons why they did not seek treatment even though they knew they had an SUD and needed treatment: 25% of respondents said fear of negative opinions among neighbors and friends and fear about potential negative effect by their employer were significant barriers to seeking care.[18] Addressing self-stigma certainly could have a profound impact on how individuals perceive their disease and the opportunities to treat it in the future. Reductions in self-stigma could motivate millions more to seek and find treatment and support their recovery.

The Language of Stigma

Language reflects our belief system. While the neurobiology of addiction has clearly demonstrated the validity of the disease approach to SUDs, the language used to describe both the condition and those affected remains rooted in our belief that people with an SUD are somehow morally flawed. Language is perpetuated by the general public, by the media, by the medical community, and even by those in the recovery community. Historically, we have used language to isolate those affected and to treat them in a less than compassionate and therapeutic way. Words like "addict," "junkie," and even "substance abuser" connote a level of moral judgment that is not done with most physical or behavioral conditions. In a highly cited study, Dr. John Kelly of the Recovery Research Institute gave nearly identical vignettes to doctoral-level mental health clinicians.[19] Use of the term "substance abuser" was shown to assign blame and to concur with a punitive response to the patient when compared with the term "substance use disorder."[19] The terms "clean" and "dirty" are still used to describe whether someone is in recovery or the results of a drug toxicology screen. Many in the recovery community still refer to their "clean time" and bear a special responsibility to use appropriate language.

Furthermore, the language included in US news media coverage of the opioid epidemic contributes to widespread public stigma toward people with SUDs. A recent study examined the content of 6,000 news stories about the opioid epidemic published in high-circulation US national and regional print outlets or aired by high-viewership television news networks from July 2008 through June 2018.[20] Over the study period, 49% of news stories about the epidemic mentioned a term that has been shown in research to be stigmatizing (e.g., addict, drug abuser) while only 2% mentioned any less-stigmatizing alternative (e.g., person with an opioid use disorder).[20]

In January 2017, the ONDCP issued guidance to all federal agencies encouraging them to use only clinically appropriate language on their websites, documents, and other public-facing communications. Unfortunately, the names of lead federal agencies (i.e., the National Institute on Drug Abuse; the Substance Abuse and Mental Health Services Administration) are set in federal authorizing language and can be changed only with congressional approval. Later in 2017, the *AP Stylebook*, which provides guidance to journalists seeking to use precise language, discouraged the use of words like "junkie," "addict," and "abuser" and encouraged reporters to replace these words with phrase like "he was addicted" or a "person with a substance use disorder."[20,21] These changes reflect a movement toward person-centered language similar to that of other disabilities (Table 5.1).

The term "medication-assisted treatment" can also connote stigma. It is arguably one of the reasons behind the relatively low uptake of medications for

TABLE 5.1. Examples of Stigmatizing Language and Less Stigmatizing Alternatives

STIGMATIZING LANGUAGE	LESS STIGMATIZING ALTERNATIVES
Addict	Person with a substance use
Junkie	disorder
Drug abuser	Person with an opioid use
Abuser	disorder
	He/she is addicted; he/she was addicted
Clean versus dirty	In recovery
Medication-assisted treatment	Treatment
	Medication for addiction treatment

treatment of opioid use disorder despite the preponderance of evidence of their efficacy over treatment without medication. In a 2016 commentary in *Practical Pain Management*, Wakeman writes that this phrase can imply that medications are somehow a "corollary to whatever the main part of treatment is" and calls on us to simply use the term "treatment."[22] The phrase "medication-assisted treatment" can also inadvertently communicate that there are two different treatments: one with medications and the other without. This division is often emphasized within the recovery community, with some individuals considering people on medications as "not really in recovery" or "replacing one addiction for another."[23] While Alcoholics Anonymous encourages people to use medications if they need them, Narcotics Anonymous still refers to medications as "drug replacement" and encourages complete "abstinence" even in the absence of an evidence base to support the efficacy of abstinence alone.[23]

Communication Strategies to Reduce Stigma

Strategic communication strategies have the potential to reduce stigma and increase support for policies to combat the epidemic, including harm reduction approaches. Harm reduction approaches such as safe or supervised consumption sites, syringe services programs, and naloxone distribution programs aim to minimize the negative health, social, and economic consequences of drug use and have been shown to reduce overdose deaths and HIV transmission and hepatitis C–related risk behaviors among individuals using drugs.[24,25] Safe consumption sites have not been implemented in the United States due in part to low public support.[26] Recent evidence suggests the potential role for strategic communication efforts to encourage public support for harm reduction and other controversial policies. Even small changes in language, known as framing effects, can sometimes shift attitudes fairly dramatically, including on controversial public health topics.[27] For example, Barry et al. surveyed representative national samples of Americans and found that only 29% of respondents were in favor of "safe consumption sites," but 45% supported them when the term "overdose prevention sites" was used instead.[28]

The use of a sympathetic narrative can also be an effective approach for stigma reduction. The use of narrative needs to be approached with some care given research showing that individual depictions can increase stigma by leading audiences to blame the affected individuals, as opposed to societal and other factors, for the problem they are experiencing.[28] In contrast, the use of narratives that blend individual depictions with contextual information about the structural factors influencing addiction can be stigma reducing. For example, one experimental study found that a short text narrative that included both an individual depiction of a pregnant woman with opioid use disorder and a description of the external barriers to treatment that she faced, such as a long waiting list for methadone treatment, increased audiences' feelings of sympathy and pity for the woman relative to a control arm and a narrative describing the same woman without discussing barriers to treatment.[29]

Similarly, Bachhuber et al. conducted an experiment to test whether support for naloxone distribution might be increased by describing the policy in terms of a sympathetic narrative about a young woman who died from a prescription opioid overdose.[30] Compared with a control group, this narrative reduced stigma and raised support for policies to train first responders to use naloxone, to provide naloxone to friends and family members of people at risk of opioid overdose, and to protect people from civil or criminal liability if they call for medical help for an opioid overdose or administer naloxone.

Summary

One cannot minimize the role that stigma continues to play in thwarting evidence-based, compassionate public policy. This will change only if we make concerted efforts to reform our language, reform our images and portrayals of those affected by addiction, and use sympathetic personal narratives. The manifestation of stigma is important as public health and health care professionals promote ways to get more individuals with SUDs into treatment. Addressing stigma will also address the way we develop public policy—for example, access to insurance coverage, or the traditional law enforcement approach to addiction such as incarceration rather than diversion to treatment. To reduce the morbidity and mortality of the current opioid crisis, public health professionals and policymakers must focus on reducing stigma and its consequences.

References

1. Shrivastava A, Johnston M, Bureau Y. Stigma of mental illness 1: Clinical reflections. *Mens Sana Monogr*. 2012; 10(1):70.
2. Bruce G, Phelan JC. Conceptualizing stigma. *Ann Rev Sociol*. 2001; 27:363–385.
3. Sartorius N. Stigmatized illnesses and health care. *Croatian Med J*. 2007; 48(3):396–397.
4. Dreyfus A. Massachusetts public opinion poll: The state of the opioid epidemic. 2018. https://www.slideshare.net/AndrewDreyfus/massachusetts-public-opinion-poll-the-state-of-the-opioid-epidemic. Accessed February 12, 2019.
5. Barry CL, McGinty EE, Pescosolido B, Goldman HG. Stigma, discrimination, treatment effectiveness and public policy support: Americans' attitudes toward persons with drug addiction and mental illness. *Psychiatr Serv*. 2014; 65(10):1269–1272.
6. Columbia University, National Center on Addiction and Substance Abuse. Behind bars: Substance abuse and America's prison population. 1998. https://www.centeronaddiction.org/addiction-research/reports/behind-bars-ii-substance-abuse-and-america%E2%80%99s-prison-population. Accessed February 12, 2019.
7. McGinty EE, Kennedy-Hendricks A, Baller J, et al. Criminal activity or treatable health condition? News media framing of opioid analgesic abuse in the United States, 1998–2012. *Psychiatr Serv*. 2016; 67(4):405–411.
8. Barry CL, Goldman HH, Huskamp HA. Federal parity in the evolving mental health and addiction care landscape. *Health Aff*. 2016; 35(6):1009–1016.
9. Barry CL, Sindelar JL. Equity in private insurance coverage for substance abuse: A perspective on the federal parity debate. *Health Aff*. 2007; 26(6):w708–w716.
10. Barry CL, Gabel JR, Frank RG, et al. Design of mental health insurance coverage: Still unequal after all these years. *Health Aff*. 2003; 22(5):127–137.
11. Barry CL, Huskamp HA, Goldman HH. A political history of federal mental health and addiction insurance parity. *Milbank Q*. 2010; 88(3):404–433.
12. Congressional Record. Keeping Alive the Work and Spirit of Paul Wellstone. US Senate, Volume 150, February 5, 2004, p. S599.
13. Van Boekel LC, Brouwers EPM, Van Weeghel J, Garretsen HFL. Stigma among health professionals towards patients with substance use disorders and its consequences for healthcare delivery: Systematic review. *Drug Alcohol Depend*. 2013;131(1-3):23–35.
14. Kennedy-Hendricks A, Busch S, McGinty E, et al. Primary care physicians' perspectives on the prescription opioid epidemic. *Drug Alcohol Depend*. 2016; 165:61–70.
15. US Government Accountability Office. Laws, Regulations, and Other Factors Can Affect Medication-Assisted Treatment Access. 2016. https://www.gao.gov/assets/690/680050.pdf. Accessed February 12, 2019.
16. Wakeman SE, Pham-Kanter G, Donelan K. Attitudes, practices, and preparedness to care for patients with substance use disorder: Results from a survey of general internists. *Subst Abus*. 2016; 37(3):635–641.
17. Matthews S, Dwyer R, Snoek A. Stigma and self-stigma in addiction. *J Bioeth Inq*. 2017;14(2):275–286.

18. US Substance Abuse and Mental Health Services Administration. National Survey on Drug Use and Health. 2016. https://www.samhsa.gov/data/sites/default/files/NSDUH-DetTabs-2016/NSDUH-DetTabs-2016.pdf. Accessed February 12, 2019.

19. Kelly JF, Westerhoff CM. Does it matter how we refer to individuals with substance-related conditions? A randomized study of two commonly used terms. *Int J Drug Policy*. 2010; 21(3):202–207.

20. McGinty EE, Stone E, Kennedy-Hendricks A, Barry CL. Stigmatizing language in news media coverage of the opioid epidemic: Implications for public health. *Prev Med*. https://doi.org/10.1016/j.ypmed.2019.03.018.

21. Freyer F. Influential word-usage guide changes the language of addiction. *Boston Globe*, June 15, 2017.

22. Wakeman SE. Commentary: A modern epidemic—The case for addiction medicine. *Internal Medicine News*, July 16, 2015.

23. Narcotics Anonymous. Narcotics Anonymous and persons receiving medication-assisted treatment. https://www.na.org/admin/include/spaw2/uploads/pdf/pr/2306_NA_PRMAT_1021.pdf. Accessed February 12, 2019.

24. Ritter A, Cameron J. A review of the efficacy and effectiveness of harm reduction strategies for alcohol, tobacco and illicit drugs. *Drug Alcohol Rev*. 2006; 25(6):611–624.

25. Rhodes T, Hedrich D. *Harm Reduction: Evidence, Impacts and Challenges*. European Monitoring Centre for Drugs and Drug Addiction. Luxembourg: Publications Office of the European Union; 2010.

26. McGinty EE, Barry CL, Stone E, et al. Public support for safe consumption sites and syringe services programs to combat the opioid epidemic. *Prev Med*. 2018; 111:73–77.

27. Barry CL, Sherman SG, McGinty EE. Language matters in combatting the opioid epidemic: Safe consumption sites versus overdose prevention sites. *Am J Public Health*. 2018; 108(9):1157.

28. Iyengar S. Framing responsibility for political issues: The case of poverty. *Pol Behav*. 1990; 12(1):19–40.

29. Iyengar S. Framing responsibility for political issues. *Ann Am Acad Pol Soc Sci*. 1996; 546:59–70.

30. Bachhuber MA, McGinty EE, Kennedy-Hendricks A, et al. Messaging to increase public support for naloxone distribution policies in the United States: Results from a randomized survey experiment. *PLoS One*. 2015; 10(7):e0130050.

31. White House Office of National Drug Control Policy. National Drug Control Budget; FY18 Funding Highlights. 2017. https://www.whitehouse.gov/sites/whitehouse.gov/files/ondcp/Fact_Sheets/FY2018-Budget-Highlights.pdf. Accessed February 12, 2019.

6 | The Neuroscience of Addiction

A PRIMER FOR PUBLIC HEALTH PROFESSIONALS

JAY C. BUTLER

FFECTIVE PUBLIC HEALTH APPROACHES to addressing the opioid crisis require an understanding of addiction as a health condition primarily involving the brain, rather than an individual's series on ongoing "bad choices" or inherent criminal tendencies that ultimately lead to poor health outcomes. Addiction has been defined as "the most severe, chronic stage of substance-use disorder, in which there is a substantial loss of self-control, as indicated by compulsive drug taking despite the desire to stop taking the drug."[1] Whether addiction is viewed primarily as a "disease"[1] or the outcome of experiential and environmental influences resulting in a "learning disorder,"[2] chronic changes that occur in the brain of the person with addiction form the scientific basis of an effective public health response. Understanding the behavioral changes driven by addiction is vital since they have a profound impact on public safety, the criminal justice system, and public health. This chapter provides an overview of the changes that occur in the brain during development of addiction and how understanding these changes can improve public health practice and policy. It complements more complete clinical and basic science reviews of the neuroscience of addiction that have been recently published.[1-4]

Neurologic Function in Health and Addiction

Dopamine is a central nervous system neurotransmitter that is crucial to normal brain function but also central to addiction development and continuation. The release of dopamine from the nucleus accumbens, an area in the ventral striatum at the base of the forebrain, produces a sensation of pleasure and reward. The physiologic release of dopamine occurs during eating or sex, both functions crucial to survival of the individual and the species. Drugs with addiction potential exert their self-reinforcing effects by triggering supraphysiologic dopamine spikes in the nucleus accumbens, producing the subjective sensation of being "high." However, unlike natural drivers of dopamine release, which usually lead to satiation, dopamine release continues and increases with drug use, leading to ongoing desire to use and compulsive patterns of consumption. Figure 6.1 illustrates the density of dopamine transporters in a healthy brain, and then at one and 14 months of abstinence (in this image, methamphetamine). Figure 6.1 also illustrates the remarkable capacity of the brain to recover from drug use, albeit in the long term (in this case, 14 months).

Opioids exert their analgesic effects primarily by binding to the *mu*-opioid receptors in the brain regions that regulate pain perception, pain-induced emotional responses, and the sense of reward.[5] Opioids not only directly stimulate receptors in these areas of the brain but also lead to the release of neurotransmitters, including dopamine as described above, that reinforce the pleasurable sensations and can lead to conditioned behaviors the amplify the desire to use opioids again. Long-lasting neurobiologic changes develop over a period of opioid use that may vary from months to years. Koob and Volkow[3] have proposed a conceptual model for understanding the progressive development of opioid addiction that involves three stages along a continuum. Initial use of opioids may be driven by voluntary behaviors, such as following a health care provider's prescription, or by impulsive actions, including drug experimentation. However, as the stages of addiction advance, the capacity for an individual to self-control is muted and the voluntary nature of drug-seeking

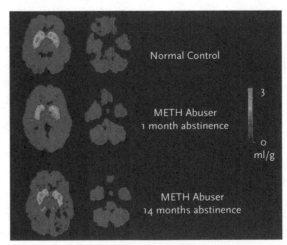

FIGURE 6.1. Brain images of the distribution volume of [¹¹C]*d-threo*-methylphenidate in a control subject and a methamphetamine abuser [*sic*].
Source: Volkow N, Wang G, et. al.[25]
(c) Journal of Neuroscience, 2001. Reproduced with permission.

behavior and drug use is lost to the compulsive desire to obtain and use opioids despite the user's awareness of catastrophic consequences.

Three Stages of Addiction

The first stage of addiction, *the binge/intoxication stage*, is characterized by the experience of intense pleasure and a sense of reward mediated through the release of dopamine. Users often describe the euphoria experienced with initial use as fleeting and unreproducible because repeated exposure to opioids will lead to downregulation of the *mu*-receptor and neurotransmitter release mechanisms. As a result, increasing doses are required to achieve that same level of dopamine release and subjective experience, including pain relief, a phenomenon known as *tolerance*. Tolerance develops more slowly in the *mu*-receptors in the respiratory drive centers of the brain stem than in the structures of the basal forebrain, increasing the risk of dangerous respiratory depression and overdose death with increasing doses.[6]

Both duration of exposure and dose appear to affect the development of tolerance. In clinical settings, the risk of tolerance is greater in persons who have experienced major trauma, in those requiring prolonged mechanical ventilation, and in pediatric patients.[7] The frequency of exposure also influences development of tolerance, with tolerance developing less rapidly with intermittent exposures. While tolerance is part of the progression of opioid use disorder to addiction, it is crucial to distinguish tolerance from addiction: Tolerance will inevitably develop in anyone who is exposed to repeated doses of opioids over a period of days to weeks, but addiction develops more slowly and in only a small proportion of those who develop tolerance.[5] Moreover, the pathophysiology of tolerance differs from that of addiction, and the effects of tolerance will resolve rapidly after discontinuation of opioid use.

In addition to creating a euphoric sensation, dopamine release stimulated through repeated use leads to neuroplastic remodeling that is an essential part of learning and creation of memory. After prolonged use, neurotransmitters may be released in anticipation of the drug-induced reward by conditioning stimuli. As a result, subtle non–drug-related experiences, such as the feeling of a needle piercing the skin during venipuncture, or environmental stimuli such as the smell of foil being heated by a flame, may trigger intense drug craving and drive behaviors that may lead to obtaining the drug. These neurologic changes and susceptibility to the resulting sensations can persist; as a result, the risk of relapse may persist for years and, for some persons, may even be lifelong.

Ongoing opioid use leads to the second stage, *withdrawal/negative affect*, manifested by irritability, malaise, and dysphoria, as well as onset of withdrawal symptoms when opioids are not used. During this stage, the major motivation to use opioids is not to experience euphoria ("get high"), but rather to avoid the dysphoria and physical manifestations of opioid withdrawal. Withdrawal symptoms include nausea, vomiting, diarrhea, rhinorrhea, lacrimation, photosensitivity, sweats and chills, piloerection, tremulousness, insomnia, and myalgias. The prominence of pain during withdrawal merits special emphasis given that patients who use opioids for chronic pain management may not be able to distinguish withdrawal pain from their pain syndrome. These symptoms vary in intensity and may last as long as two weeks depending on the type of opioid used. With progressive use, the sense of reward naturally stimulated by activities such as eating, sex, and activities of daily life is diminished, resulting in weight loss, strained relationships, and generally diminished physical health and psychosocial function.

The final stage of opioid addiction, *preoccupation/anticipation*, is characterized by loss of salience (assignment of relative values) in preference for use of the drug. Continued downregulation of dopamine signaling and interruption of other neurotransmitters dulls the function of the prefrontal cortex, the center of executive function in the brain, essential to goal-directed behavior. As a result, committing a crime becomes simply a path to obtaining the drug, and sensory input that normally would be prioritized for immediate reaction, such as a child crying, becomes secondary to behavior needed to maintain drug use. Persons with a genuine desire to discontinue drug use are often unable to follow through, and ongoing drug use becomes an essentially involuntary behavior.

Implications for Public Health Practice and Policy

While the current epidemic of opioid misuse, addiction, and overdose deaths has been created by a "perfect storm" of social, economic, and health care factors, the initial cause was iatrogenic: an untoward effect of the increased prescribing of opioid analgesics in a wide variety of clinical settings that began in the late 1990s.[8] While the amount of opioids dispensed has declined in recent years, these medications are still prescribed at much higher rates than they were prior to the beginning of the crisis. Heroin and fentanyl and other synthetic opioids have played an increasing role in opioid addiction and overdose deaths during the second decade of the twenty-first century, but the significance of oral prescription painkillers in the ongoing crisis must not be minimized.

The 2017 National Survey on Drug Use and Health indicates that more than 11 million Americans aged 12 years and older, over 4% of the population, misuse opioids, and are thus at high risk of opioid use disorder and addiction.[9] The vast majority of those who misuse opioids are taking prescription opioids, and of those who use heroin, the majority first became addicted through misuse of prescription opioids. Thus, reducing inappropriate prescribing of opioid pain relievers or dispensing them in dosages or counts greater than needed is an important opportunity for prevention. Given the risks of opioid use, as well as the emerging data on the comparative efficacy of non-opioid analgesia for acute and chronic pain,[10,11] policies that help clinicians improve their skills in pain management through educational opportunities are needed.[12] However, better training for providers alone will not address the problem of overprescription of opioids. Third-party reimbursement reforms are needed so that coverage of non-opioid and nonpharmacologic approaches to managing acute and chronic pain are adequately reimbursed and evidence-based multimodal care of patients with pain is advanced.[13]

Adolescence represents a critical time of susceptibility because of the neurologic changes that normally occur beginning in preadolescence and continuing into the mid-20s. Drug use during adolescence is associated with more intensive and chronic use, resulting in greater risk of substance use disorder and addiction than is seen after initiation at older ages. Prolonged opioid use and misuse has been associated with prescribed opioids following sports injuries in student athletes and after procedures that are common among teens and young adults, such as wisdom tooth extraction, appendectomy, and orthopedic repairs.[14,15] Therefore, pain management strategies that minimize pain and that maximize patient safety and public health benefit are particularly important in the pediatric/young adult age group.

Treatment of opioid addiction and maintenance of recovery will be more successful if initiated early in the progression of the stages of addiction outlined in this chapter when altered brain structure and function is less "hard-wired" and difficult to reverse. The neurologic changes induced by substance use and leading to addiction develop over time; reversal of these changes should not be expected to occur rapidly. Management strategies and reimbursement plans that address addiction as a chronic condition and that provide for prolonged treatment are more likely to be successful than short-term therapies or simple "detox." Understanding and communicating the long-term and sometimes lifelong neurologic effects of addiction will help family members and loved ones to better provide support for persons seeking recovery. Clearer conceptualization of how addiction affects that brain will help patients, family members, and policymakers understand that opioid replacement therapy with opioid agonists, such as methadone or buprenorphine, helps address the pathologic processes and is not merely "replacing one addiction with another."

The neuroscience of addiction provides the evidence base to destigmatize opioid addiction. Stigma creates disincentives to seeking treatment and often creates additional barriers during treatment and maintenance of recovery. Most mental illnesses have been recognized as worthy of coordinated advocacy; however, the opioid user is often blamed for the poor health outcomes caused by opioid misuse and addiction even when initial use was based on advice of a trusted health care provider. Public health officials are well placed to change the opioid addiction dialogue by avoiding and discouraging use of negative terminology when speaking on the topic.[16] Public health agencies have the opportunity to avoid unintentionally reinforcing stigma when prevention messages conflate drug misuse and criminal behavior.[17]

Misperception of opioid addiction as primarily a criminal justice issue has been used in the past to justify inaction on the part of lawmakers and health agencies in providing harm reduction services such as syringe and needle service programs, increasing access to naloxone, and making treatment widely available to those in need. Incarcerated persons with opioid addiction have been particularly ignored, not receiving effective treatments for substance use disorders or screening and treatment for hepatitis C virus infections caused by self-injection drug use, despite evidence of high risk of relapse and overdose death from untreated addiction after release and data indicating the cost-effectiveness of addressing hepatitis C in prisons.[18,19] Emerging data from Rhode Island indicate that providing effective treatment during incarceration and care during transition back to the community after release improves outcomes.[20]

Primary prevention of opioid addiction requires addressing both the supply of and demand for opioids, as wells as other substances with potential for misuse and addiction. The supply side of the opioid market equation can be transformed through good opioid stewardship in clinical practice and disrupting illicit drug trafficking. Addressing the demand side will require addressing the social determinants that drive substance use, including racism, inequities in economic opportunity, and adverse childhood experiences (ACEs). The neurologic changes that occur from ACE-related toxic stress in childhood may account for the epidemiologic association between ACEs and opioid misuse and highlight the need to prevent ACEs and mitigate their effects through primary prevention efforts such as home visitation programs.[21,22]

Finally, there is much that is still not known about how to solve the current opioid crisis in North America. Funds for basic science, translational, clinical, and epidemiologic research are needed. New and better modalities are needed to reverse opioid overdose, treat opioid addiction, and provide effective, nonaddictive alternatives for management of pain.[23] Improved and standardized epidemiologic methods and practices are required to accurately track the evolution of the epidemic and to assess the effectiveness of control measures. Robust evaluation of new laws, policies, and public health interventions are needed to ensure that steps taken to address the current crisis have a minimum of unanticipated consequences.

Summary

While our understanding of addiction as a chronic health condition primarily involving the brain has progressed rapidly in recent years, public health and clinical practice have lagged behind the neuroscience of addition, and there is still much left to learn. We know little of the neuroscience of recovery, including the specific neural pathways that should be targeted for therapeutic intervention and the relative roles of restitutive healing and development of compensatory mechanisms that drive behaviors toward entering and maintaining successful recovery.[24] Genetics likely plays a role in susceptibility to addictions, but clinically useful tools for genetic markers that could guide risk assessment and decisions about pain management are yet to be developed. Biomarkers for risk, such as those that exist for infectious diseases, atherosclerotic heart disease, and certain types of cancer, are lacking but sorely needed.

What is most important about understanding the neuroscience of addiction is that the "addicted" brain does not function like the nonaddicted brain. Programs and policies that assume individuals with opioid use disorder can "just stop" fail to recognize the complexity of how brains are changed through substance use and the different phases of addiction. Public health practitioners should be aware of the neuroscience of addiction and the different ways that individual behaviors are influenced by substance use. Understanding addiction as a chronic health condition rather than a moral failing is essential to developing effective policies and programs to prevent it and end the current crisis.

References

1. Volkow ND, Koob GF, McLellan AT. Neurobiologic advances from the brain disease model of addiction. *N Engl J Med*. 2016; 374(4):363–371.
2. Lewis M. Brain changes in addiction as learning, not disease. *N Engl J Med*. 2018; 379(16):1551–1560.
3. Koob GF, Volkow ND. Neurobiology of addiction: A neurocircuitry analysis. *Lancet Psych*. 2016; 3(8):760–773.
4. Volkow ND, Morales M. The brain on drugs: From reward to addiction. *Cell*. 2015; 162:712–725.
5. Volkow ND, McLellan AT. Opioid abuse in chronic pain—Misconceptions and mitigation strategies. *N Engl J Med*. 2016; 374(13):1253–1263.
6. Boyer EW. Management of opioid analgesic overdose. *N Engl J Med*. 2012; 367(2):146–155.
7. Martyn JAJ, Mao J, Bittner EA. Opioid tolerance in critical illness. *N Engl J Med*. 2019; 380(4):365–378.
8. Jones MR, Viswanath O, Peck J, et al. A brief history of the opioid epidemic and strategies in pain medicine. *Pain Ther*. 2018; 7:13–21

9. Bose J, Hedden SL, Lipari RN, Park-Lee E. Key substance use and mental health indicators in the United States: Results from the 2017 National Survey on Drug Use and Health (HHS Publication No. SMA 18-5068, NSDUH Series H-53). Center for Behavioral Health Statistics and Quality, U.S. Substance Abuse and Mental Health Services Administration. 2018. https://www.samhsa.gov/data/report/2017-nsduh-annual-national-report. Accessed January 30, 2019.

10. Busse JW, Wang L, Kamaleldin M, et al. Opioids for chronic non-cancer pain: A systematic review and meta-analysis. *JAMA*. 2018; 320(23):2448–2460.

11. Chang AK, Bijur PE, Esses D, Barnaby DP, Baer J. Effect of a single dose of oral opioid and nonopioid analgesics on acute extremity pain in the emergency department: A randomized clinical trial. *JAMA*. 2017; 318(17):1661–1667.

12. Ashburn MA, Levine RL. Pennsylvania state core competencies for education on opioids and addiction. *Pain Med*. 2017; 18(10):1890–1894.

13. Heyward J, Jones CM, Compton WM, et al. Coverage of nonpharmacologic treatments for low back pain among US public and private insurers. *JAMA Netw Open*. 2018; 1(6):e183044.

14. Harbaugh CM, Nalliah RP, Hu HM, et al. Persistent opioid use after wisdom tooth extraction. *JAMA*. 2018; 320(5):504–506.

15. Harbaugh CM, Lee JS, Hu HM, et al. Persistent opioid use among pediatric patients after surgery. *Pediatrics*. 2018;141(1):e20172439.

16. Botticelli MP, Koh H. Changing the language of addiction. *JAMA*. 2016; 316(13):1361–1362.

17. Corrigan P, Schomerus G, Smelson D. Are some of the stigmas of addiction culturally sanctioned? *Br J Psychiatry*. 2017; 210:180–181.

18. Binswanger IA, Blatchford PJ, Mueller SR, Stern MF. Mortality after prison release: Opioid overdose and other causes of death, risk factors, and time trends from 1999 to 2009. *Ann Intern Med*. 2013; 159(9):592–600.

19. He T, Kan L, Roberts MS, et al. Prevention of hepatitis C by screening and treatment in U.S. prisons. *Ann Intern Med*. 2016; 164(2):84–92.

20. Green TC, Clarke J, Brinkley-Rubinstein L, et al. Postincarceration fatal overdoses after implementing medications for addiction treatment in a statewide correctional system. *JAMA Psychiatry*. 2018; 75(4):81–83.

21. Dube SR, Felitti VJ, Dong M, et al. Childhood abuse, neglect, and household dysfunction and the risk of illicit drug use: The Adverse Childhood Experiences Study. *Pediatrics*. 2003; 111(3):564–572.

22. Gardner AS. Home visitation and the biology of toxic stress: Opportunities to address early childhood adversity. *Pediatrics* 2013; 132(2):S65–S73.

23. Volkow ND, Collins FS. The role of science in addressing the opioid crisis. *N Engl J Med*. 2017; 377(4):391–394.

24. Humphreys K, Bickel WK. Toward a neuroscience of long-term recovery from addiction. *JAMA Psychiatry*. 2018; 75(9):875–876.

25. Volkow ND, Chang L, Wang G-J, et al. Loss of dopamine transporters in methamphetamine abusers recovers with protracted abstinence. *Neuroscience*. 2001; 21(23):9414–9418.

II | Connecting Clinical Perspectives and Public Health Practice

7 | Non-Opioid Alternatives to Managing Chronic Pain

AN OVERVIEW FOR PUBLIC HEALTH PRACTITIONERS

VANILA M. SINGH AND RACHEL KATONAK

WHILE PUBLIC HEALTH PRACTITIONERS generally focus on the primary prevention of illness and disease by developing programs and policies that promote health and well-being, an understanding of chronic pain and its treatment is important for public health professionals working to address the opioid crisis in the United States. There are unintended consequences of well-intentioned policies that may restrict prescribing behavior or otherwise interrupt or change access to opioids. For example, one consequence of expanding state prescription drug monitoring programs has been concern by providers that "legitimate" pain patients may be subjected to increased suspicion and stigma and not able to obtain needed medications. State and federal efforts to shut down "pill mills" are vital to addressing diversion and criminal behavior, but pain patients who are also seen in these clinics may have an interruption in their treatment or access to medication. Understanding chronic pain treatment, and non-opioid alternatives to pain management, is an important part of developing sound public health policies to prevent opioid use disorder and its sequelae.

Pain affects an estimated 50 million people in the United States.[1] This includes about 19.6 million adults that have "high-impact" chronic pain (pain that lasts more than three months and limits activities such as ability to work outside the home, attend school, or perform household chores). There is a higher prevalence of both chronic pain and high-impact chronic pain reported among women, older adults, previously but not currently employed adults, adults living in poverty, adults with public health insurance, and rural residents. Chronic pain costs the nation an estimated $560 billion each year in medical treatment and lost work productivity.[2]

Chronic pain is defined by the International Association for the Study of Pain as "an unpleasant sensory and emotional experience associated with actual or potential tissue damage or described in terms of such damage."[3] Pain is a general

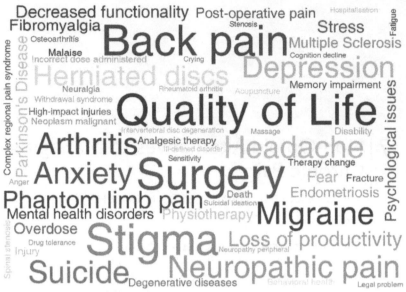

FIGURE 7.1. Illustrative representation of public comments on the Pain Management Best Practices Inter-Agency Task Force draft report. U.S. Department of Health and Human Services (2019). Pain Management Best Practices Inter-Agency Task Force Report: Updates, Gaps, Inconsistencies, and Recommendations. Retrieved from https://www.hhs.gov/ash/advisory-committees/pain/reports/index.html.
Source: https://commons.wikimedia.org/wiki/File:Children%27s_pain_scale.JPG

term used to refer to dozens of various, often complex, medical conditions and pain syndromes, including neurologic disorders, musculoskeletal conditions, and inflammatory diseases. The goal of pain management is to address the patient's symptoms in order to restore functional abilities and overall quality of life.

The approach for diagnosis and treatment of pain would benefit from a consideration of the biopsychosocial model of health. The biopsychosocial model could be used by clinicians to systematically assess the relative contribution that three factors (biologic etiology, psychological etiology, and social context etiologies) make to a particular patient's experience of chronic pain. Contemporary pain management involves multidisciplinary approaches to pain care and an appreciation of the vital need for various treatment modalities. A collaborative, multimodal, and interdisciplinary patient-centered approach to treatment for various chronic pain syndromes is essential to good clinical outcomes and to preventing potential opioid addiction. Continuous reconsideration and reevaluation are essential throughout the management of pain syndromes to ensure treatment goals are reached. As such, multidisciplinary teams of many different types of specialists play important roles in educating and treating patients and their families.

Multimodal approaches for treatment are needed now more than ever given that federal, state, and local officials, in addition to the community, physicians, and other health care providers, are working to end the opioid overdose crisis while balancing the ability of those living with pain to work with their physicians and/or health care providers to develop and implement an individualized integrative pain treatment plan that improves functional status, quality of life, and work productivity outcomes. Because of the complexity of concerns related to the multifaceted opioid crisis, there is a concerted movement toward applying various pain therapy modalities that are effective and result in limited opioid exposure only when clinically indicated. For certain patients with chronic pain, opioids may continue to be a part of their treatment plan of care when the benefits outweigh the risks.

As described in the Foreword to this volume, the US Department of Health and Human Services (HHS) has a multipronged public health approach to address the opioid crisis that includes advancing pain management. A component of the overall five-point HHS plan is "better pain management":

Better pain management: HHS is overseeing and coordinating numerous concerted efforts to support evidence-based pain management. The Pain Management Best Practices Inter-Agency Task Force is working to propose updates to best practices and issue recommendations that address gaps or inconsistencies for managing chronic and acute pain. HHS is overseeing this effort along with the U.S. Department of Veterans Affairs and U.S. Department of Defense. The [US] National Institutes of Health (NIH) funds the Centers of Excellence in Pain Education (CoEPEs), providing pain management curriculum resources to improve how health care professionals are taught about pain and its treatment. In addition, the National Pain Strategy was developed to transform the way we think about pain. The strategy calls for a better understanding of pain in order to treat it more appropriately, with focus areas on population research, prevention and care, disparities, service delivery and reimbursement, professional education and training, and public awareness and communication.

Advancing better pain management encompasses addressing various neurologic disorders, cancers, and musculoskeletal and inflammatory conditions. Such underlying medical conditions can lead to providers' consideration of the biopsychosocial model, which allows for better capture of other aspects to chronic pain, including social determinants, that if addressed can improve outcomes. Symptoms may change over time and experiences with pain differ person to person. Some chronic pain conditions are not clearly understood, such as complex regional pain syndrome and fibromyalgia. Furthermore, data on the incidence, prevalence, and consequences of pain are not reliable or comprehensive partly because in many cases pain is treated as a symptom of a disease or condition and is often not reported in and of itself.[2]

Treatment modalities for pain includes various classes of medications; interventional pain procedures such as nerve blocks, steroid injections, and neuromodulation; behavioral health interventions; psychological counseling; rehabilitative and physical therapy; and complementary and integrative health approaches. More long-term research on pain management strategies, including those examining nonpharmacologic approaches, is essential to better implement effective strategies to the individualized patient. The rest of the chapter summarizes some of the most common nonpharmacologic and non-opioid pharmacologic treatments that are used to manage common pain conditions and that could be considered as part of a multimodal treatment plan. It is important to develop an individualized, patient-centered plan of care with the patient in order to achieve a therapeutic alliance, as well as to address the public health goals of preventing addiction and reducing the supply of opioids in communities. The efficacy of these treatment approaches will be described briefly; the goal is not to provide a comprehensive review but rather to inform readers about non-opioid alternatives that could be considered by health care and public health providers.

Nonpharmacologic Approaches to Pain Management

Exercise Therapy/Physical Therapy

Therapeutic exercise is physical activity that improves aerobic ability, strength, and/or flexibility. A therapy program can be designed specifically for each patient depending on the patient's injury and the physician's ability, and the specific disorder or illness associated with the patient's pain. Physical activities that can help relieve certain pain conditions and improve function include cardiovascular exercise, strength training, yoga, and tai chi. Exercise therapies can be safe and beneficial, although some require learning new movements and postures.

Physical therapy, along with other movement therapies, is an essential part of managing acute and/or chronic pain conditions, including rehabilitation after joint replacement, fibromyalgia, osteoarthritis, and back pain.[4,5] Physical therapists and other professionals are able to develop a highly individualized plan of care from a vast toolbox of treatment modalities and conduct thorough patient assessments. Physical therapy can play a significant role in treating acute and/or chronic pain when combined with other treatment modalities. For example, physical therapy is the mainstay of treatment for complex regional pain syndrome and may be beneficial for acute flares in chronic conditions such as multiple sclerosis and Parkinson disease.

Manual Therapies

Manual therapies, including massage, are recommended for pain management in conjunction with other therapies or alone. Such interventions prove to be safe and clinically effective. There are various studies on different types of massage, including Swedish, Thai, and myofascial. Small study sizes and their short-term nature contribute to the insufficient evidence.

Psychological Approaches to Chronic Pain

Chronic pain is often associated with decreased quality of life and functional ability and may contribute to depression, which in turn can intensify pain perception. Cognitive-behavioral therapies (CBT) are approaches that can be conducted over multiple sessions in an individual or group setting and can include teaching relaxation techniques, pain-related coping skills, scheduling activities to minimize pain, and improving sleep patterns.[6] Several studies reveal the efficacy of CBT for treating pain, alone or in conjunction with other treatments.[7] Patient acceptance may be a barrier to such behavioral therapies due to patients not wanting a psychological treatment for what is perceived as a physical problem. The field of pain psychology, including self-management, coping skills, and/or addressing comorbid conditions, can play a significant role in a multidisciplinary treatment approach for chronic pain and yield improved outcomes for patients.

Mindfulness Meditation

Mindfulness-based stress reduction is a program that incorporates mindfulness skills training to enhance one's ability to manage and reduce pain. Mindfulness enables an attentional stance of removed observation and is characterized by concentrating on the present moment with openness, curiosity, and acceptance. This allows for a change in one's point of view of the pain experience. Studies on such programs support statistically significant beneficial effects for pain, but the evidence thus far is of low quality.

Acupuncture

Acupuncture is a Traditional Chinese Medicine technique involving the insertion of fine needles at specified points or combinations of points on the body. Acupuncture is rapidly evolving as an effective therapeutic modality within the framework of modern American medicine. A physician who is trained and licensed in Western biomedicine may receive additional training in medical acupuncture. Acupuncture is effective in treating musculoskeletal, headache, and osteoarthritis pain. The effects of treatment are found to persist over time, with a small decrease in effect after about one year.[8] Studies on acupuncture and preventing migraines show similar benefits to prophylactic medications, but with fewer adverse effects.

Interventional Treatments

Interventional pain treatments are invasive techniques, including percutaneous and image-guided procedures. A broad array of treatments are available in this category, such as joint injections, Botox injections, ultrasound-guided nerve blocks, facet blocks, spinal cord stimulators, neuromodulation, and intrathecal injections. Interventional techniques are localized, targeting the specific area of pain. Epidural steroid injections are the most frequently used interventional technique for radicular type of pain. Botox injections are used for migraine headaches when other therapies have failed.

Specific training is required to perform each of these procedures and in the management of potential complications. An interventional pain anesthesiologist is certified in both anesthesiology and pain management. This type of physician can treat all levels of pain through minimally invasive techniques such as injection therapy, radiofrequency ablation, or spinal cord stimulation. Interventional procedures should be based on the patient's clinical pain syndrome and specific clinical indications, following appropriate procedural guidelines. Psychological screening should be done prior to procedures and surgeries in order to identify mental health comorbidities; if needed the patient can be referred to a multidisciplinary team with a better multimodal plan for the perioperative and postoperative period.

Non-opioid Pharmacologic Treatments for Pain

A number of non-opioid pharmacologic treatments have been found to be effective in treating many chronic pain conditions. However, a recent narrative review illustrated a lack of high-quality studies and the need for rigorous and standardized research methodologies to improve evidence-based pain care.[9] Most studies examine only short-term outcomes, so it is difficult for physicians and health care providers to determine the best plan of care for their chronic pain patients. A comprehensive approach to pain management includes combining pharmacologic and nonpharmacologic treatments because their differing mechanisms of action may further the success of the treatment plan, depending both on the pain syndrome and the individual patient response.

Acetaminophen

Acetaminophen (paracetamol) is the most commonly used drug to treat various pain conditions worldwide and is recommended by the World Health Organization as a first-line therapy. Acetaminophen is considered to be safe within the recommended doses. Liver damage is a risk when taken in higher-than-recommended doses or with other potentially hepatotoxic substances; this risk can be elevated in patients with underlying medical conditions such as chronic hepatitis.

Nonsteroidal Anti-inflammatory Drugs

Nonsteroidal anti-inflammatory drugs (NSAIDs), including aspirin, ibuprofen, and indomethacin, reduce pain and inflammation. They can be effective in treating low back pain, osteoarthritis, and other pain conditions. Cyclooxygenase-2 (COX-2) inhibitors, such as celecoxib, are thought to cause fewer upper gastrointestinal adverse effects than conventional NSAIDs. Topical NSAIDs, such as topical diclofenac and ketoprofen, can significantly reduce chronic musculoskeletal pain.

Muscle Relaxants

Muscle relaxants provide relief for a number of musculoskeletal conditions, such as chronic low back and neck pain. Examples of skeletal muscle relaxants are baclofen, tizanidine, chlorzoxazone, and cyclobenzaprine. These medications can cause drowsiness and sedation and should be used with extreme caution, if at all, with opioid pain relievers.

Anticonvulsants/Antiepileptics

Anticonvulsants can be used to treat neuropathic pain, which is caused by damaged, dysfunctional nerves and fibromyalgia. Examples of conditions involving nerve pain include diabetic neuropathy and trigeminal neuralgia. Gabapentin, pregabalin, and carbamazepine are common drugs prescribed for neuropathic pain. Medications for neuropathic pain do have some risk of misuse.

Antidepressants

Numerous antidepressants are used to treat chronic pain unrelated to depression, although the mechanisms of how these medications help with pain are not fully understood. Several weeks of treatment may be needed before relief occurs. Tricyclic antidepressants are thought to be the most effective group of antidepressants for managing pain, although selective serotonin and norepinephrine reuptake inhibitors (SNRIs) are increasing in popularity because they have fewer adverse effects than the tricyclics. For example, studies show that duloxetine is effective for treating neuropathic pain conditions as well as low back pain.[10]

NMDA-Receptor Antagonists

N-methyl-D-aspartate (NMDA)-receptor antagonists may be used for patients experiencing hyperalgesia, neuropathic pain, and/or complex pain syndromes. Hyperalgesia is a condition where patients have a hypersensitivity to pain caused by pain medications, including opioids. There are a number of NMDA-receptor antagonists available for treating pain, including ketamine, methadone, memantine, amantadine, and dextromethorphan. The severity and frequency of adverse effects of such drugs vary and include hallucinations, an out-of-body sensation, dizziness, lightheadedness, and fatigue. In the case of methadone, opioid overdose is an additional risk.

Capsaicin Creams and Patches

Capsaicin (capsicum), derived from chili peppers, is the active ingredient in topical creams and lotions used for temporary relief of muscle or joint pain and neuralgia. These topical medications treat pain locally and are available over the counter and/or with a prescription. Moderate evidence supports their effectiveness.

Additional Considerations to Treating Chronic Pain

In addition to various treatment modalities, health care and public health practitioners should also consider two cross-cutting issues related to treating chronic pain and policies that support non-opioid alternatives to pain management. These are the risks or adverse effects of several approaches, and barriers to accessing pain treatment exist. Addressing barriers in patient access to care is an essential public health service and is an area where public health practitioners and health care providers have tremendous opportunities in the future.

Risks or Adverse Effects of Approaches

Patient-specific risk factors need to be considered when selecting non-opioid analgesics.[11] Possible adverse effects of non-opioid pain medications include kidney, gastrointestinal, and liver problems; bleeding/bruising problems (with NSAIDs); anxiety; drowsiness; lightheadedness; and abnormal heart rate. Physicians and health care providers need to be aware of the patient's comorbidities, cognitive and functional status, and social/environmental factors, such as social/family support, when prescribing medications to older adults. This patient population is at an increased risk for toxicity related to long-term use of NSAIDs.

Barriers to Accessing Treatment for Chronic Pain

There are a number of barriers related to accessing pain management treatment. These include health care system barriers, such as health plan coverage and benefits design, payer network adequacy, and a shortage of pain specialists. Barriers are also specific to individual prescribers, including physicians and other health care providers who may not feel equipped to properly treat pain and may have limited access to pain specialty consultations. Opioid stewardship includes continuing medical education for prescribers on alternative approaches to pain. In addition, medical schools and other graduate-level health professional schools are moving toward providing a greater understanding of pain mechanisms and diagnosis and treatment in their curricula. However, much more education is needed at the various levels of education for physicians and other members of the health profession.

Many treatments may be unfeasible for patients with chronic pain due to socioeconomic constraints or underinsurance, or lack of any insurance coverage for pain treatment. Furthermore, health insurance benefits vary in what is covered and limit the implementation of multimodal treatment strategies as well as multidisciplinary collaboration. Although coordination of multidisciplinary care is recommended, health insurance benefits do not reimburse physicians for the extra time and efforts spent to implement these best practices.

Summary

Effective pain management ideally involves active patient participation in the plan of care. An assessment of patient health outcomes, including functional and quality-of-life goals, is paramount to achieving quality pain care. Patient needs, costs, and level of convenience and accessibility must be considered when implementing treatment strategies. It is vital to provide patient education and to be responsive to individual patient preferences and sociocultural backgrounds. Physicians and other health care providers can help educate patients and set realistic expectations and goals.

Improved collaboration between public health practitioners, pain specialists, and other clinicians and primary care providers can result in a better understanding of the chronic pain that a patient is suffering and the patient's biopsychosocial needs. Earlier treatment plans are likely to result in improved health outcomes through decreasing the severity of symptoms and supporting improved function. Telemedicine offers an additional method of delivering care to remote areas for improved access to care coordination. An innovative program, Project ECHO, initiated at the University of New Mexico and now used at the state and regional level across the United States, uses telehealth technologies to provide case-based learning for community clinicians enhancing their ability to treat pain in the primary care versus specialty setting.[12] The program fosters learning specific to pain and addictions and offers no-cost continuing medical education credit. Project ECHO and similar programs have the potential to expand workforce capacity to treat more patients sooner, using existing resources.

Increasing education of physicians and other healthcare providers and training in and awareness of pain treatment modalities, including a multidisciplinary approach, will be essential to improving patient health outcomes. Improving provider education and lowering patient barriers to non-opioid alternatives for treating chronic pain will be essential to helping people living with pain to access a multidisciplinary, patient-centered, compassionate, and empathetic treatment plan. Non-opioid alternatives should be considered when clinically indicated in order to limit unnecessary exposure to opioids while improving patient outcomes, including quality of life, activities of daily living, and functionality. This will not only potentially improve pain management outcomes but will also address the public health community's goals of preventing opioid misuse and other substance use disorders.

References

1. Dahlhamer J, Lucas J, Zelaya C, et al. Prevalence of chronic pain and high-impact chronic pain among adults—United States, 2016. *MMWR*. 2018; 67:1001–1006.
2. Institute of Medicine (IOM). Relieving pain in America: A blueprint for transforming prevention, care, education and research. 2011. http://www.nationalacademies.org/hmd/Reports/2011/Relieving-Pain-in-America-A-Blueprint-for-Transforming-Prevention-Care-Education-Research.aspx. Accessed September 11, 2018.
3. International Association for the Study of Pain (IASP). IASP terminology. http://www.iasp-pain.org/Education/Content.aspx?ItemNumber=1698. Accessed September 11, 2018.
4. Ojha HA, Wyrsta NJ, Davenport TE, Egan WE, Gellhorn AC. Timing of physical therapy initiation for nonsurgical management of musculoskeletal disorders and effects on patient outcomes: A systematic review. *J Orthop Sports Phys Ther*. 2016; 46(2):56–70.
5. Lemmon R, Hampton A. Nonpharmacologic treatment of chronic pain: What works? *J Fam Pract*. 2018; 67(8):474–483.
6. Knoerl R, Lavoie Smith EM, Weisberg J. Chronic pain and cognitive behavioral therapy: An integrative review. *West J Nurs Res*. 2016; 38(5):596–628.
7. Barrett K, Chang YP. Behavioral interventions targeting chronic pain, depression, and substance use disorder in primary care. *J Nurs Scholarsh*. 2016; 48(4):345–353.
8. Vickers AJ, Vertosick EA, Lewith G, et al. Acupuncture for chronic pain: Update of an individual patient data meta-analysis. *Pain*. 2017;19(5):455–474.
9. Nicol AL, Hurley RW, Benzon HT. Alternatives to opioids in the pharmacologic management of chronic pain syndromes: A narrative review of randomized, controlled, and blinded clinical trials. *Anesth Analg*. 2017; 125(5):1682–1703.
10. Chou R, Deyo R, Friedly J, et al. Systemic pharmacologic therapies for low back pain: A systematic review for an American College of Physicians clinical practice guideline. *Ann Intern Med*. 2017; 166(7):480–492.
11. Merlin JS, Bull HW, Vucovich LA, et al. Pharmacologic and non-pharmacologic treatments for chronic pain in individuals with HIV: A systematic review. *AIDS Care*. 2016; 28(12):1506–1515.
12. University of New Mexico, School of Medicine. Project ECHO: A Revolution in Medical Education and Health Care Delivery. https://echo.unm.edu/. Accessed March 17, 2019.

8 | The Role of Community Pharmacy in Addressing and Preventing Opioid Use Disorder

NICHOLAS E. HAGEMEIER

WHILE PHARMACISTS ARE ACTIVELY engaged in providing patient care across multiple practice settings, the community pharmacist, defined as the pharmacist responsible for ensuring the accuracy and appropriateness of medications dispensed in outpatient settings, arguably has the most opportunity to engage in activities that mitigate opioid use disorder (OUD) and downstream morbidity and mortality. US Drug Enforcement Administration (DEA) regulations state that "the responsibility for the proper prescribing and dispensing of controlled substances is upon the prescribing practitioner, but a corresponding responsibility rests with the pharmacist who fills the prescription."[1] Failure to assume this responsibility can result in criminal penalties and loss of the ability to practice pharmacy. Community pharmacists' roles have also been expanded in some states to include conducting and being reimbursed for comprehensive medication reviews, administering injections (e.g., immunizations, long-acting antipsychotics), and prescribing through collaborative practice agreements with physicians. All of these expanded roles potentially have OUD-related implications.

These expanded practice authorities highlight the need to strengthen understanding of pharmacists' engagement in public health interventions.[2] Given the role of pharmaceuticals in public health interventions (e.g., immunizations, antimicrobial prophylaxis) and the accessibility of community pharmacies across the nation, determining ways to effectively and efficiently connect the public health and pharmacy professions to improve patient and population health is warranted. Pharmacy education accreditation standards have incorporated aspects of public health and require that pharmacy education include "[e]xploration of population health management strategies, national and community-based public health programs, and implementation of activities that advance public health and wellness."[3] Likewise, the American Public Health Association has developed policy specific to the role of pharmacists in public health.[4]

As described by Butler in Chapter 3 of this volume, public health prevention interventions can be categorized across three levels: primary, secondary, and tertiary prevention.[5] Specific to opioid-related morbidity and mortality, these levels can be operationalized on a continuum of non-use of opioids to overdose death.[6] Pharmacist interventions to mitigate nonmedical use of prescription opioids and OUD fit within each of these three levels and are applicable across the continuum. Importantly, actions at the community pharmacy level do not exist in a vacuum. Short-sighted pharmacist (and pharmacy staff) judgments, behaviors, and interventions have unintended negative consequences for public health. This chapter describes current and potential community pharmacist interventions across the levels of public health prevention. While not exhaustive, the listed interventions describe the role of pharmacists in preventing opioid misuse and, more importantly, challenge the status quo regarding pharmacists' roles in decreasing morbidity and mortality associated with opioid use.

Overview of Prevention of Opioid Misuse Morbidity and Mortality by Pharmacists

Operationalizing Corresponding Responsibility

Pharmacists have a responsibility to ensure that controlled substances, including prescription opioids, are issued for a legitimate medical purpose in the usual course of a prescriber's professional practice. In the traditional community pharmacy where patient and prescriber information used to inform prescribing is not routinely available to the pharmacist, ensuring that a prescription is legitimate and is issued in the usual course of a prescriber's professional practice can be quite difficult. However, the professional responsibility of the pharmacist to foster interprofessional communication between the prescriber and the dispenser presents an opportunity for prevention. Interprofessional communication is necessary across prevention levels; however, operationalizing corresponding responsibility is not without controversy as it routinely evokes a perception among prescribers that pharmacists are questioning their prescribing behaviors. Research in this area indicates that collaborative working relationships between prescribers and dispensing pharmacists can indeed be established, and that rapport-building, patient-centered communication is a key ingredient.[7] Such relationships could facilitate evidence-based patient care that minimizes the risks associated with opioids across prevention levels.

Patient Counseling and Education

Providing drug information and patient counseling at the point of dispensing is a key intervention opportunity at all prevention levels. During the patient counseling process, pharmacists can ask open-ended questions to gain an understanding of a patient's prior history with prescription opioids, concerns the patient may have, and what the patient knows about prescription opioids. Patient-centered counseling approaches (i.e., approaches that elicit information from the patient to inform and target counseling) are the gold standard in the profession. While state-specific administrative rules will inform topics to be covered in patient counseling, questions specific to the interventions listed in this chapter would be appropriate in the context of opioid-related patient counseling.

The US Indian Health Service's (IHS) *Three Prime Questions* model is one with which many pharmacists are familiar.[8] At the point of dispensing, pharmacists ask the following questions:

What did the doctor tell you the medicine was for?
How did the doctor tell you to take the medicine?
What did the doctor tell you to expect?

The model also uses a final verification statement: "Just to make sure I didn't leave anything out, please tell me how you are going to use your medicine." Pharmacists can use this approach to gather information from the patient specific to opioids, including information about nonmedical use of opioids or OUD. While data specific to opioids are not available, use of patient-centered communication among pharmacists has been associated with improved patient outcomes, including improved medication adherence, medication safety, and overall health status.

Primary Prevention of Opioid Misuse Morbidity and Mortality

Primary prevention interventions are done before health effects occur and emphasize optimizing environmental controls and social determinants of health to reduce self-medication, decrease access to addictive substances, and promote protective factors.[5] While in most cases pharmacy-based primary prevention interventions target the patient specifically, opioid-related interventions can impact both the patient and those who may have access to the patient's opioid medication.

Prescription Drug Monitoring Program (PDMP) Queries

PDMPs serve as a source of information about recent and concurrent controlled substance prescribing and dispensing. State-specific PDMPs are the norm in the United States, and increasingly states are able to exchange information with other states. While PDMPs can be used as a tool across all prevention levels, the ability to identify prescribing and dispensing patterns early in the continuum from non-use to overdose death aligns well with primary prevention of opioid-related morbidity and mortality. In many states, pharmacists are required to query the PDMP prior to dispensing a new opioid prescription, prior to dispensing any opioid prescription, or on an annual or semiannual basis when opioid prescriptions continue to be dispensed. In other states, PDMP queries are conducted on an as-needed or voluntary basis using professional judgment. Research indicates that use of and robustness of PDMPs is associated with reduced opioid overdoses, reduced opioid prescribing, and reduced high-dose prescribing/dispensing.[9,10] It is important to note, however, that PDMPs are a decision support tool for pharmacists. They should inform the decision rather than make the decision for the pharmacist. Pharmacists should use PDMP data in addition to information obtained from the patient/caregiver and the patient's prescriber to inform both dispensing behaviors and nonmedical use/OUD prevention behaviors.

Drug Storage

Lack of knowledge regarding appropriate medication storage is common.[11] Therefore, promoting and equipping patients to store prescription opioids in an appropriate manner has the potential to minimize the extent to which prescription opioids are used nonmedically (i.e., other than how they were prescribed to be used). Pharmacists can promote appropriate drug storage by selling and/or providing medication safes to patients, directing patients to places they can obtain medication safes (e.g., anti-drug coalitions), or providing access to other mechanisms that secure prescription opioids, such as locking prescription vials.

Drug Disposal

Prescription medications with abuse potential are often maintained in patients' possession for years after being prescribed,[12] and over half of the prescription opioids prescribed and dispensed for dental surgeries go unused.[13] Importantly, unused and inappropriately secured prescription opioids serve as a common access point for individuals seeking to use opioids nonmedically. As the most common point of dispensing, community pharmacists are uniquely positioned to champion returning of dispensed medications for appropriate disposal. It was not too long ago that DEA regulations prohibited pharmacies from collecting controlled substances for disposal. However, changes to DEA regulations that took effect in October 2014 allow pharmacies to serve as "collectors," and many pharmacies have subsequently installed disposal receptacles through which unwanted, expired, and unused controlled (and non-controlled) substances can be disposed. Ideally, every pharmacy that dispenses prescription opioids would also serve as a disposal site. Moreover, every patient dispensed a prescription opioid should know how and when to dispose of unused prescription opioids. Newer technologies such as drug disposal pouches and inactivating agents should also be promoted or provided to patients to facilitate convenient and timely drug disposal. Text Box 8.1 describes legislation passed in Washington state requiring pharmaceutical manufacturers to sponsor a statewide prescription drug disposal program.

Drug Utilization Reviews

Drug utilization reviews (DURs) are "behind the scenes" medication evaluations commonly conducted by pharmacy computer systems and pharmacists. The goal of a DUR is to identify potential "red flags" caused by

---

TEXT BOX 8.1 WASHINGTON STATE'S MEDICATION TAKE-BACK PROGRAM

Andy Baker-White, JD

In 2018, the Washington state legislature passed, and the governor signed, a law requiring pharmaceutical manufacturers to establish a program for the collection and disposal of unwanted or unused prescription drugs within the state. The take-back program is to include a drug collection system, as well as systems for handling and properly disposing of the drugs. The pharmaceutical manufacturers are required to identify the entities that will collect and provide collection sites for the unused medications, as well as the entities that will transport and dispose of them. Ensuring the security of any patient information on packaging is also required. The manufacturers must also promote the take-back program as well as safe storage practices through public education and outreach.

The take-back program is overseen by the Washington State Department of Health, which reviews and approves program proposals, audits and inspects program activities, and ensures program compliance. The program's administration and operational costs are to be paid for the manufacturers; however, they may not recoup the costs of the program through any sort of sales or collection fee. The manufacturers are also to cover the costs of the state's administration and oversight through established fees.

Source: Washington Revised Code §§ 69.48.010-.200. A link to the legislation can be found here: https://app.leg.wa.gov/RCW/default.aspx?cite=69.48&full=true

dispensing a medication to a patient that may exist when considering a patient's current medication profile and past medical/medication history. DURs look for contraindications to the medication prescribed (e.g., the medication causes an allergic reaction in the patient), therapeutic duplications (e.g., the patient is already taking the same or a similar medication), drug–drug interactions (e.g., the patient is taking another medication that will interact negatively with the prescription opioid, such as a benzodiazepine), and multiple other potentially negative effects of the medication. Pharmacy computer systems are designed to facilitate the pharmacist's review and to address red flags identified through DURs. However, pharmacists can be overwhelmed by a large number of minor or irrelevant red flags. Better methods of identifying and addressing safety concerns identified through the DUR process are needed.

Neonatal Abstinence Syndrome Prevention

Neonatal abstinence syndrome (NAS; also known as neonatal opioid withdrawal syndrome) involves a cascade of withdrawal symptoms resulting from a baby becoming dependent on opioids via transplacental exposure while in utero, followed by cessation of exposure at the time of delivery. From a primary prevention perspective, pharmacists have a role to play given that rates of unintentional pregnancy are two to three times greater in women using prescription opioids nonmedically as compared to the general population.[14] Research also indicates that women with a diagnosed substance use disorder are less likely to use contraceptives.[15] At the point of prescription opioid dispensing to women of childbearing age, pharmacists are positioned to inquire about the patient's pregnancy status and to educate patients on the use of contraceptive approaches, including the use of voluntary, long-acting reversible contraception methods. Research indicates that pharmacist conversations regarding contraceptive use are more the exception than the norm, however.[16] It is notable that several states are now allowing pharmacists to dispense hormonal contraceptives via standing order or to prescribe some hormonal contraceptives. Therefore, pharmacists can engage in the prevention of NAS by preventing unintended pregnancies in patients using opioids.

OUD Risk Assessment

Even patients who have never taken a prescription opioid in the past may be at increased risk of developing an OUD based on both personal and family histories. Tools such as the Opioid Risk Tool (ORT) can be used to quantify risk.[17] As is the case with all assessment tools, the ORT is not perfect. The ORT is a tool that should be used to inform provider professional judgment and provider–patient conversations. Unfortunately, unpublished research conducted by the author indicates that the use of the ORT is more the exception than the norm in pharmacy as well as primary care settings.

Secondary Prevention of Opioid Misuse Morbidity and Mortality

Secondary prevention interventions seek to identify and treat diseases in the earliest stages before disease progresses to life-threatening complications. Pharmacists are positioned to identify nonmedical use of prescription opioids and the early stages of an OUD.

Screening, Brief Intervention, and Referral to Treatment (SBIRT)

The overarching goal of the SBIRT model is to intervene early by identifying risky substance use behaviors and using an evidence-based communication approach to either discourage risky behaviors or refer a patient to an appropriate OUD treatment program. Commonly used assessments include the NM-ASSIST, the CAGE-AID, and the DAST-10. A negative screen presents an opportunity to provide patient-specific education about the risks and benefits of prescribed opioids as well as primary prevention approaches to keep others safe.

If risky opioid use behaviors are identified, pharmacists should use motivational interviewing techniques to elicit information about the patient's substance use and intervene appropriately. The intervention could include educating patients on the risks of opioid use, advising patients to avoid risky use, and educating patients on types of OUD treatment available. If an OUD is identified, the pharmacist would refer the patient to an evidence-based treatment program. Pharmacists, therefore, need to have a working knowledge of how to best refer patients and to whom they should be referred. In some situations, this may involve contacting the patient's primary care provider. In others, it may involve calling a treatment facility or reputable buprenorphine prescriber on behalf of a patient. Importantly, an appropriate referral to treatment is not simply refusing to dispense a controlled substance or telling patients that they need some help or need to talk with their health care provider. To the extent possible, pharmacists should directly connect patients who need treatment to treatment providers.

While the multistep SBIRT model has been studied extensively and shown to be associated with positive outcomes specific to alcohol use disorder, evidence for its effectiveness specific to risky opioid-taking behavior is less clear.[18] A catalog of SBIRT resources (see www.samsha.gov/sbirt/resource) is maintained by the US Substance Abuse and Mental Health Services Administration (SAMHSA), including available training programs for health professionals.

Medication-Assisted Treatment (MAT)

The Drug Addiction Treatment Act of 2000 (DATA 2000) significantly changed the extent to which community pharmacists are involved in the management of OUD. Prior to that time, dispensing medications for an OUD was simply not allowed in community pharmacies. Today, however, pharmacists are intimately involved in dispensing buprenorphine products prescribed by providers who meet the requirements of DATA 2000. Despite the change in regulation, several barriers exist that keep pharmacists from fully engaging in buprenorphine dispensing, based on the author's work in South Central Appalachia. First, many pharmacists (and other health care providers) harbor stigma toward OUD that may manifest as a refusal to provide care for patients being prescribed buprenorphine. Second, many pharmacists were not adequately trained on OUDs and the use of buprenorphine as MAT during their pharmacy education. Third, controlled substance inventory and ordering limits, including buprenorphine limits, can make it difficult for pharmacists to accept new patients, given an inability to receive adequate supplies of controlled substances from their distributors (Figure 8.1).

Pharmacists may be put in a position to weigh legal constraints in addition to risks and benefits to the patient when dispensing some buprenorphine

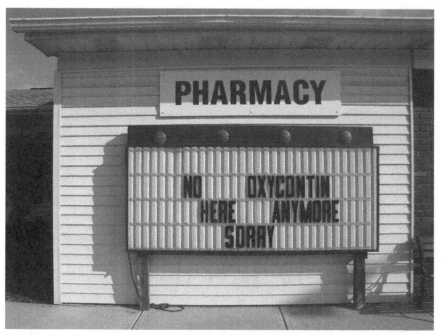

FIGURE 8.1. Example of a pharmacy no longer stocking opioids.

Source: https://motherboard.vice.com/en_us/article/jppbxk/how-big-pharma-hooked-america-on-legal-heroin; https://thenewdirectionoftime.files.wordpress.com/2012/04/pharmacy1.jpg

prescriptions. Pharmacists are encouraged to participate in DATA 2000 waiver courses, offered for free to providers seeking the waiver. While completion of the courses does not currently grant pharmacists buprenorphine-prescribing privileges, it does equip pharmacists to better understand the role of buprenorphine in MAT and to engage buprenorphine prescribers in conversations regarding evidence-based practice. Buprenorphine prescribers are encouraged to establish collaborative working relationships with community pharmacists to optimize patient care. Likewise, pharmacists are encouraged to establish relationships with their patients prescribed buprenorphine and to invest in their recovery by providing patient-centered care. Opportunities also exist for pharmacists to support patients and providers through providing injections for products such as naltrexone as allowed by state statutes and regulations.

Tertiary Prevention of Opioid Misuse Morbidity and Mortality

Tertiary prevention focuses on prevention of life-threatening health events.[5] The point of dispensing is an opportune time for pharmacists to engage patients in conversations focused on harm reduction interventions to prevent overdose deaths and to prevent transmission of HIV and hepatitis C virus infection associated with injection drug use.

Naloxone Dispensing

Opioid use disorder, like many diseases, is characterized by chronicity and relapse. Therefore, naloxone has a role to play in decreasing morbidity and mortality for patients with OUDs, regardless of whether the patients are being treated for their OUDs. Conversations about co-dispensing of naloxone with MAT medications should be routine in community pharmacy settings. These conversations may be with the patient and/or may involve caregivers.

Importantly, overdoses can also occur in individuals for whom opioids were not prescribed. For example, a child could overdose on prescription opioids by intentionally or unintentionally ingesting a parent's medication. Naloxone could prevent death in such a situation. Likewise, some patients legitimately prescribed and managed on opioid medications may be at increased risk of respiratory depression from taking opioids. One risk assessment tool that pharmacists can use to evaluate the risk of respiratory depression associated with prescription opioids is the Risk Index for Overdose or Serious Opioid-Induced Respiratory Depression (RIOSORD).[20] RIOSORD takes into consideration patient factors such as chronic pulmonary disease, chronic kidney disease, sleep apnea, and the type of opioid prescribed. The risk assessment tool has demonstrated solid predictive accuracy in retrospective studies.[20] Such a tool can be used to facilitate pharmacist conversations about co-dispensing of naloxone in patients who may not be perceived to be, or may not perceive themselves to be, at risk of opioid-related morbidity and mortality. A recent pilot study has explored employing an "opt-out" approach to naloxone dispensing where naloxone is routinely provided based on predetermined risk criteria rather than the current "opt-in" model where the responsibility for requesting naloxone is passed to the prescribing provider or to the patient.[19]

It is important to note that a majority of states allow pharmacists to prescribe naloxone and/or dispense naloxone via a standing order. Whereas naloxone is routinely considered a reviving agent for patients with an OUD, mortality risk is not limited to this population. Pharmacists are therefore positioned to increase access to naloxone for use across all prevention levels.

Nonprescription Syringe Dispensing

While syringes can be dispensed with a valid prescription just like medications, the community pharmacist's legal authority to dispense syringes without a prescription as a harm reduction approach varies by state. Additionally, there is significant variation in pharmacists' perceptions of the appropriateness and legality of dispensing syringes to people who inject drugs. The connection between injection drug use and prescription opioids gained national attention when injection of prescribed opioids resulted in an HIV outbreak in Scott County, Indiana, in 2015. The US Centers for Disease Control and Prevention (CDC) subsequently conducted an analysis that modeled the risk for HIV or hepatitis C outbreaks related to injection drug use by county.[21] Access to sterile syringes was a factor in that model. While syringe exchange programs or syringe service programs (SEPs/SSPs) are an approach to reducing OUD morbidity and mortality, the reach of SEPs/SSPs is limited in rural and urban areas alike. Community pharmacies, however, are easily accessible in many areas of the United States and thus present an opportunity to engage in harm reduction through syringe dispensing as allowed by law. Pharmacists could also educate patients on how to appropriately dispose of used syringes and where to find access to health care resources that might be warranted (e.g., HIV/hepatitis C testing). Although some health care professionals have ideological objections to providing harm reduction services, there is a significant body of literature that supports the effectiveness of such interventions. Pharmacists are well positioned to prevent HIV/hepatitis C transmission related to injection drug use.

Summary

While not intended to be an exhaustive list of potential interventions, this chapter highlights some of the major roles community pharmacists can play in mitigating the opioid crisis and ways to collaborate with governmental public health agencies. A common theme across most, if not all, pharmacist-delivered public health interventions is interpersonal communication. George Bernard Shaw said, "[T]he single biggest problem with communication is the illusion that it has taken place." Pharmacists, as well as other health professionals, are called to reflect on default communication behaviors and to adjust them as needed to provide patient-centered care. It is important to note that there are pockets of excellence across the United States: Some pharmacists are already engaging in most if not all of the prevention interventions mentioned. However, a crisis calls for widespread, evidence-based action. Given the extent to which they are integrated in patient care provision nationwide, pharmacists are well positioned to come alongside public health professionals and to champion primary, secondary, and tertiary prevention efforts.

References

1. US Drug Enforcement Administration. Purpose of issue of prescription. 2005; 21 CFR 1306.04.
2. DiPietro Mager NA, Farris KB. The importance of public health in pharmacy education and practice. *Am J Pharm Educ.* 2016; 80(2):18.
3. Accreditation Council for Pharmacy Education. Accreditation Standards and Key Elements for the Professional Program in Pharmacy Leading to the Doctor of Pharmacy Degree. 2015. https://www.acpe-accredit.org/pdf/Standards2016FINAL.pdf. Accessed February 13, 2019.
4. American Public Health Association. The Role of the Pharmacist in Public Health, Policy Number 200614. 2006. https://www.apha.org/policies-and-advocacy/public-health-policy-statements/policy-database/2014/07/07/13/05/the-role-of-the-pharmacist-in-public-health. Accessed February 13, 2019.
5. Butler JC. 2017 ASTHO president's challenge: Public health approaches to preventing substance misuse and addiction. *J Public Health Manag Pract.* 2017; 23(5): 531–536.
6. Mathis SM, Hagemeier N, Hagaman A, et al. A dissemination. and implementation science approach to the epidemic of opioid use disorder in the United States. *Curr HIV/AIDS Rep.* 2018; 15(5):359–370.
7. Snyder ME, Zillich AJ, Primack BA, et al. Exploring successful community pharmacist–physician collaborative working relationships using mixed methods. *Res Social Adm Pharm.* 2010; 6(4):307–323.
8. Lam N, Muravez SN, Boyce RW. A comparison of the Indian Health Service counseling technique with traditional, lecture-style counseling. *J Am Pharm Assoc.* 2015; 55(5):503–510.
9. Haffajee RL, Mello MM, Zhang F, et al. Four states with robust prescription drug monitoring programs reduced opioid dosages. *Health Aff.* 2018; 37(6):964–974.
10. Pardo B. Do more robust prescription drug monitoring programs reduce prescription opioid overdose? *Addiction.* 2017; 112(10):1773–1783.

11. Maeng DD, Snyder RC, Medico CJ, et al. Unused medications and disposal patterns at home: Findings from a Medicare patient survey and claims data. *J Am Pharm Assoc.* 2016; 56(1):41–46.e46.
12. Gray JA, Hagemeier NE. Prescription drug abuse and DEA-sanctioned drug take-back events: Characteristics and outcomes in rural Appalachia. *Arch Intern Med.* 2012; 172(15):1186–1187.
13. Maughan BC, Hersh EV, Shofer FS, et al. Unused opioid analgesics and drug disposal following outpatient dental surgery: A randomized controlled trial. *Drug Alcohol Depend.* 2016; 168:328–334.
14. Heil SH, Jones HE, Arria A, et al. Unintended pregnancy in opioid-abusing women. *J Subst Abuse Treat.* 2011; 40(2):199–202.
15. Terplan M, Hand DJ, Hutchinson M, et al. Contraceptive use and method choice among women with opioid and other substance use disorders: A systematic review. *Prev Med.* 2015; 80:23–31.
16. Hagemeier NE, Click IA, Flippin H, et al. Pharmacists' and prescribers' neonatal abstinence syndrome (NAS) prevention behaviors: A preliminary analysis. *Int J Clin Pharm.* 2018; 40(1):20–25.
17. Webster LR, Webster RM. Predicting aberrant behaviors in opioid-treated patients: Preliminary validation of the Opioid Risk Tool. *Pain Med.* 2005; 6(6):432–442.
18. Saitz R, Palfai TA, Cheng DM, et al. Screening and brief intervention for drug use in primary care: The aspire randomized clinical trial. *JAMA.* 2014; 312(5):502–513.
19. Skoy E. A pilot evaluation of incorporating "opt-out" naloxone dispensing within a chain community pharmacy. *Res Social Adm Pharm.* 2018 [Epub ahead of print]. doi:10.1016/j.sapharm.2018.11.006.
20. Zedler BK, Saunders WB, Joyce AR, et al. Validation of a screening risk index for serious prescription opioid-induced respiratory depression or overdose in a US commercial health plan claims database. *Pain Med.* 2018; 19(1):68–78.
21. Van Handel MM, Rose CE, Hallisey EJ, et al. County-level vulnerability assessment for rapid dissemination of HIV or HCV infections among persons who inject drugs, United States. *J Acquir Immune Defic Syndr.* 2016; 73(3):323–331.

9 | Screening, Brief Intervention, and Referral to Treatment (SBIRT) as a Public Health and Prevention Strategy to Address Substance Misuse and Addiction

ALEXANDRA NOWALK AND JANICE PRINGLE

SCREENING, BRIEF INTERVENTION, AND referral to treatment (SBIRT) is a comprehensive and integrated public health approach that aims to address hazardous and harmful substance use in patients through universal screening for substance misuse risk and the subsequent delivery of appropriate evidence-based interventions to reduce this risk.[1] Although SBIRT was not officially recognized as an evidence-based practice until the late 1990s, the foundation of SBIRT began in 1981 when the World Health Organization (WHO) launched the development of the first reliable screening tools.[1,2] The Alcohol Use Disorder Identification Test (AUDIT)[3,4] and the Drug Abuse Screening Test (DAST)[5,6] were subsequently designed, tested, and validated as effective tools for identifying individuals' risky substance use.

Additionally, throughout the 1980s and 1990s, clinical trials were performed to assess the efficacy of providing brief interventions in patients with risky substance use.[7,8] These patients were identified using screening tools in emergency rooms and primary care practices.[1] The clinical trials found that alcohol use of patients who received brief interventions significantly decreased compared to those who did not receive brief interventions.[9–11] Due to the success of these clinical trials, especially with alcohol use, and the perceived positive impact of implementing universal screening, researchers started planning ways to apply SBIRT in various medical settings and address potential implementation barriers.

By the early 2000s, the WHO had begun partnering with researchers around the world to create plans for SBIRT implementation programs within health care systems in developed and developing countries, including the United States, the European Union, Brazil, South Africa, and Australia.[1,2] In 2003, the US Substance Abuse and Mental Health Services Administration (SAMHSA) awarded grants to states seeking to implement SBIRT to establish a program for sustained use within various medical settings throughout the United States. In 2008, SAMHSA began delivery of SBIRT training curricula to educate diverse groups of health care providers to create systems and organizational changes to support the integration of SBIRT into routine clinic practices.

Today, SBIRT has been implemented throughout all 50 states in a wide variety of medical settings, including hospitals, emergency departments, family medical practices, and primary care facilities.[12] Thus far, over one million people across the country have been screened for substance use using SBIRT practices. SBIRT has also been implemented in over 18 countries in Europe, Asia, North America, South America, and Australia.[12–14]

SBIRT is predicated on the premise that, like other chronic diseases, substance use falls along a clinical spectrum ranging from low to high risk. As an example, Figure 9.1 illustrates each risk category for both diabetes and substance use and presents a correlating disease category. Patients with a normal body mass index (BMI) and normal blood glucose levels are at low risk for developing diabetes. Similarly, patients who abstain from or engage in minimal substance use are at low risk for developing a substance use disorder (SUD). Patients with pre-diabetes or harmful/hazardous substance use do not meet the diagnostic criteria for diabetes or SUD, respectively, but are engaging in behaviors that would place them at an elevated risk for developing these disorders. Patients at high risk are those that can be diagnosed with a disorder, whether it be based on established clinical benchmarks (i.e., A1C levels ≥ 6.5) or designated diagnostic criteria (i.e., those in the *Diagnostic and Statistical Manual of Mental Disorders*).[1,15] Thus, patient substance use can be stratified

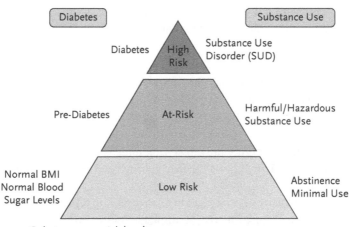

FIGURE 9.1. Substance use risk levels.

TABLE 9.1. Disease Categories, Risk Level, and Intervention

DISEASE CATEGORY	RISK LEVEL	INTERVENTION
Abstinence/Minimal Use	Low Risk	Positive Feedback
Harmful/Hazardous Use	At Risk	Brief Intervention
Substance Use Disorder	High Risk	Referral to Treatment

across increasing risk levels that correlate with an appropriate disease state extending from abstinence to a diagnosable SUD.

As a public health practice, SBIRT is unique in that it provides a truly comprehensive framework with embedded pathways that links individuals to a targeted intervention based on their risk for substance-related harms, as seen in Table 9.1.

SBIRT involves the application of an evidence-based intervention matched to each patient's identified substance use risk level. Patients identified through universal screening procedures to be low risk are provided positive feedback on their substance use behaviors by a health care professional. From a public health perspective this is considered to be primary prevention, as the goal of educating patients about their substance use is preventing patients from developing a SUD before it occurs.

Patients who are at risk for developing a SUD due to harmful/hazardous substance use are provided a brief intervention by a health care professional for the purpose of increasing the patient's understanding of his or her risk level and motivating the patient to change his or her behaviors associated with elevated substance use risk. The brief interventions last about 5 to 15 minutes and involve the use of motivational interviewing principles.[16,17] Brief interventions are a form of secondary prevention as they aim to reduce the impact of patients' substance misuse that is already occurring by encouraging patients to adopt positive behaviors and prevent further clinical escalation to a diagnosed SUD.

When a patient with a potential SUD is identified, referral to treatment is considered to be tertiary prevention as SUD treatment programs help patients manage their SUD and provide long-term strategies for preventing relapses. More recent applications of SBIRT combine the use of a brief intervention with the referral-to-treatment component, where the principles of providing the brief intervention are used to facilitate the patient's motivation to access SUD treatment.[18] In addition, most SBIRT initiatives prescribe the use of "warm handoffs" in the referral process. "Warm handoffs" are defined as facilitated care coordination between two members of a patient's health care team that directly links the patient to SUD treatment at the time of the patient's initial appointment. They are associated with increased rates of patient SUD treatment access.[19]

Traditionally, substance use has been framed as a separate behavioral health issue best addressed in specialty treatment settings. This mindset is reflected in the lack of substance use education and training embedded within the standard curricula of most medical schools and other health care professional education programs. Because of this education gap, many health care providers fail to recognize substance use as a medical issue and lack the skills to effectively discuss and manage substance use with their patients. Past approaches to managing substance use have focused on primary prevention efforts, such as Drug Abuse Resistance Education (DARE) programs in schools, or tertiary prevention, increasing patient access to a specialty field such as SUD treatment. However, these approaches fail to identify and address at-risk individuals at an earlier stage in their substance use prior to the development of a SUD. SBIRT provides a framework that fully integrates these approaches into a single continuum of care, allowing for earlier identification of and interventions for at-risk patients engaging in hazardous/harmful substance use. Ultimately, SBIRT is a systems-change initiative that requires health care professionals to reconceptualize how substance use problems are understood, redefine how they are identified, and redesign how they are treated.

While SBIRT efforts have primarily focused on alcohol consumption, there have been an increasing number of more recent studies that have examined its impact on drug use. While many of these studies have reported a negative association between brief interventions and prevention of drug use,[20,21] a few have reported a positive association.[22–24] More recent studies have yielded promising results with respect to the effectiveness of SBIRT in addressing illicit and prescription drug misuse, including opioids. Overall, screening patients for substance use as a discrete event has been demonstrated to have a positive effect on patients' substance use behaviors.[25] Furthermore, brief interventions have been shown to reduce patients' risk for overdose and improve their screening results.[26,27] In addition, brief interventions conducted by peer educators with opiate users have led to decreases in opiate use.[23] Finally, brief interventions conducted in hospital emergency departments have been demonstrated as a successful means for initiating buprenorphine/naloxone treatment for opioid-dependent patients.[28]

SBIRT Components

Screening

SBIRT screening involves the universal administration of validated screening instruments to quickly assess a patient's substance use risk and subsequently identify an appropriate level of intervention. Substance use screening is an evidence-based practice that can be easily integrated into preexisting clinical

TABLE 9.2. Patient Substance Use Prevalence by Clinical Setting

PRIMARY CARE		EMERGENCY DEPARTMENTS	
Alcohol	3–5%	Alcohol	>15%
Illicit Drugs	5–39%	Illicit Drugs	>24%

workflows and provides an opportunity for health care providers to identify substance use prevalence and behavioral patterns putting their patients at increased risk for physical, mental, and social harms. These behavioral patterns correlate with diagnostic criteria for SUDs in the *Diagnostic and Statistical Manual for Mental Disorders, Fifth Edition* (DSM-V) and can help detect patients with a potential SUD. However, while substance use prevalence varies between clinical settings and patient populations, overall, the majority of patients (80–85%) screened for substance use in health care settings screen negative. Table 9.2 presents the prevalence rates of alcohol and illicit drug use in different clinical settings.

Screening Tools

Screening tools can be categorized as either initial screens or full screens, depending on their purpose within the clinical workflow. Initials screens are brief triage questions that quickly assess patient substance use risk and identify patients who need further assessment. Using an initial screen helps filter out patients who would otherwise screen negative on a full screen, thus eliminating the need to complete a full screen with every patient and reducing the time burden on clinical staff. The most common initial screening tools include the US National Institutes of Health's National Institute of Alcoholism and Alcohol Abuse (NIAAA) single-question screen for alcohol misuse,[29] the National Institute of Drug Abuse (NIDA) single-question screen for drug misuse,[30] and the three-question Alcohol Use Disorder Identification Test—Consumption (AUDIT-C).[3] Because of their brevity, these initial screening tools can be easily incorporated into a clinical workflow.

Full screening tools are used to further assess the severity of patient substance use risk if the initial screen is positive. Different tools can be used when screening for specific substances (e.g., alcohol, tobacco, prescription drugs, marijuana, and other drugs). Common full screening tools include the Alcohol, Smoking and Substance Involvement Screening Test (ASSIST),[8] the AUDIT,[3] and the DAST.[5] Specific screening tools for special populations also exist, including adolescents[31] and pregnant women.[32,33]

Principles

As a practice, screening should be universal, brief, and indicative of next steps.

Universality implies that all patients are screened as part of routine medical care. This increases the acceptability of screening among patients and normalizes assessment of substance use as a medical issue among health care providers. While screening for substance use is not yet routinely applied across all clinical settings, health care providers already employ various screening methods designed to prevent, manage, and treat other chronic health conditions, such as cancer, blood pressure, BMI, cholesterol, and diabetes. SBIRT for alcohol use in adults aged 18 and over has received a "B" rating by the US Preventive Services Task Force,[34] meaning that the task force concludes, based on currently available data, that there is high certainty that the net benefit of screening is moderate or that there is moderate certainty that the net benefit is moderate to substantial. Other screenings with a "B" rating by the task force include those for depression, obesity, diabetes, and lung and breast cancer.

Second, screening patients for substance use should be brief in that administering both the triage and full screening tools should take only a few minutes (less than one minute for initial screens, one to five minutes for full screens).

Finally, because the screening tools result in a score that is associated with an appropriate intervention based on the patient risk level obtained from the screen, this scoring process should be easy for health care providers to perform.

Application

Patients should be screened for substance use at every medical visit as individual risk for substance misuse can change at any given time (Text Box 9.1).[18] Examples of possible circumstances that could trigger an individual to engage in risky substance misuse include separation from a child or partner, changes in employment, financial difficulties, death of a loved one, changes in mental or physical health status, and trauma exposure. While administering an annual substance use screening can be useful in establishing a clinical baseline for substance use prevalence, screening patients at every visit allows health care providers to more accurately monitor and capture changes in the substance use behavior patterns of patients over time.

In addition, while research indicates that most patients eventually feel comfortable discussing substance use with their health care providers,[35] some patients, particularly those who engage in illicit drug use, may be more reluctant to disclose this information, especially early in their relationship with the health care provider. Patients report past negative experiences with health care providers, an overall lack of trust, stigmatization experiences, confidentiality concerns, and fear of legal ramifications as reasons for withholding substance use information during the screening process. However, screening patients at every visit helps to establish substance use as a medical issue and creates a safe environment where patients feel more comfortable discussing their substance

TEXT BOX 9.1 CASE STUDY: UNIVERSAL SCREENING AT EMPOWER³ CENTER FOR HEALTH®

The EMPOWER³ Center for Health® in Blair County, Pennsylvania, takes a different approach to health care delivery, offering a direct-pay primary care model. Patients pay one monthly fee and receive unlimited access to services, including primary care, pharmacy, radiology, chronic disease management, telehealth, SBIRT, and other healthcare specialists. EMPOWER³ screens every patient for substance use at every visit, because clinical staff recognize that their patients' substance use behaviors can change at any time and health care providers play a critical role in normalizing conversations with patients surrounding substance use. By normalizing the conversation, clinical staff have seen patients become more comfortable discussing their substance use over time. One patient did not reveal 15 years of opioid use until the patient's fifth screening at EMPOWER³. The patient remarked they began to feel more comfortable over time and realized the clinical staff were truly concerned with providing all their patients with the best health care possible. Previously, the patient had been scared by legal consequences and confidentiality issues. After repeated screenings, the patient felt the conversation had been normalized and they had not been judged or pressured on disclosing their regular opioid use. The health care provider noted that nothing in the patient's medical or social history would have otherwise prompted this conversation. Upon receiving SBIRT services, the patient was successfully enrolled in medication-assisted treatment (MAT) for opioid use and has been in recovery since September 2017.

---

use with their providers as a routine part of medical care. In addition, the use of motivational interviewing principles, provided in an open, transparent and non-stigmatizing manner, will also improve the chances that patients will be honest about behaviors such as illicit substance use.[36–38]

A substance use screening process can be easily integrated within preexisting clinical workflows using established processes such as "lean" methodology for quality improvement (Text Box 9.2).[1,18,39–41] SBIRT screening tools can be administered with minimal training by medical assistants, nurses, health care educators, and other health care professionals to patients as part of a lifestyle behaviors review during a triage intake or within a more comprehensive review-of-systems interview. Incorporating the SBIRT triage (one question) screening questions into a general lifestyle questionnaires, healthy habits surveys, or triage intake screens has been found to increase patients' receptivity to the entire screening process.[35,42] Full screens can then be administered via interviews with clinical staff (e.g., nurses, physicians, advanced practice professionals), providing an opportunity for clinical staff to build rapport with patients and evoke more truthful responses. While screening tools can be administered on paper, most tools have also been validated for electronic use

TEXT BOX 9.2 CASE STUDY: INTEGRATING SBIRT WITHIN CLINICAL WORKFLOWS

Many models exist for successfully integrating SBIRT within clinical workflows. The Systems Transformation Framework (STF), developed by Pringle, is one such model. Rooted in continuous quality improvement (CQI) principles, including Lean[40,41,60] and the Toyota Rules in Use,[61] specific steps in the implementation framework include (1) assembling an executive committee or planning team for project oversight, (2) identifying a site champion, (3) conducting an organizational health assessment and current condition analysis through an initial site walkthrough (A3 Process),[62] (4) developing highly specified SBIRT clinical workflow protocols, (5) conducting clinical trainings, and (6) developing evaluation and performance measurements to ensure implementation fidelity.

The STF has been used to successfully guide implementation of SBIRT protocols in various health care settings, including emergency departments,[63] pharmacies,[39] and primary care. Key informant interviews with clinical staff from primary care sites throughout Pennsylvania who have used the STF to implement SBIRT reveal that the most common implementation barriers were lack of time and clinical burden on staff performing SBIRT services. During the onset of implementation, SBIRT was commonly viewed as a separate form of care removed from the preexisting clinical workflow and screened 60% of patients. Staff indicated that this barrier was overcome by the development and utilization of the highly specified SBIRT workflow protocol that was tailored to each site. The highly specified roles allowed the staff to become comfortable with the process and individual responsibilities.

Furthermore, as part of the STF, the executive committee would review project data for specific indicators, compare results to established benchmarks, identify areas where the project was or was not meeting the ideal, and provide technical assistance as needed to improve the clinical SBIRT workflow. During meetings, the committee would discuss implementation progress, CQI activities, and evaluation results to ensure fidelity to the STF. Site champions were able to share CQI results with clinical staff during daily huddles or regular staff meetings, which motivated staff to improve service delivery.

Over time, staff involved with care began to realize firsthand how SBIRT directly benefits patients: "Some people just need to be asked if they are having a problem. Then they will actually open up to you. Therefore, we could get people actually help that wanted help." Now, SBIRT is viewed as a normalized, routine part of clinical care at these sites and 90+% of patients are screened at every visit, every time. One staff member remarked, "I think there was some unwillingness initially by the staff . . . but then, very quickly it just became part of the routine. And now everybody does it."

and are readily available within electronic health records (EHRs). Electronic use can also help with data collection, patient outcome tracking, and documentation for billing and reimbursement purposes.

Brief Intervention

All patients who screen positive for substance misuse risk should receive a brief intervention from a health care provider to explore their motivations for reducing their risk.[1,34] Brief interventions provide health care professionals with the opportunity to provide patients with feedback on the risks associated with their substance use, explore positive and negative behaviors related to their substance use, and set realistic goals with specific action steps the patient is willing to take to reduce his or her risk. Rooted in the spirit of motivational interviewing, brief interventions work by addressing a patient's internal ambivalence and connecting change to something the patient values. Research has demonstrated that successful brief interventions can lead to long-term reductions in alcohol and other substance use,[43–46] harmful physical consequences and mortality,[44,47] adverse social consequences of use,[22] sick days and missed work,[22,48,49] and hospitalization/health care utilization.[46,49–51] However, as noted previously, research regarding the effectiveness of brief interventions to reduce substance use has primarily focused on alcohol use. Depending on the clinical setting, approximately 15% to 20% of patients will score positive for a brief intervention during the screening process.

Brief Intervention Models

Feedback–Listening–Options

The US Centers for Disease Control and Prevention (CDC) recommends Feedback–Listening–Options (F-L-O) as a model for counseling patients on the risks of alcohol misuse.[52] The F-L-O process involves:

1. Providing simple, factual feedback regarding the individual's risk for harm related to substance use
2. Listening to the individual verbalize his or her personal motivations for changing the substance use behaviors
3. Providing options for behavior change that are realistic and important to the individual.

When providing feedback, health care professionals should ask the patient for permission to provide feedback and briefly disclose their concern for the patient's risk level and disease state using a collaborative, patient-centered approach. Listening is the most vital component of the F-L-O process and allows health care professionals to understand the patient's perspective, motivation, and struggles with change; to build trust; and to strengthen rapport with the patient. The F-L-O process ends with creating a specific, relevant, and realistic plan for behavior change by listing options the patient verbalizes.

Brief Negotiated Interview

The Brief Negotiated Interview (BNI), originally developed by D'Onofrio, Bernstein, Bernstein, and Rollnick,[53] is a semistructured interview process based on motivational interviewing that can be completed in five to 15 minutes. Steps in the BNI process include:

1. Building rapport with the patient by raising the subject and exploring the pros and cons of use
2. Providing the patient with feedback on the substance use
3. Building the patient's readiness to change through motivational interviewing principles
4. Negotiating a plan for change where the patient's input is central to the conversation.

When engaging a patient during a BNI, the health care professional should begin with general conversation and ask the patient permission to discuss his or her substance use. If the patient agrees, the health care professional should move the BNI forward by discussing the pros and cons of the patient's substance use behaviors. The health care professional can then provide feedback by asking the patient permission to provide information, discuss the patient's screening results, and link the patient's substance use behaviors to any known medical consequences.

Principles

Health care professionals should recognize that effective brief interventions are not simple "one-time fixes" to a patient's alcohol or drug use. Rather, success should be measured by incremental reductions in harm over time. During the brief intervention, the health care professional should employ motivational interviewing principles to evoke realistic, measurable goals for change from the patient. "Realistic" implies the patient can readily achieve the goal given his or her motivations, confidence, and social circumstances. Measurable goals are quantifiable and serve to hold patients accountable. For example, instead of having the patient simply state, "I will cut back on my drug use," have the patient vocalize how much he will cut back by (quantity) and how many times he will use (frequency). This harm reduction approach will increase the patient's confidence and commitment to longer-term behavior change and reduce the likelihood of relapse.

Patient Engagement and Referral to Treatment

As part of the "quadruple aim" in health care, health care professionals strive to help their patients achieve optimal health and well-being, while reducing overall costs.[54] For many patients, this may involve complete abstinence from substance use. However, complete abstinence may not be a realistic goal for all patients, and it can even be dangerous for some (i.e., sudden cessation of certain substances could cause patients to go into withdrawal). An essential principle of effective brief interventions is respecting and supporting patients' autonomy to make informed choices about their health, including their decision to engage in risky substance use.

When engaging patients in brief interventions, it is important to remember that accepting a patient's lack of abstinence does not imply the health care professional is condoning the patient's behaviors. Rather, effective brief interventions are about meeting patients where they are and having patients voice their own personal motivations for wanting to change their substance use behaviors. For example, a patient who reports regular injection of heroin during a brief intervention with a provider may be unwilling to enter treatment or quit using as possible behavior changes. From the perspective of the health care professional, drug treatment may be the ideal scenario. However, the patient accepting a referral to specialty treatment may not be realistic at the time of intervention, given the patient's reluctance.

Exploring alternative options for behavior change that the patient would be willing to accept could include carrying naloxone, using sterile needles, refraining from polysubstance use, and agreeing not to use alone. While the patient may not have agreed to enter treatment, adopting one of these alternative harm reduction strategies will significantly reduce the patient's risk for overdose and potentially save his or her life. Regardless of how small the change may be, securing the patient's commitment to realistic and specific change is essential to effective brief interventions.

Brief interventions are meant to last five to 15 minutes and can occur over a series of visits (usually up to 12). Clinical staff who are effectively trained in motivational interviewing principles will be best equipped to conduct brief interventions, and personnel who could receive training include physicians, physicians' assistants, certified registered nurse practitioners, social workers, mental health counselors, or behavioral health specialists. With regard to opioid use, the primary goal of a brief intervention is to increase patients' motivation toward making realistic behavioral changes to improve medication adherence and reduce their risks for overdose and downstream health effects of opioid misuse. Specific outcomes addressing downstream, longer-lasting impacts of opioid use include providing at-risk patients with access to naloxone and educational materials to prevent overdose and facilitating referrals for patients in need of opioid use disorder treatment via warm handoffs to local specialty treatment providers (as noted earlier in the chapter, a warm handoff is a facilitated linkage between two members of a health care team with the goal of directly connecting a patient to treatment services).[55]

Referral to treatment involves actively assisting or linking patients to the appropriate level of SUD treatment and recovery support when warranted. These patients will be identified during the screening process as high risk and could have a potential SUD (see Table 9.1). While high-risk patients receive a brief intervention from a health care professional, the goal of the brief intervention is to engage the patient in specialty SUD treatment. When introducing the need for a referral, health care professionals should (1) connect the patient's screening results and current office visit to the need for specialized treatment; (2) set the tone by displaying genuine interest with active listening; (3) display a nonjudgmental demeanor; (4) and explain their role and concern as the patient's health care provider.

For patients who agree to enter treatment, direct linkages in the form of warm handoffs can further improve care coordination and patients' engagement with treatment. In the warm-handoff referral, the health care professional directly introduces the patient to the treatment provider at the time of the patient's office visit. It is a collaborative effort between two members of a patient's health care team with the purpose of improving the connection and reducing gaps in services that the patient will receive. Health care professionals with a specialized understanding of SUD treatment can be involved with the warm handoff process, including certified SUD counselors and clinicians, psychologists with SUD experience, clinical social workers, behavioral health specialists, peer navigators, or certified peer recovery specialists. Evidence strongly indicates that warm handoffs are dramatically more successful than passive referrals.[19,55]

Rather than simply handing the patient an appointment card, warm handoffs can help patients navigate the complex SUD treatment system and overcome additional barriers that would otherwise prevent them from connecting with treatment providers. Common barriers to accessing treatment include unreliable transportation, lack of child care, issues with health care access, unstable living conditions, and unavailability of culturally appropriate treatment services. Thus, warm handoffs can also help patients gain access to additional wraparound social services that will improve their initial engagement in SUD treatment, length of stay, and treatment outcomes.

Billing and Reimbursement

SBIRT services are reimbursable in a fee-for-services structure in many states. The US Centers for Medicare and Medicaid Services (CMS) has been reimbursing for SBIRT (the SBI portion of services) since the early 2000s. The billing Medicare billing codes include G0396 (SBI for 15 minutes: $29.42) or G0397 (SBI for 30 minutes: $57.69). Medicaid billing codes exist for SBIRT services: H0049 (brief SBI: $24) or H0050 (per every 15 minutes of SBI services: $48). However, each state Medicaid entity or the Medicaid managed care organization recognized by the state must recognize these codes and support reimbursement by qualified entities. Currently, approximately 16 states' Medicaid offices recognize the SBIRT billing codes.[56,57] SBIRT billing codes also exist for commercial insurance use. There are two Current Procedural Terminology (CPT) codes, the 99408 (SBI for 15 to 30 minutes: $33.41) and the 99409 (SBI for greater than 30 minutes: $65.51). Approximately 31 states have at least one commercial insurer that will reimburse SBI services using these codes. SBIRT services can also be accomplished via billing codes that involve similar services. The CPT codes involving Health Behavior Assessment/Intervention (assessment and reassessment: 96150, 96151; intervention: 96152-55) have been used by many providers throughout the country for the provision of SBIRT services. Moreover, many providers report that these codes are more often reimbursed by managed care organizations and at rates that are higher than the codes specifically designed for SBIRT services.

Despite the fact that these reimbursement codes have been available and even activated for over 10 years, most states have reported that their use is relatively low.[58,59] As many states move to address issues such as the opioid use disorder crisis, the desire for improving SBIRT use among health care professionals has resulted in a closer examination of why the billing codes are infrequently used. From these examinations, it has been learned that embedding SBIRT within EHRs in a way that supports ease of use, providing effective training and technical assistance to users, and providing monetary incentives to providers that exceed the reimbursement rates evident in the billing codes have been successful alone or in combination to boost SBIRT billing rates.

The addition of the Unhealthy Alcohol Use Screening and Follow-Up (ASF) measure as part of the Health Effectiveness Data Information Set 2018 (HEDIS) is expected to provide an additional incentive to managed care organizations to provide incentives and support to providers in the use of SBIRT for the purpose of identifying especially alcohol misuse among their patients. Many managed care organizations may choose to provide lucrative bundled rates in which SBIRT services are required as part of the service array as well as value-based incentives to their health care providers to encourage SBIRT service provision both for the purpose of meeting the new ASF HEDIS measure and to improve identification of patients who may require additional specialty services and/or changes in clinical management strategies, such as pain patients who are receiving unnecessarily high opioid dosages.

Future Directions

SBIRT is an effective practice that can be used to help identify patients who are engaging in hazardous and unhealthy alcohol and other substance use, help patients reduce their alcohol use via brief conversations involving motivational interviewing principles, and help patients who are engaging in likely unhealthy alcohol and other drug use to access additional clinical assessment and treatment services. More work is needed to provide efficient and effective SBIRT training to health care professionals as well as appropriate reimbursement of SBIRT services throughout the US healthcare system. In addition, more work is needed to ensure that patients who receive referrals via the SBIRT process for specialty assessment and care can effectively access that care in as close to real time as possible. Only after we are assured that the vast majority of health care providers are implementing at least the SBI service portion with all patients every time they are seen will we realize whether SBIRT service provision can truly reduce population SUD risk over time.

References

1. Babor TF, McRee BG, Kassebaum PA, et al. Screening, brief intervention, and referral to treatment (SBIRT): Toward a public health approach to the management of substance abuse. *Subst Abus.* 2007; 28(3):7–30.
2. Babor TF, Saunders J, Grant M. *AUDIT: The Alcohol Use Disorders Identification Test: Guidelines for Use in Primary Health Care.* Geneva: World Health Organization; 1989.
3. Babor TF, Higgins-Biddle JC, Saunders JB, Monteiro MG. *The Alcohol Use Disorders Identification Test: Guidelines for Use in Primary Care.* 2d ed. Geneva: World Health Organization; 2001.
4. Saunders JB, Aasland OG, Babor TF, et al. Development of the Alcohol Use Disorders Identification Test (AUDIT): WHO collaborative project on early detection of persons with harmful alcohol consumption—II. *Addiction.* 1993; 88(6):791–804.
5. Skinner HA. The Drug Abuse Screening Test. *Addict Behav.* 1982; 7(4):363–371.
6. Gavin DR, Ross HE, Skinner HA. Diagnostic validity of the Drug Abuse Screening Test in the assessment of DSM-III drug disorders. *Br J Addict.* 1989; 84(3):301–307.
7. WHO Brief Intervention Study Group. A cross-national trial of brief interventions with heavy drinkers. *Am J Public Health.* 1996; 86(7):948–955.
8. World Health Organization. The Alcohol, Smoking and Substance Involvement Screening Test (ASSIST): Development, reliability and feasibility. *Addiction.* 2002; 97(9):1183–1194.
9. Bien TH, Miller WR, Tonigan JS. Brief interventions for alcohol problems: A review. *Addiction.* 1993; 88(3):315–335.
10. Kahan M, Wilson L, Becker L. Effectiveness of physician-based interventions with problem drinkers: A review. *CMAJ.* 1995; 152(6):851–859.
11. Wilk AI, Jensen NM, Havighurst TC. Meta-analysis of randomized control trials addressing brief interventions in heavy alcohol drinkers. *J Gen Intern Med.* 1997; 12(5):274–283.
12. Bray JW, Del Boca FK, McRee BG, et al. Screening, brief intervention and referral to treatment (SBIRT): Rationale, program overview and cross-site evaluation. *Addiction.* 2017; 112(Suppl 2):3–11.

13. Vendetti J, Gmyrek A, Damon D, et al. Screening, brief intervention and referral to treatment (SBIRT): Implementation barriers, facilitators and model migration. *Addiction.* 2017; 112(Suppl 2):23–33.
14. World Health Organization. Brief Intervention for Substance Use: A Manual for Use in Primary Care. https://www.who.int/substance_abuse/activities/en/Draft_Brief_Intervention_for_Substance_Use.pdf. Accessed March 7, 2019.
15. Association AP. *Diagnostic and Statistical Manual of Mental Disorders (DSM-5).* Washington, DC: American Psychiatric Publishing; 2013.
16. O'Donnell A, Anderson P, Newbury-Birch D, et al. The impact of brief alcohol interventions in primary healthcare: A systematic review of reviews. *Alcohol Alcoholism.* 2014; 49(1):66–78.
17. US Department of Health and Human Services (HHS), Office of the Surgeon General. *Facing Addiction in America: The Surgeon General's Report on Alcohol, Drugs, and Health.* 2016. Washington, DC: HHS; 2016.
18. Babor TF, Del Boca F, Bray JW. Screening, brief intervention and referral to treatment: Implications of SAMHSA's SBIRT initiative for substance abuse policy and practice. *Addiction* 2017; 112(Suppl 2):110–117.
19. Mussulman LM, Faseru B, Fitzgerald S, et al. A randomized, controlled pilot study of warm handoff versus fax referral for hospital-initiated smoking cessation among people living with HIV/AIDS. *Addict Behav.* 2018; 78:205–208.
20. Saitz R, Palfai TP, Cheng DM, et al. Screening and brief intervention for drug use in primary care: The ASPIRE randomized clinical trial. *JAMA.* 2014; 312(5):502–513.
21. Roy-Byrne P, Bumgardner K, Krupski A, et al. Brief intervention for problem drug use in safety-net primary care settings: A randomized clinical trial. *JAMA.* 2014; 312(5):492–501.
22. Madras BK, Compton WM, Avula D, et al. Screening, brief interventions, referral to treatment (SBIRT) for illicit drug and alcohol use at multiple health-care sites: Comparison at intake and 6 months later. *Drug Alcohol Depend.* 2009; 99(1–3):280–295.
23. Bernstein J, Bernstein E, Tassiopoulos K, et al. Brief motivational intervention at a clinic visit reduces cocaine and heroin use. *Drug Alcohol Depend.* 2005; 77(1): 49–59.
24. Baker A, Lee NK, Claire M, et al. Brief cognitive behavioural interventions for regular amphetamine users: A step in the right direction. *Addiction.* 2005; 100(3):367–378.
25. Deutekom M, Vansenne F, McCaffery K, et al. The effects of screening on health behaviour: A summary of the results of randomized controlled trials. *J Public Health.* 2011; 33(1):71–79.
26. Banta-Green CJ, Coffin PO, Merrill JO, et al. Impacts of an opioid overdose prevention intervention delivered subsequent to acute care. *Inj Prev.* 2018 [Epub before print]. doi: 10.1136/injuryprev-2017-042676.
27. Humeniuk R, Ali R, Babor T, et al. A randomized controlled trial of a brief intervention for illicit drugs linked to the Alcohol, Smoking and Substance Involvement Screening Test (ASSIST) in clients recruited from primary health-care settings in four countries. *Addiction.* 2012; 107(5):957–966.
28. D'Onofrio G, O'Connor PG, Pantalon MV, et al. Emergency department-initiated buprenorphine/naloxone treatment for opioid dependence: A randomized clinical trial. *JAMA.* 2015; 313(16):1636–1644.

29. Smith PC, Schmidt SM, Allensworth-Davies D, Saitz R. Primary care validation of a single-question alcohol screening test. *J Gen Intern Med.* 2009; 24(7):783–788.

30. Smith PC, Schmidt SM, Allensworth-Davies D, Saitz R. A single-question screening test for drug use in primary care. *Arch Intern Med.* 2010; 170(13):1155–1160.

31. Knight JR, Sherritt L, Shrier LA, et al. Validity of the CRAFFT substance abuse screening test among adolescent clinic patients. *Arch Pediatr Adolesc Med.* 2002; 156(6): 607–614.

32. Kennedy C, Finkelstein N, Hutchins E, Mahoney J. Improving screening for alcohol use during pregnancy: The Massachusetts ASAP program. *Matern Child Health J.* 2004; 8(3):137–147.

33. Sokol RJ, Martier SS, Ager JW. The T-ACE questions: Practical prenatal detection of risk-drinking. *Am Journal Obstet Gynecol.* 1989; 160(4):863–870.

34. Moyer VA, US Preventive Services Task Force. Screening and behavioral counseling interventions in primary care to reduce alcohol misuse: U.S. Preventive Services Task Force recommendation statement. *Ann Intern Med.* 2013; 159(3):210–218.

35. Miller PM, Thomas SE, Mallin R. Patient attitudes towards self-report and bio-marker alcohol screening by primary care physicians. *Alcohol Alcoholism.* 2006; 41(3):306–310.

36. Yang LH, Wong LY, Grivel MM, Hasin DS. Stigma and substance use disorders: An international phenomenon. *Curr Opin Psychiatry.* 2017; 30(5):378–388.

37. Birtel MD, Wood L, Kempa NJ. Stigma and social support in substance abuse: Implications for mental health and well-being. *Psychiatry Res.* 2017; 252:1–8.

38. Miller WR, Rollnick S. *Motivational Interviewing: Helping People Change.* 3rd ed. New York: Guilford Press; 2013.

39. Pringle JL, Boyer A, Conklin MH, et al. The Pennsylvania Project: Pharmacist intervention improved medication adherence and reduced health care costs. *Health Aff.* 2014; 33(8):1444–1452.

40. Ahmed S, Manaf NH, Islam R. Effects of Lean Six Sigma application in healthcare services: A literature review. *Rev Environ Health.* 2013; 28(4):189–194.

41. D'Andreamatteo A, Ianni L, Lega F, Sargiacomo M. Lean in healthcare: A comprehensive review. *Health Policy.* 2015; 119(9):1197–1209.

42. Akin J, Johnson JA, Seale JP, Kuperminc GP. Using process indicators to optimize service completion of an ED drug and alcohol brief intervention program. *Am J Emerg Med.* 2015; 33(1):37–42.

43. Tanner-Smith EE, Lipsey MW. Brief alcohol interventions for adolescents and young adults: A systematic review and meta-analysis. *J Subst Abuse Treat.* 2015; 51:1–18.

44. Chi FW, Weisner CM, Mertens JR, et al. Alcohol brief intervention in primary care: Blood pressure outcomes in hypertensive patients. *J Subst Abuse Treat.* 2017; 77:45–51.

45. Edwards SH, Humeniuk R, Ali R, et al. *Brief Intervention for Substance Use: A Manual for Use in Primary Care. (Draft Version 1.1 for Field Testing).* Geneva: World Health Organization; 2003.

46. Fleming MF, Mundt MP, French MT, et al. Brief physician advice for problem drinkers: Long-term efficacy and benefit-cost analysis. *Alcohol Clin Exp Res.* 2002; 26(1):36–43.
47. Barbosa C, Cowell A, Bray J, Aldridge A. The cost-effectiveness of alcohol screening, brief intervention, and referral to treatment (SBIRT) in emergency and outpatient medical settings. *J Subst Abuse Treat.* 2015; 53:1–8.
48. Osilla KC, de la Cruz E, Miles JN, et al. Exploring productivity outcomes from a brief intervention for at-risk drinking in an employee assistance program. *Addict Behav.* 2010; 35(3):194–200.
49. Gentilello LM, Ebel BE, Wickizer TM, et al. Alcohol interventions for trauma patients treated in emergency departments and hospitals: A cost benefit analysis. *Ann Surg.* 2005; 241(4):541–550.
50. Pestka E, Nash V, Evans M, et al. Assessment of family history of substance abuse for preventive interventions with patients experiencing chronic pain: A quality improvement project. *Int J Nurs Prac.* 2016; 22(2):121–128.
51. Nicolson NG, Lank PM, Crandall ML. Emergency department alcohol and drug screening for Illinois pediatric trauma patients, 1999 to 2009. *Am J Surg.* 2014; 208(4):531–535.
52. U.S. Centers for Disease Control and Prevention, National Center on Birth Defects and Developmental Disabilities. *Planning and Implementing Screening and Brief Intervention for Risky Alcohol Use: A Step-by-Step Guide for Primary Care Practices.* Atlanta: CDC; 2014.
53. D'Onofrio G, Bernstein E, Rollnick S. Motivating patients for change: A brief strategy for negotiation. In: Bernstein E, Bernstein J, eds. *Emergency Medicine and the Health of the Public.* Boston: Jones and Bartlett; 1996:51–62.
54. Bodenheimer T, Sinsky C. From triple to quadruple aim: Care of the patient requires care of the provider. *Ann Fam Med.* 2014; 12(6):573–576.
55. Richter KP, Faseru B, Mussulman LM, et al. Using "warm handoffs" to link hospitalized smokers with tobacco treatment after discharge: Study protocol of a randomized controlled trial. *Trials.* 2012; 13:127.
56. U.S. Substance Abuse and Mental Health Services Administration. Paying for Primary Care and Behavioral Health Services Provided in Integrated Care Settings. 2018. https://www.integration.samhsa.gov/financing/billing-tools#billing%20 worksheets. Accessed February 12, 2019.
57. Institute for Research Education & Training in Addictions (IRETA). SBIRT Reimbursement—select your state. https://my.ireta.org/sbirt-reimbursement-map. Accessed March 9, 2019.
58. Winkle J. The Story Behind Oregon's SBIRT Incentive Measure and Its Impact on Implementation. https://my.ireta.org/sites/ireta.org/files/Winkle%20webinar%20 handouts.pdf. Accessed March 9, 2019.
59. Anderson T, Bhang E. Medicaid Reimbursement for Screening and Brief Intervention: Massachusetts' Preparations. 2009. https://www.integration.samhsa.gov/clinical-practice/sbirt/Medicaid_Reimbursement_for_screening_and_brief_intervention.pdf.

60. Abdallah A. Implementing quality initiatives in healthcare organizations: Drivers and challenges. *Intl J Health Care Qual Assur.* 2014; 27(3):166–181.
61. Liston DE, Richards MJ, Karl HW. Adapting the Toyota production model to teach systems-based practice to anesthesiology fellows. *J Clin Anesth.* 2017; 38:87–88.
62. Manojlovich M, Chase VJ, Mack M, et al. Using A3 thinking to improve the STAT medication process. *J Hosp Med.* 2014; 9(8):540–544.
63. Pringle JL, Kelley DK, Kearney SM, et al. Screening, brief intervention, and referral to treatment in the emergency department: An examination of health care utilization and costs. *Med Care.* 2018; 56(2):146–152.

10 | Expanding Access to Treatment and Recovery Services Using a Hub-and-Spoke Model of Care

ANNE VAN DONSEL, ANTHONY FOLLAND, AND MARK LEVINE

VERMONT'S HUB-AND-SPOKE SYSTEM OF care for treatment of opioid use disorders (OUD), also known as the Care Alliance for Opioid Addiction, was developed in response to the increasing use of heroin and other opioids in Vermont. The vision of the Care Alliance was to create a system that would not only address the clinical care needs of patients but would also assist those in treatment in building the skills needed to address other aspects of well-being, such as self-care, parenting, and employment. Vermont's hub-and-spoke system is bidirectional and provides supports for both the treatment providers participating in the system and patients receiving medication-assisted treatment (MAT) from them. Vermont's model was based on other medical models of chronic disease management, such as the patient-centered medical home, that emphasize a continuum of care provided within an integrated care system. The program is a collaborative effort of the state's Medicaid program, the Department of Health, substance abuse treatment providers, and primary care practices. Support from communities struggling with the impact of opioid use disorders and state leadership, including the governor, was also essential to fund and implement the system.

The elements of the hub-and-spoke system were recently described in detail by the American Association for the Treatment of Opioid Dependence[1] and Brooklyn and Sigmon.[2] The goals of the system were to increase total access to care, decrease the risk of overdose and transmission of infectious disease, normalize care for substance use disorder, and link patients to other needed services. The hub-and-spoke model limits disruptions in care through thoughtful and intentional placement of services in communities, by adjusting services to meet the patients' needs, and through promoting stable long-term recovery by integrating with existing primary care networks. In Vermont,

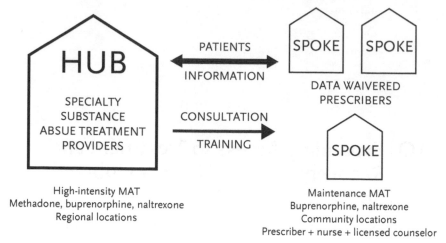

High-intensity MAT
Methadone, buprenorphine, naltrexone
Regional locations

Maintenance MAT
Buprenorphine, naltrexone
Community locations
Prescriber + nurse + licensed counselor

FIGURE 10.1. Vermont's hub-and-spoke system of care.

hub-and-spoke treatment networks comprise regionally based, specialized MAT opioid treatment programs ("hubs") and office-based opioid treatment providers ("spokes"; Figure 10.1). Both hubs and spokes use evidence-based MAT to treat OUD. Individuals for whom MAT is not desired or indicated may receive non-MAT residential, intensive outpatient, or outpatient treatment, as well as a wide array of recovery support services.

Regional hubs are addiction specialists providing centralized core services to individuals with OUD. Regional hubs also provide consultation and training to individual spoke offices and induct patients on methadone, buprenorphine, or naltrexone. Stabilized patients receiving buprenorphine or naltrexone in a hub can be transferred to spokes for ongoing treatment, while those who are on the more complex end of the OUD continuum, and all patients requiring methadone, remain in a hub. Spokes are staffed by community Drug Addiction Treatment Act (DATA)-waivered prescribers (physicians, nurse practitioners, or physician assistants) supported by a team consisting of one nurse and one credentialed counselor for every 100 patients receiving MAT. The hubs and spokes make up an integrated care system that allows for bidirectional flow from specialty services to primary care, and if a patient being seen in a spoke has needs that exceed the spoke's capacity, that patient may be transferred back to the hub for intensive services and stabilization. As with other chronic disease, such as diabetes or congestive heart failure, this model efficiently distributes OUD treatment resources by providing a concentration of specialty care resources at the hub and more routine and/or maintenance-level care in the spokes.

Vermont's Experience

Vermont has a unique Medicaid 1115 waiver that caps federal Medicaid funding available to the state and in return allows the state flexibility in service provision and coverage design. Vermont's preexisting patient-centered medical home infrastructure was developed by the state's Blueprint for Health,[3] which is a state Medicaid-funded program with goals of improving the health of the population and controlling health care costs by promoting health maintenance, prevention, and care coordination and management in an integrated system of care. Regional Blueprint Community Health Teams provide comprehensive, coordinated, and accessible patient-tailored primary care and act as models for spoke providers. Historically, Medicaid substance abuse treatment services were provided in specialty substance abuse treatment programs overseen by the state Department of Health, which also functioned as the State Opioid Treatment Authority. Medicaid-covered substance abuse treatment services predated the implementation of the hub-and-spoke model, including OUD treatment with methadone in opioid treatment programs. Some regions in the state did not have an opioid treatment program, and there were long waits for services in regions that did; capacity was capped based on available funding as well as program site and workforce limitations.

Expansion of opioid agonist treatment to general medical practice was made possible with passage of the federal Drug Addiction Treatment Act of 2000 (DATA), allowing the US Drug Enforcement Agency (DEA) to "waiver" qualified physicians to prescribe buprenorphine to treat OUD in an office setting that would otherwise require separate DEA registration. Waivered providers are authorized to treat patients using specifically approved schedule III, IV, or V narcotic medications. However, even with the DATA training, many physicians felt uncomfortable identifying patients who were appropriate for office-based opioid treatment services, so the state developed an induction program in 2004. The induction center used addiction medicine specialty staff to determine appropriate doses of buprenorphine and to monitor patients until they were sufficiently stable for transfer to an office-based opioid treatment prescriber for ongoing care.

This induction service was not available statewide, so the state explored additional methods to expand care and offer primary care physicians incentives to participate through the following: incentive payments of $500 to reimburse for time spent to become a DATA-waivered prescriber; regional care coordination support of the equivalent of one full-time coordinator per region to provide continued patient engagement; capitated Medicaid rates for induction, stabilization, and maintenance stages of treatment; and enhanced rates for those prescribing to 10 or more patients. Response to these incentives varied in successfully motivating physicians. The reimbursement for training and access to regional care coordination services were well accepted, although prescribers reported that a single coordinator per region was insufficient to support increases in patient caseload and the need for outreach and engagement to these patients. Capitated payments and enhanced rates were not successful because most prescribers were salaried employees of health care networks and consequently did not receive additional compensation for the additional work. Despite the challenges, the number of individuals receiving office-based opioid treatment services with buprenorphine rapidly surpassed the number receiving methadone in an opioid treatment program. The opioid treatment and office-based opioid treatment programs grew as separate systems through 2011, when the number of people receiving MAT stabilized, despite increasing demand for care. Several office-based opioid treatment prescribers treating large numbers of patients discontinued services and newly waived prescribers could not make up for the loss in capacity. These issues prompted the need to find a better way to care for individuals with OUD.

Hub-and-Spoke System Development Work Streams

Individuals with OUD use more health care resources than typical patients because they visit emergency departments more frequently and are more likely to have other health conditions such as depression, attention-deficit/hyperactivity disorder, anxiety, hepatitis C virus infection, as well as tobacco and other substance use.[4] People with OUD were cycling through hospital detoxification programs and the specialty substance abuse treatment system but achieved limited success in non–medication-based outpatient, intensive outpatient, and residential services. As demand for care and costs of care escalated, Vermont's Medicaid and Department of Health leadership began exploring potential solutions to address the needs of OUD patients in a more comprehensive and effective manner.

Simultaneously, there was growing awareness in the state that opioid misuse also impacted families, employers, communities, and government, all areas of concern to the legislature and then Governor Peter Shumlin. This concern resulted in the Governor Shumlin and the state's legislature providing high-level support for the hub-and-spoke system. Identifying and supporting dedicated and consistent project leadership was essential to success. Leaders engaged individuals with expertise in clinical best practice, system development and implementation, payment reform, finance, data analytics, billing procedures, and quality in developing and implementing the project. Leaders set regular team meetings and solicited input from federal, regional, and state-wide stakeholders to build buy-in and momentum. Planning for the hub-and-spoke system began in late 2011, implementation occurred region by region between January 2013 and January 2014, and it continues to mature today. Four simultaneous work streams were identified in system development: clinical, community relations, funding, and regulatory. Each work stream is described in more detail below.

Clinical Work Stream

This work stream comprised three work groups:

1. A clinical/operations work group to develop procedures for admission, assessment, and treatment planning, and for operationalizing the health home services
2. A physician work group to develop a method for matching patients to appropriate pharmacotherapy and to develop guidelines for medical screenings and dosing structure
3. A work group focused on identifying the resources and needs of pregnant women.

System development required a wide range of tools, policies, and procedures, including the following:

- *Screening and assessment tools*. In addition to standard assessment tools, methodology was needed to determine which level of care (hub or spoke) was appropriate for the patient seeking treatment. The University of Vermont–licensed Treatment Needs Questionnaire[2] makes placement recommendations based on various domains of psychosocial functioning and prioritizes locus of treatment over specific medication. However, physicians provided recommendations and guidelines for selecting the most appropriate medication for those treated in hubs.
- *Selection of the type of buprenorphine to be used*. The sublingual film formulated in conjunction with naloxone was selected as the preferred format, based on both the reduced likelihood of misuse and diversion and the availability of Medicaid pharmacy rebates. Combination tablets may be used for individuals with negative reactions to the film and buprenorphine mono-product for individuals with naloxone sensitivity and when medically indicated. Dosing schedules and dispensing methods had to be determined for each format. For instance, with sublingual film in hubs, witnessed dissolving ensures the medication is fully absorbed and prevents diversion. Double dosing with buprenorphine in hubs on Monday and Wednesday, with triple dosing on Friday, reduced patient travel and still afforded frequent opportunities for clinical services.
- *Releases.* Releases that meet all regulatory requirements were needed to share patient information between hubs, spokes, and other providers.
- *Prior authorization requirements.* Overly restrictive prior authorization requirements often result in high administrative burden for both providers

and the state and may result in delays in care; these had to be mitigated as the system was developed.

- *Urine testing standards and processes.* Urinalysis drug testing costs escalated when the hub-and-spoke system began. The program had to develop standards for testing frequency, substances in the test panel, and confirmation testing requirements, recognizing these may change over time. Providers needed to be trained on how best to use test results to inform care. Over time it was learned that confirmation testing is typically not indicated (a positive result is often sufficient) and provided there no adverse consequences, patients often admit to substance use, allowing further discussion and clinical response.

- *Consequences of continued substance use or other aberrant behavior while in treatment.* Individuals with substance use disorders often have challenging life situations, and the chronic relapsing nature of addiction can result in treatment setbacks. The system had to develop responses consistent with the risk to the patient and provider, but with the overall goal of continuing treatment, such as transferring a patient to a higher level of care, increasing clinical and support services, or decreasing take-home doses. This was complicated because patient use of other substances while in treatment is common.

- *Addressing the needs of high-risk specialty populations.* A system of care for pregnant women on MAT includes trained obstetricians and hospitals and must address the needs of both the mother and baby. Identification of such women early in pregnancy allowed integration of substance use disorder care with high-risk obstetric care to reduce the incidence of severe neonatal abstinence syndrome. Child protection policies must ensure that women are not at risk of losing custody of their children solely because they are receiving MAT. In addition, providers' roles must be clarified when treating individuals with both OUD and complex conditions such as severe and persistent mental illness, chronic debilitating medical conditions, or developmental disabilities to ensure that all services are fully coordinated. Providers also needed standard procedures for identifying and referring people for care for infectious diseases, such as hepatitis C or HIV, which are more common among people who inject drugs. Building linkages with the harm reduction agencies and syringe services programs in each region helped ensure a clinical referral pathway to treatment for those at risk. Finally, people leaving corrections custody are at very high risk for overdose after release. A corrections release planning process was implemented to include pre-release medication induction with direct referral for continuing care within the hub-and-spoke system.

- *Guest dosing procedures*. A system-wide process for provision of hub guest dosing to accommodate patients with this need, such as those who occasionally work in one region and live in another and were not yet eligible for take-home doses, was developed.
- *Learning opportunities for providers*. Learning collaboratives,[5] which are facilitated, short-term, multi-agency quality improvement projects, allowed provider staff to address emerging challenges as the system grew. This helped to develop both the clinical and office workforce and to optimize workflow in facilities.
- *Recruiting staff.* Workforce was one of the largest and ongoing system challenges, especially recruiting and retaining licensed clinicians and registered nurses. Entry-level salaries for clinicians is low, the work is challenging, and many of those currently providing care are nearing retirement. Clinicians often attain the two years of experience needed for independent licensure in the hubs and then accept higher-paying positions in other parts of the system or pursue private practice. There are national shortages of registered nurses, giving those in the field a wide variety of opportunities, and few are drawn to the addictions field. This issue remains a critical challenge for system development.

Community Work Stream

Prior to implementing the hub-and-spoke model, all existing Medicaid-funded MAT providers were encouraged to take on new patients to address demand and long waits for treatment. Caseload modeling was used to estimate capacity needed by region and drive-time maps were used to identify regions without convenient access to opioid treatment services. Because patients are often required to visit the clinic daily, accessibility is a key consideration in siting. In addition, barriers to overcome in engaging communities were identified as the system was developed. Concerns about crime and drug diversion, and beliefs that MAT was substituting one drug for another, had to be addressed by both understanding the community concerns and sharing best practice and the scientific basis for MAT. Proactively working with the community by involving individuals and family members willing to discuss how access to MAT helped themselves or their loved ones, convening business owners to discuss the impact of drug-related retail theft on their businesses, and engaging police and first responders to discuss their experiences responding to overdose calls highlighted the importance of access to care and how it supported community priorities. Community involvement was a key part of identifying potential sites with access to public transportation and other services, and also helped acknowledge the problems of social isolation and lack of adequate transportation options present in this population.

Recruiting new DATA-waivered prescribers and increasing prescriber census remained challenging. Many providers did not feel qualified to treat people with OUD, and some worked within health systems that were not supportive of MAT. State representatives visited individual practices and health systems, listened to concerns, and explained the system and supports the model offered to assist with patient care. This was a slow but effective process. As the system matured, community leadership began to urge resistant health system providers to make spoke services available. These efforts were helped by the realization that patients were already in many primary care practices and that tremendous gratification can come from caring for patients whose lives have been transformed by treatment and who successfully engage in recovery supports and community engagement efforts.

Regulatory Work Stream

The Medicaid statute is vague on required services beyond hospital, physician, and skilled nursing facility care,[6] so one of the most important steps was for the Medicaid authority to designate MAT for OUD as a service available to anyone eligible to enroll in Medicaid. Federal regulations vary by treatment structure. OTPs are governed by 42 CFR Part 8, which is a highly prescriptive regulation. Opioid treatment programs must also be licensed by the DEA as Narcotic Treatment Programs. Office-based opioid treatment prescribers are licensed under the authority of the DATA Act. Because of the different regulatory structures, opioid treatment programs are the licensed entity and have no cap on the number of patients that may be treated, while in office based treatment programs, prescribers are independently responsible for their patients' care and subject to maximum patient loads based on experience. The state also enacted rules applicable to office-based programs to establish minimum standards of professional care and assurance of patient protections in the use of MAT.[7] Methadone patients continued to be served only in hubs to comply with federal regulations associated with the use of methadone for treating OUD.[8]

An additional regulatory challenge included the limited technological capacity of many specialty substance abuse treatment providers. These providers were not eligible for Affordable Care Act of 2010 (ACA) funding to implement or upgrade electronic medical records, and substance abuse patient confidentiality protections in 42 CFR Part 2 are more stringent than those of the Health Insurance Portability and Accountability Act (HIPAA) confidentiality requirements for medical care. Simply put, with HIPAA, patients agree to sharing information related to their care unless they specifically opt out of sharing with a specific entity and 42 CFR Part 2 requires that patients specifically identify any provider with whom information will be shared. Patient information sharing processes and releases, and data systems needs in general, must both be addressed in the implementation process.

Funding Work Stream

Vermont's hub-and-spoke system is supported by funding streams from multiple sources. Financial modeling was used to build a monthly hub case rate based on personnel, materials, administrative, and facility costs. Methadone is a negligible expense in the overall cost of care and was included in the case rate. Buprenorphine and naltrexone intramuscular injections are expensive, so they are billed separately in a mechanism that supports continued receipt of Medicaid Drug Rebate Program funds. The Medicaid Drug Rebate Program is a program that helps to offset the federal and state costs of most outpatient prescription drugs dispensed to Medicaid patients.[9] Funding for the hub-and-spoke system's underlying supportive services provided by nurses and licensed clinicians was accessed through ACA Section 2703, and optional Centers for Medicare & Medicaid Services (CMS) Medicaid State Plan Health Home benefit to coordinate care for Medicaid recipients with chronic conditions. Substance use disorder was identified as a chronic condition eligible for health home services and, through an approved Medicaid State Plan Amendment, provided an enhanced match rate of 10% state funds and 90% federal funding for a period of eight quarters per Medicaid enrollee receiving services.

In addition to Medicaid funds, hubs also receive Substance Abuse Prevention and Treatment Block Grant funds for services and medication provided to uninsured and Medicare patients, as Medicare did not pay for MAT services provided by some substance use disorder treatment service types at the time the system was developed. Third-party payers pay for opioid treatment programs and office-based opioid treatment services, and hub providers have worked with insurers to align third-party billing with Medicaid, including reimbursement for the enhanced services. Negotiations are ongoing to require third-party payers to contribute funds to support spoke staff.

Impact of Vermont's Hub-and-Spoke System

Vermont's hub-and-spoke system of care has had a significant positive impact in the state. The number of people receiving MAT increased more than 125% between January 2014 and January 2018. An evaluation of the hub-and-spoke system[10] showed positive outcomes for those receiving services. Study participants reported statistically significant reductions in the use of alcohol and illicit drugs except for cannabis/marijuana, which remained unchanged. A comparison sample of people with OUD who were not in treatment reported no significant changes in any measure. Family conflict and feelings of depression, anxiety, and anger decreased, and participants reported being more satisfied with their lives when being treated in the hub-and-spoke system. Hub-and-spoke participants viewed medication as more important than counseling to their treatment and recovery. Those treated in spokes perceived their improvement more positively and appreciated being treated like any other patient at a primary care provider's office. Participants reported decreases in emergency department visits, illegal activities, and police stops/arrests, and none had overdosed in the 90 days before the evaluation interview compared with 25% who had overdosed before entering treatment. There were no significant differences in outcomes found between males and females, or those treated at hubs or spokes. An early evaluation[4] of Medicaid utilization of recipients receiving hub-and-spoke services suggested the system is associated with reduced general health care expenditures and utilization, such as inpatient hospital admissions and outpatient emergency department visits. Research, quality improvement, and evaluation activities to better understand the results of system implementation are ongoing and should be a core component of new hub-and-spoke efforts in other states.

Summary

The success of the hub-and-spoke system was based on its grounding in a health home model of care and the existence of a framework for health reform in the state, including Vermont's Blueprint for Health. In implementing a hub-and-spoke model, Vermont learned that there must be a clear understanding of the coordinated roles of the hubs and spokes and the bidirectional transfer process in to order to increase clinician comfort with managing OUD as a chronic disease. Strong systems development leadership was key to successful implementation, as was political, provider, and community engagement. State leadership roles included coordinating the clinical, regulatory, funding, and community work streams and identifying individuals with the skills needed to support those work streams statewide. After initial implementation, the focus of the hub-and-spoke model changed to refining processes, providing technical assistance and training, and surmounting challenges such as adding new locations and staff to increase treatment capacity and avoid waitlists while continuing to provide quality care. Vermont's experience demonstrated that barriers to treatment expansion can be overcome though thoughtful and efficient deployment of resources. The State's experience also highlighted issues to be aware of when establishing such systems in other states, and things to consider in future expansions.

References

1. Casper KL, Storti S, Walters V. *Models of Integrated Patient Care through OTPs and DATA 2000 Practices*. Submitted by the American Association for the Treatment of Opioid Dependence in partial fulfillment of contract #HHSP233201400268P. February 22, 2016.

2. Brooklyn JR, Sigmon SC. Vermont hub-and-spoke model of care for opioid use disorder: Development, implementation, and impact. *J Addict Med.* 2017; 11(4):286–292.

3. Department of Vermont Health Access. *Vermont Blueprint for Health Manual.* October 1, 2017. http://blueprintforhealth.vermont.gov/implementation-materials. Accessed July 30, 2018

4. Mohlman MK, Tanzman B, Finison K, et al. Impact of medication-assisted treatment for opioid addiction on Medicaid expenditures and health services utilization rates in Vermont. *J Subst Abuse Treat.* 2016; 67:9–14.

5. Joly BM, Booth M, Shaler G, Conway A. Quality improvement learning collaboratives in public health. *J Public Health Manag Pract.* 2012; 18(1):87–94.

6. *42 U.S.C.—The Public Health and Welfare.* 2010. §1396a, pp. 3281–3366. Washington, DC: US Government Publishing Office.

7. *Rules Governing Medication-Assisted Therapy for Opioid Dependence.* 2017. Chapter 8, Alcohol and Drug Abuse; Subchapter 6. Burlington, VT: Vermont Department of Health.

8. *Federal Guidelines for Opioid Treatment Programs.* 2015. HHS Publication No. (SMA) PEP15-FEDGUIDEOTP. Rockville, MD: Substance Abuse and Mental Health Services Administration.

9. U.S. Centers for Medicare & Medicaid Services, Medicaid Drug Rebate Program. https://www.medicaid.gov/medicaid/prescription-drugs/medicaid-drug-rebate-program/index.html. Accessed August 14, 2018.

10. Rawson RA. Vermont hub-and-spoke model of care for opioid use disorders: An evaluation. 2017. http://www.healthvermont.gov/sites/default/files/documents/pdf/ADAP_Hub_and_Spoke_Evaluation_2017_1.pdf. Accessed July 31, 2018.

11 | Engaging Payers to Transform Treatment of Substance Use Disorders

SAMANTHA ARSENAULT

WHILE PUBLIC HEALTH PROFESSIONALS often focus on the primary prevention of substance use disorder (SUD), an understanding of the way public and commercial insurance cover and pay for treatment and recovery services is important to a comprehensive approach to ending the opioid crisis. Scientific evidence demonstrates that addiction is a chronic disease of the brain that can be effectively treated using the same types of individualized, evidence-based medical practices that are effective in treating other chronic illnesses such as diabetes or heart disease. The SUD treatment industry, however, has been slow to adopt a chronic disease approach. Hindered by fragmentation and antiquated infrastructure, many treatment programs continue to offer only acute care or regimented programmatic services with limited effectiveness rather than patient-specific biopsychosocial treatment.

An important element in improving addiction treatment services and increasing patient access to more effective care is changing treatment reimbursement policies. Currently, several aspects of the payment system for SUD treatment services perpetuate outdated care models through perverse incentives that hinder adoption of best practices—for example, fee-for-service payments that incentivize high-intensity acute treatment episodes rather than chronic disease management. Fortunately, however, these payment practices are undergoing scrutiny and many changes have already begun, spurring transform in treatment policies and improving outcomes by moving toward evidence-based treatment of SUD and applying current knowledge and evidence to the treatment of patients with opioid use disorder (OUD).

Private insurance currently pays for roughly 16% of SUD treatment services in the United States.[1] While this is far below the proportion private insurers pay for general health care, it represents a marked increase from just 6% prior to 2009. Insurance coverage for addiction treatment expanded under the Mental Health Parity and Addiction Equity Act (the Parity Act) and the Patient Protection and Affordable Care Act (ACA). The ACA required third-party payers to cover addiction services (most plans had not done so previously) at parity with coverage rates and provisions in place for comparable physical illnesses. The rationale for this dramatic change was based on the science of addiction as a chronic disease and it was also influenced by findings from health economic research showing the substantial financial and societal benefits of providing evidence-based care for SUD, including decreased health care utilization, increased worker productivity, and reduced crime.[2,3]

Recognizing a turning point for the engagement of third-party payers and an impetus for progressive payment reform, Shatterproof, a national nonprofit organization, in collaboration with leaders of its Substance Use Disorder Treatment Task Force, identified partnering with health insurers as a critical step to advance the SUD treatment system in the United States. The first deliverable of the task force was an agreement to identify, promote, and reward care that aligns with Shatterproof's National Principles of Care for SUD Treatment, which has been publicly signed by 19 large insurance providers collectively covering over 248 million lives (Text Box 11.1).

TEXT BOX 11.1 SHATTERPROOF SUBSTANCE USE DISORDER TREATMENT TASK FORCE: PAYER REPRESENTATIVES

Aetna
AmeriHealth Caritas Family of Companies
Anthem, Inc.
Beacon Health Options
Blue Cross Blue Shield of Massachusetts
Blue Cross Blue Shield of North Carolina
CareOregon
CareSource
Centene Corporation
Cigna
Commonwealth Care Alliance
Envolve Health
Highmark Health Plan
Horizon Blue Cross Blue Shield of New Jersey
Magellan Health
Molina Healthcare, Inc.
UnitedHealth Group
UPMC Insurance Division
WellCare

The agreement represented a commitment by insurers to manage addiction with the same urgency and respect as other chronic diseases and to align financial incentives with best clinical practices. Shatterproof's Principles comprise eight core components of SUD treatment that have been demonstrated to improve patient outcomes, derived and summarized directly from the 2016 Surgeon General's Report on Alcohol Drugs and Health:[4]

1. Universal screening for SUDs across medical care settings
2. Personalized diagnosis, assessment, and treatment planning
3. Rapid access to appropriate SUD care
4. Engagement in continuing long-term outpatient care with monitoring and adjustments to treatment based on monitoring results
5. Concurrent, coordinated care for physical and mental illness
6. Access to fully trained and accredited behavioral health professionals
7. Access to medications approved by the US Food and Drug Administration (FDA)
8. Access to non-medical recovery support services

With this agreement, the task force began working to move toward identifying practical payer strategies to improve access and incentivize high-quality care based on the Principles (Text Box 11.2). These strategies fall into several domains, including reimbursement, coverage, benefit design, utilization management, payment models, and policies that directly address barriers to high-quality addiction treatment. As of today, payers are beginning to experiment with these strategies to improve the quality of addiction treatment and support implementation of the Principles within their organizations.

Coverage

SUD and addiction treatment services have not been covered by insurance to the same degree as other health conditions. While the Parity Act and the ACA require mental health and addiction services be covered at parity with medical and surgical services, disparity remains in the scope of coverage for each, and opportunity exists to reduce current restrictions and barriers to care for the former. To improve access to care, coverage should be aligned with evidence-based medical practices outlined in the Principles. This alignment requires removing arbitrary annual or lifetime coverage limitations; eliminating waiting periods for care; lessening restrictions on the scope, type, or duration of treatment; and ending excessive utilization review requirements.

Payers should also cover all medications approved by the FDA to treat OUD, with products, including each medication, offered at the lowest cost-sharing tier, and with dosage and duration determined by prevailing

TEXT BOX 11.2 ABOUT SHATTERPROOF (WWW. SHATTERPROOF.ORG)

Shatterproof's Substance Use Disorder Treatment Task Force developed the National Principles of Care, a standard for addiction treatment based on proven research. With this agreement, we are closer than ever to ensuring that every American with a substance use disorder has access to quality, evidence-based treatment. Shatterproof also takes on federal and state advocacy battles, mobilizing families affected by addiction and providing them with a platform to make their voices heard. Advocacy support has helped 15 states pass life-saving legislation: broadening access to lifesaving naloxone, strengthening prescription drug monitoring programs, and ensuring prescriber practices align with CDC guidance on opioids. Joining forces with advocacy groups across the country, we have supported federal laws like the Comprehensive Addiction and Recovery Act (CARA) and the 21st Century Cures Act. We are also passionately advocating to protect insurance coverage for substance use disorders, joining the federal health care fight whenever the issue is raised. To shatter the deadly stigma of addiction, we have built a Community Alliance program with nearly 500 local ambassadors, providing education and supporting advocacy efforts. And we have created the largest peer-focused addiction event series, the Shatterproof Rise Up Against Addiction 5K Walk/Run, which unites families, media partners, and corporations across the country to raise funds and help erase the stigma of this disease.

guidelines set by the FDA, the US Centers for Disease Control and Prevention (CDC), the US Substance Abuse and Mental Health Service Administration (SAMHSA), and specialty medical associations (such as the American Society of Addiction Medicine). Additionally, coverage should include pre-prescription evaluation (clinical and laboratory testing) as well as coverage for adjunctive evidence-based behavioral therapies applied by appropriately trained clinicians.

To promote "engagement in continuing long-term outpatient care with monitoring and adjustments to treatment" (Principle Four), reimbursement could incentivize repeated patient evaluations during outpatient treatment in order to monitor patient symptoms and functional improvements and to guide the nature and intensity of continuing care. Addiction treatment, like all other forms of chronic care, is enhanced when an individual's housing, employment, and family or social relationships support the health care objectives and the patient's treatment plan. While support services may not be provided directly in health care settings, it is important that access to, referral to, and engage-ment in these social and community services are part of SUD treatment and discharge planning.

Cost Sharing

When copays are a condition of services, patients are more likely to defer or discontinue services.[5] This is particularly relevant for treatment of OUD, where gaps in service utilization may result in increased risk for relapse and where some courses of treatment require frequent or even daily visits, resulting in the accumulation of high out-of-pocket expenses for patients with copays. Therefore, copays and co-insurance requirements for the evidence-based addiction treatment modalities described in the Principles, including pharmacotherapies or medication-assisted treatment (MAT), and medical and behavioral health services, should be examined as a strategy for supporting access and treatment retention.[6]

Cost sharing as a barrier to treatment should especially be examined around the use of methadone for OUD treatment. While buprenorphine is promising in treating OUD, methadone remains a critical and underused tool in treating patients.[7] Under federal law, methadone can only be provided by opioid treatment programs, which are federally certified facilities (regulated through a trifurcated system by SAMHSA, DEA, and the state) that provide methadone for individuals diagnosed with OUD.[8] Since methadone is only offered at opioid treatment programs, and not through pharmacies, it is considered by health insurers to be a medical treatment service, not a pharmaceutical benefit, thus impacting payer structures. In addition, unlike buprenorphine or naltrexone, which can be administered semiweekly or even monthly, methadone is usually administered daily and often requires the patient to be observed by a provider when taking the medication.[9] Some insurance plans cover methadone maintenance therapy, but not all do. Currently, 14 state Medicaid programs do not cover it.[10] Even when methadone maintenance therapy is covered, if there is a daily copay for the service it may actually result in higher costs in copays than in direct payment.

This may be a contributing factor to the fact that a substantial portion of opioid treatment programs (35%) do not accept private insurance and instead operate on state funding or out-of-pocket payments. The dearth of treatment facilities accepting insurance creates several challenges and reduces the impact of payer financial incentives that can be used to drive quality improvement. Moving forward, value-based cost-sharing strategies should be explored. These strategies could incentivize individuals to use evidence-based, cost-effective, quality addiction services by lowering cost sharing around higher-value, higher-quality services, such as the ones outlined in the Principles.[11(p143)] This includes reducing copays or co-insurance for SUD treatment modalities that are evidence-based, including pharmacy (MAT drugs), medical, and behavioral health services.[6] It also includes offering formulations of each FDA-approved medication for MAT at the lowest cost-sharing tier to ensure that patients and physicians do not experience barriers to accessing the most effective treatment to meet individual needs.

Carve-outs and Fragmentation

Payers have typically covered addiction services through separate payment and administrative mechanisms in "carved-out" behavioral health management plans, which differ from medical and pharmaceutical health benefits administration.[12] In the public market, this separate payment and administration may be delivered by another state agency or contracted out to a managed-care behavioral health organization. In the commercial or private market, some payers administer an enrollee's entire benefit while others separate the administration of the behavioral health benefit by either having separate lines of business for their behavioral, medical, and pharmacy benefits or contracting with payers that specialize in behavioral health services. The approach to covering benefits varies by the target geographic area of the plan and the payers providing services in that area.

The push for integrated care coordination as a cost-containment strategy has resulted in a move away from carve-outs as providers and payers push for collaboration across administrative areas. This trend is evidenced by the decrease in the number of state Medicaid carve-outs from 17 in 2013 to 11 in 2017.[13] However, the separate delivery of behavioral health care remains prevalent in both the public and private insurance markets. There are 24 states that manage at least a portion of their behavioral health care through a carve-out,[14] and approximately 85% of private insurance plans use a behavioral health carve-out.[15] This practice is also common among employers who contract with multiple payers to deliver benefits. Engagement with payers around comprehensive behavioral health, medical, and pharmaceutical strategies to combat the opioid crisis has highlighted that separate delivery systems for these services creates significant administrative barriers to coordination and challenges to comprehensive treatment.

Regardless of the mechanism, we observe that carved-out administrative plans exacerbate the clinical segregation of addiction and mental health service from medical care and continue to foster uncoordinated care. Notable among these challenges is the lack of data integration. Even when payers administer all three benefits, data are sometimes not integrated across different lines of business, leading to substantial data fragmentation by benefit type. For example, aspects of MAT could theoretically be paid by three separate entities: the physician visit under the medical benefit, counseling under the behavioral health benefit, and the medication under the pharmacy benefit. Second, payers and researchers alike do not have access to the comprehensive data necessary for predictive analytic tools that measure expected health care utilization and other potential areas of interest such as opportunities for early interventions. Finally, limited data integration restricts research and innovation focused on treatment protocols that span the medical, behavioral, and pharmaceutical benefits, including protocols for comprehensive OUD care.

High Out-of-Network Utilization and Payer Network Adequacy

Plan networks are required by state and federal laws to have an adequate number of providers actively accepting new patients within each evidence-based treatment modality and in all the geographic areas they serve. Many researchers and stakeholders have pointed out the lack of treatment capacity for OUD nationwide, but the assessment of network adequacy by payers themselves is very limited. To determine network adequacy, payers should assess disease incidence and prevalence, overdose rates, density of clinicians authorized to prescribe and actively prescribing buprenorphine for the treatment of OUD, the availability of methadone maintenance, the number and type of credentialed behavioral health providers and their ability to take on new patients, and the availability of ancillary support services.

These assessments should be used to identify areas for network enhancement through telemedicine or partnering with other providers to develop innovative strategies. Payers and states should work jointly to establish enhanced mechanisms for patients to report access problems to payers and departments of insurance in order to help ensure compliance with existing state and federal parity laws. A recent report found that out-of-network utilization of behavioral health services was roughly three to five times higher than out-of-network utilization of medical/surgical benefits.[16] This was found to be true for inpatient care, outpatient facility services, and outpatient office visits. This elevated level of out-of-network use for behavioral health services may be due to a variety of factors, such as in-network service challenges (whereby providers cannot reach an agreement with plans to join the network), supply-side challenges (where there may not be enough providers), or patients' decisions to seek treatment from out-of-network providers.

Many third-party payer representatives on the Shatterproof Task Force have discussed out-of-network utilization as a major area of concern for SUD treatment because it removes mechanisms designed to ensure that beneficiaries receive care from high-quality, qualified providers. In many cases, payers report that there is no indication of an individual struggling with SUD until claims for payment are submitted for admission to residential treatment, and sometimes these are at out-of-network and out-of-state destination facilities. Overuse of residential rehabilitation as a primary treatment modality represents a lost opportunity for more appropriate and effective care. While residential treatment may be an appropriate first step in addiction treatment for some individuals based on their disease severity and co-occurring conditions, it is a misunderstanding that 28-day residential rehabilitation is or should be the norm or first option for treating addiction. In fact, data show that residential rehabilitation is not the appropriate course of care for all patients[17] and is rarely adequate by itself for most patients.[18] More effective and more continuous addiction treatment may be encouraged through the use of insurance mechanisms that foster better awareness and understanding of addiction among their primary care provider networks and the enhancement of mechanisms that connect primary care providers with expanded in-network SUD providers.

The stigma around addiction, and the misconception that it is a moral failing rather than a medical disease, may cause individuals to seek self-care via the internet or personal recommendations from friends or colleagues instead of seeking a referral from their primary care provider or an addiction specialist or reaching out to their insurance provider. This represents another lost opportunity to promote quality, evidence-based care. For individuals with employer-sponsored health care, fear of losing one's job should their company become aware of their SUD may prevent them from seeking care through their employer's insurance company. These individuals may instead feel compelled to pay high out-of-pocket costs for out-of-network care. In addition to administrative and payment reforms, culture change is needed by employers to ensure their employees feel comfortable accessing care for SUD and by insurers and providers to promote an understanding that it is a chronic and treatable disease.

Some third-party payers are taking steps to mitigate use of out-of-network services by publishing materials on evidence-based SUD treatment, providing information on in-network services to beneficiaries who may request out-of-network coverage, and using technology to connect individuals to preferred providers. For example, Optum has launched a Substance Use Treatment Helpline where its beneficiaries can be connected 24 hours a day, seven days a week with a substance use recovery advocate to provide information on appropriate treatments, arrange a clinical evaluation, and connect the individual with service providers within Optum's preferred SUD network. The Optum provider network has been vetted by the organization and participants have been determined to provide clinically appropriate, evidence-based care.

Adequate Rates and Timely Payment

There is an imbalance between the high demand for addiction treatment and the supply of providers offering evidence-based treatments across the United States. One cannot examine the many contributing factors to this supply-side problem without looking at reimbursement rates. The Milliman report referenced above also found that behavioral health providers were paid roughly 20% less on average than medical and surgical providers for similar billing codes.[16] Similarly, insurance company payments to providers for SUD services may be delayed, causing financial strains on providers. These payment discrepancies may reduce incentives to enter the SUD treatment market compared to other higher-paying medical specialties or may create challenges for existing SUD treatment programs. Specialty addiction treatment providers may have limited budgets and limited ability to absorb payment delays. For this reason, special efforts need to be made to assess reimbursement requests and ensure they are managed rapidly. Closing this gap may support providers in delivering evidence-based care and keeping their doors open.

More information is needed to assess the variation in reimbursement rates across different market segments, addiction treatment services, and insurer service lines. Because commercial payment rates are proprietary, specific costs and reimbursements for care are not easily available for analysis. While a landscape assessment across payer plans would illuminate areas for change, large variations in reimbursement rate calculation methods and formulary design by plans within each carrier limit the applicability of a universal survey instrument. A proposed alternative is to obtain median reimbursement rates or ranges for each type of service, an understanding of which could then be used to promote change in both the reimbursement and SUD treatment domains.

Alternative and Value-Based Payment Models

Modifying payment models for addiction treatment services has the potential to transform this system to meet current patient needs by incentivizing delivery of care that improves patient outcomes. Historically, addiction treatment has been delivered in acute-care episodes, despite the fact that SUDs are chronic conditions, leading to a perception that SUD treatment is ineffective. Additional research is needed to determine how best to align SUD payment with the chronic disease model. Specifically, this research must assess the percentage of patients who remain in long-term SUD care, evaluate which strategies are most effective to promote continued engagement in care, and identify which providers offer quality long-term care. These efforts should be implemented in collaboration with payers to create, implement, and evaluate a chronic disease payment model that pays for performance.

In conjunction with a shift toward chronic care for SUD, a change in payment models needs to occur as well. Existing fee-for-service payment structures, which reimburse providers for volume of services provided, incentivize the use of as many services as possible. These pay-for-volume systems generally create little incentive for quality care or care coordination. Moving away from fee-for-service toward value-based or pay-for-performance payment models would create increased incentives for improved access, quality, and care coordination of SUD treatment services.

In promoting higher-quality care, payers may also choose to develop bundled payments for comprehensive treatment of SUDs. Unlike traditional fee-for-service insurance payments, bundled payment programs usually provide a single payment for all the services a patient receives during one episode of care.[19] As an example, bundled payments for MAT for OUD typically include two payment types: one for treatment initiation (evaluating, diagnosing, and planning treatment of the patient) and one for treatment maintenance (ongoing medication administration and wraparound services) rather than a payment for every visit a patient makes for care.[20] Bundled payments disincentivize volume-based use of services and may encourage providers to treat otherwise complex patients because their reimbursement is adequate and requires less administrative burden than fee-for-service models.[21] Thus, bundled payments have the potential to improve the quality of care while simultaneously encouraging efficiency.[22] Bundled payments may also reduce cost sharing by allowing a single copay for individuals whose treatment plan requires multiple visits in a specified time rather than a copay for every visit.

One proposed bundled payment for MAT for OUD is the Patient-Centered Opioid Addiction Treatment (P-COAT) alternative payment model developed by the American Society of Addiction Medicine and the American Medical Association.[23] The P-COAT model is designed to support high-quality, office-based treatment that utilizes buprenorphine as well as psychological and social treatment services.

Payers could determine bundled rates for services such as those outlined in the P-COAT model or other high-quality evidence-based services outlined in the Principles and link those payments with measures to ensure quality care is maintained.[24] While there has been some evaluation of bundled payments among Medicaid programs,[25] conclusive data are lacking at this time. Additional evaluation of the impact of bundled payments, including cost savings, patient outcomes, and provider participation, may increase uptake of these models. The creation of a federal bundled payment code would also improve adoption and standardization of the bundled payment approach on a larger scale.[26]

Sharing Data for Clinical Care and Public Health Surveillance

One area where there is a great deal of interest by both public health practitioners and payers is how to better leverage treatment and care data for more accurate disease surveillance in the area of SUD. A great deal of effort has been placed on setting up state-based prescription drug monitoring programs to identify patients receiving multiple prescriptions for controlled substances and the physicians or other providers who prescribe them. These systems, however, do not always easily integrate into the clinical workflow and may or may not be tied to payer information technology systems. By linking clinical data with public health data, payers could leverage advances in technology that support provider decision making, reduce provider burden, improve and streamline care coordination, and identify high-risk individuals while meeting state requirements relating to public health surveillance.[27] Payer support for integrated systems could include updates, enhancements, and modifications to prescription drug monitoring programs, electronic health records, state and regional health information exchanges, and other technologies, including alerts and data sharing. These advances could rapidly reduce prescribing of dangerous drug combinations by multiple prescribers, promote providers to talk to patients about medications, and alert that a patient should be screened or treated for a substance use disorder. In the meantime, there should be continued efforts to promote discussions between patients and providers about the risks of opioids and effective treatment options for OUD. The National Safety Council has made free "Opioids: Warn Me" labels (Figure 11.1), for individuals to add to their insurance cards in order to prompt these such discussions until they are part of daily practice.

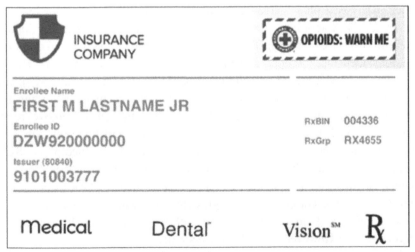

FIGURE 11.1. "Opioids: Warn Me" label for use on individual insurance cards. The National Safety Council developed this sticker for individuals to add to their insurance cards to signal their desire to be informed about opioid misuse and addiction if their health care provider prescribes an opioid.
Source: National Safety Council. https://www.nsc.org/home-safety/safety-topics/opioids/treating-chronic-noncancer-pain

Utilization Management

Utilization management is a set of techniques used by payers to decrease health care utilization, reduce costs, and prevent fraud by reviewing patient and provider decisions about the appropriateness of care.[11(p155)] For SUD treatment, utilization management often takes the form of prior authorization, step therapy, fail-first requirements, or similar policies. While these techniques may limit fraud and waste, they have also been shown to create barriers and/or delays to effective treatment for SUD and may conflict with or delay a prescribed course of treatment from a licensed health care professional.[28]

In particular, prior authorization (also known as preauthorization) has been identified by providers, patients, and payers as a barrier to timely access to evidence-based treatment for OUD.[29,30] When prior authorization is required, a player representative reviews the patient's claim and must deem the services to be appropriate before agreeing to reimburse for those services, except in the case of an emergency.[30] Health insurers typically have distinct prior authorization requirements for each of the three FDA-approved medications to treat OUD and for the varying levels of care for addiction treatment. Regardless of variation in complexity and time demands, providers often find the requirements burdensome and report that prior authorization creates arbitrary care delays and additional administrative burden on their practices; most importantly, it delays and/or interrupts patient access to timely treatment.[31]

Some national payers, including Aetna, Anthem, and Cigna, among other state-based plans, have begun to streamline or remove prior authorization for FDA-approved medications for SUD treatment. The President's Commission on Combatting Drug Addiction and the Opioid Crisis Report[32] recommended that the operating divisions of the US Department of Health and Human Services (HHS), including the Centers for Medicaid and Medicare and the Indian Health Service, as well as non-HHS agencies including the Veterans Administration (including Tricare), and the DEA, remove reimbursement and policy barriers (such as patient limits, fail-first protocols, and frequent prior authorizations) that impede access to evidence-based SUD treatment modalities. The Commission also recommended that federal and state regulators use a standard tool that requires health plans to document and disclose their compliance strategies for non-quantitative treatment limitations parity, including stringent prior authorization and medical necessity requirements.[32] However, no tool currently exists.

In addition, there are external initiatives and campaigns aiming to end utilization review and promoting parity in mental health and medical care through education of consumers, providers, and policymakers and policy reform. Parity at 10 is a three-year, multi-organization campaign to establish effective models for robust enforcement of the Parity Act in 10 states and to disseminate those models across the country. The campaign's goal is to ensure that insurance carriers and state Medicaid programs offer fully parity-compliant substance use and mental health benefits. Currently, enforcement is often "complaint-driven" and requires a consumer to advocate for care. The campaign seeks pre-market compliance reporting by health plans and compliance reviews by regulators. The campaign is being spearheaded by the Legal Action Center (LAC), the Kennedy Forum, the Center on Addiction, the Partnership for Drug-Free Kids, and the Public Health Management Corporation.[30]

Summary

Payers have recognized and are now taking steps to address the many barriers associated with access to and quality improvements in addiction treatment. As the treatment sector continues to grow to meet burgeoning demand, the role of payers becomes even more critical. Any public health efforts aimed at increasing access to or improving the quality of SUD treatment should consider the role of payers in each of the areas highlighted in this chapter and identify pertinent focus areas based on the concerns and needs of the community the effort will serve. Both public and private payers have taken steps to address supply and demand factors that will strengthen the response to the opioid epidemic, but more is needed to accelerate these efforts.

Acknowledgments

The author wishes to acknowledge the editorial support of Caroline Davidson, MPH, reviewer A. Thomas McLellan, PhD, and research partner Daniel Polsky.

References

1. US Substance Abuse and Mental Health Services Administration (SAMHSA). *Projections of National Expenditures for Treatment of Mental and Substance Use Disorders, 2010–2020.* 2014. Rockville, MD: SAMHSA.
2. US National Institutes of Health, National Institute on Drug Abuse (NIDA). https://www.drugabuse.gov/publications/principles-drug-addiction-treatment-research-based-guide-third-edition/frequently-asked-questions/how-effective-drug-addiction-treatment. Published January 2018. Accessed October 10, 2018.
3. McLellan AT, Lewis DC, O'Brien CP, Kleber HD. Drug dependence, a chronic medical illness: Implications for treatment, insurance, and outcomes evaluation. *JAMA.* 2000; 284(13):1689–1695.
4. Shatterproof Substance Use Disorder Treatment Task Force. National Principles of Care. 2018. http://shatterproof.prod.acquia-sites.com/sites/default/files/2018-02/Principles-of-Care-General-Audience-wbleeds.pdf. Accessed September 18, 2018.

5. Goldman DP, Joyce GF, Zheng Y. Prescription drug cost sharing: Associations with medication and medical utilization and spending and health. *JAMA*. 2007; 298(1):61–69.

6. Elitzer J, Tatar M. Why health plans should go to the "MAT" in the fight against opioid addiction. California Health Care Foundation (CHCF). 2017. https://www.chcf.org/publication/why-health-plans-should-go-to-the-mat-in-the-fight-against-opioid-addiction/. Accessed February 13, 2019.

7. Kampman K, Jarvis M. American Society of Addiction Medicine (ASAM) national practice guideline for the use of medications in the treatment of addiction involving opioid use. *J Addict Med*. 2015; 9(5):358–367.

8. US Substance Abuse and Mental Health Services Administration (SAMHSA). Methadone. September 2015. https://www.samhsa.gov/medication-assisted-treatment/treatment/methadone. Accessed September 18, 2018.

9. US Library of Congress, Congressional Research Service (CRS). Opioid Treatment Programs and Related Federal Regulations. 2018. https://fas.org/sgp/crs/misc/IF10219.pdf. Accessed February 13, 2019.

10. Kaiser Family Foundation. Medicaid's role in addressing the opioid epidemic. 2018. https://www.kff.org/infographic/medicaids-role-in-addressing-opioid-epidemic/. Accessed February 13, 2019.

11. Committee on Developing Evidence-Based Standards for Psychosocial Interventions for Mental Disorders, Board on Health Sciences Policy. Chapter 6—Quality Improvement. In: England MJ, Butler AS, Gonzalez ML, eds. *Psychosocial Interventions for Mental and Substance Use Disorders: A Framework for Establishing Evidence-Based Standards*. Washington, DC: National Academies Press; 2015:143.

12. Mandros A. The landscape of behavioral health carve-ins. September 2015. https://www.openminds.com/market-intelligence/executive-briefings/are-you-prepared-for-the-behavioral-health-carve-in/. Accessed September 18, 2018.

13. Mandros A. Medicaid behavioral health carve-outs—11 Remain. January 2017. https://www.openminds.com/market-intelligence/executive-briefings/are-we-watching-the-demise-of-the-behavioral-health-carve-out/. Accessed September 18, 2018.

14. Mandros A. Understanding the Medicaid behavioral health carve-out map—Step one in health plan contracting. April 2017. https://www.openminds.com/market-intelligence/executive-briefings/understanding-the-medicaid-behavioral-health-carve-out-map-step-one-in-health-plan-contracting/. Accessed September 18, 2018.

15. Horgan CM, Stewart MT, Reif S, et al. Behavioral health services in the changing landscape of private health plans. *Psychiatr Serv*. 2016; 67(6):622–629.

16. Melek SP, Perlman D, Davenport S. Addiction and mental health vs. physical health: Analyzing disparities in network use and provider reimbursement rates. 2017. http://www.milliman.com/uploadedFiles/insight/2017/NQTLDisparityAnalysis.pdf. Accessed February 13, 2019.

17. Reif S, George P, Braude L, et al. Residential treatment for individuals with substance use disorders: Assessing the evidence. *Psychiatr Serv*. 2014; 65(3):301–312.

18. McFarland B. Outpatient versus residential treatment comparison for pregnant substance abusers. AHRQ MCC Research Network. 2013. https://www.ahrq.gov/sites/default/files/wysiwyg/professionals/prevention-chronic-care/decision/mcc/mcfarland_r21grant.pdf. Accessed February 13, 2019.

19. American Hospital Association (AHA). Bundled payment. https://www.aha.org/bundled-payment. Accessed September 18, 2018.
20. LaPointe J. AMA, ASAM create alternative payment model for opioid use disorder. April 2018. https://revcycleintelligence.com/news/ama-asam-create-alternative-payment-model-for-opioid-use-disorder. Accessed September 18, 2018.
21. Shih T, Chen LM, Nallamothu BK. Will bundled payments change health care? Examining the evidence thus far in cardiovascular care. *Circulation*. 2015; 131(24):2151–2158.
22. Hutchens L. Innovations in hospital payment models: The pros and cons of bundled payments. Michigan Health Lab Blog. January 2017. https://labblog.uofmhealth.org/industry-dx/innovations-hospital-payment-models-pros-and-cons-of-bundled-payments. Accessed September 18, 2018.
23. American Society of Addiction Medicine (ASAM), American Medical Association (AMA). Patient-centered opioid addiction treatment (P-COAT)—Alternative payment model (APM). 2018. https://www.asam.org/docs/default-source/advocacy/asam-ama-p-coat-final.pdf?sfvrsn=447041c2_2.
24. Mechanic D. Seizing opportunities under the Affordable Care Act for transforming the mental and behavioral health system. *Health Aff*. 2012; 31(2):376–382.
25. Walker LS, Sheng Y, Cunningham P, Barnes A. Virginia Commonwealth University (VCU). Many buprenorphine users receive no other services for addiction disorders. 2018. https://hbp.vcu.edu/media/hbp/policybriefs/pdfs/HBP_ARTSIssue02_030718_website.pdf. Accessed March 9, 2019.
26. Gruessner V. Private payers follow CMS lead, adopt value-based care payment. Health Payer Intelligence. https://healthpayerintelligence.com/news/private-payers-follow-cms-lead-adopt-value-based-care-payment. October 17, 2016. Accessed September 18, 2018.
27. Laverdiere D, Pereyda M, Silva J. California Health Care Foundation (CHCF). Changing course: The role of health plans in curbing the opioid epidemic. 2016. https://www.chcf.org/publication/changing-course-the-role-of-health-plans-in-curbing-the-opioid-epidemic/. Accessed September 18, 2018.
28. American Medical Association (AMA). Model Bill—Ensuring Access to Medication Assisted Treatment Act. 2015. https://www.asam.org/docs/default-source/advocacy/ama-model-bill-ensuring-access-to-medication-assisted-treatment-act.pdf.
29. Madara JL, American Medical Association (AMA). To: Jim McPherson and the Honorable George Jepsen. February 2017. https://searchlf.ama-assn.org/letter/documentDownload?uri=%2Funstructured%2Fbinary%2Fletter%2FLETTERS%2FAMA-Letter-re-AG-SChneiderman-MAT-FINAL.pdf.
30. US Centers for Medicare and Medicaid Services, healthcare.gov. Glossary: Preauthorization. https://www.healthcare.gov/glossary/preauthorization/. Accessed September 18, 2018.
31. American Society of Addiction Medicine (ASAM). Advancing access to addiction medications. a project of the American Society of Addiction Medicine—The voice of addiction medicine. https://www.asam.org/docs/default-source/advocacy/aaam_implications-for-opioid-addiction-treatment_final. Accessed March 9, 2019.
32. White House, Office of National Drug Control Policy. The President's Commission on Combating Drug Addiction and the Opioid Crisis. 2017. https://www.whitehouse.gov/sites/whitehouse.gov/files/images/Final_Report_Draft_11-15-2017.pdf. Accessed March 17, 2019.

12 | Collaborating to Address Substance Use Disorder in Correctional Settings

THE RHODE ISLAND EXPERIENCE

ROSEMARIE A. MARTIN, NICOLE ALEXANDER-SCOTT, JOSEPH WENDELKEN, AND JENNIFER G. CLARKE

SUBSTANCE USE DISORDER (SUD) in general, and opioid use disorder (OUD) in particular, are among the gravest public health threats facing the United States today. The crises are particularly acute in New England, including Rhode Island. In 2016, Rhode Island had the ninth highest rate of drug overdose deaths in the nation, with 336 Rhode Islanders dying from an overdose. However, Rhode Island has started to make progress in reducing overdose deaths. While many states have continued to see increases in drug overdose deaths, Rhode Island saw a 6.5% decrease in 2018 from 2016.

A comprehensive state strategic plan has guided this progress (preventoverdoseri.org). This strategic plan was developed by Governor Gina M. Raimondo's Overdose Prevention and Intervention Task Force. The task force is a working group composed of experts inside and outside of state government, including people in recovery, clinicians, insurers, pharmacists, law enforcement personnel and other first responders, legislators, and many more. Governor Raimondo convened the task force shortly after coming into office in 2015 with the aim of creating a cross-agency, cross-sector group that would be able to come together to prevent overdoses and save lives throughout the state.

The four focus areas of the task force's strategic plan are prevention, treatment, rescue, and recovery. Many jurisdictions throughout the country have developed action plans of similar scope, but what differentiates Rhode Island's work has been its focus on the socioeconomic and environmental determinants of health in establishing priority populations for interventions. Initial data reviews in Rhode Island made clear that the single most significant socioeconomic or environmental determinant of health when it came to an individual's vulnerability to overdose was recent interaction with the criminal justice system—more specifically, recent incarceration. For example, 21% of all people in Rhode Island who died of drug overdoses in 2014 and 2015 had been incarcerated at some point in the two years before their deaths. A review of state data also indicated that every year, more than 250 individuals were entering the Rhode Island Department of Corrections (RIDOC) on medication for addiction treatment (MAT) and were either withdrawn (if on methadone) or provided no taper schedule (if on buprenorphine) (Tables 12.1).

TABLE 12.1. Characteristics and Number of Deaths from Accidental Overdose in Rhode Island, Overall and Among Individuals With Recent Incarceration

Characteristic	# OF DECEDENTS WITH RECENT INCARCERATION (%)		OVERALL # OF DECEDENTS (%)	
	First 6 mo of 2016 (n = 26)	First 6 mo of 2017 (n = 9)	First 6 mo of 2016 (n = 179)	First 6 mo of 2017 (n = 157)
Sex				
Male	24 (92.3)	7 (77.8)	123 (68.7)	94 (59.9)
Female	2 (7.7)	2 (22.2)	56 (31.3)	63 (40.1)
Race/ethnicity				
White	25 (96.2)	8 (88.9)	168 (93.9)	137 (87.3)
Other	1 (3.8)	1 (11.1)	11 (6.1)	20 (12.7)
Age, in years				
18–29	8 (30.8)	2 (22.2)	43 (24.0)	23 (14.6)
30–39	9 (34.6)	4 (44.4)	34 (19.0)	54 (34.4)
40–49	6 (23.1)	3 (33.3)	40 (22.3)	35 (22.3)
≥50	3 (11.5)	0 (0.0)	62 (34.6)	45 (28.7)
Died of overdose attributed to fentanyl	16 (61.5)	8 (88.9)	92 (51.4)	92 (58.6)
Months of incarceration, median (IQR)	30 (4–70)	23 (9–113)	NA	NA
Days since release from incarceration to death, median (IQR)	112 (12–223)	190 (49–241)	NA	NA
Died within 30 days of release from incarceration	10 (38.5)	1 (11.1)	NA	NA

For years, advocates in Rhode Island, including many individuals on staff at RIDOC, had been envisioning a criminal justice system that did not perpetuate the crises of SUD and overdose and instead helped address them through treatment and recovery supports. With the involvement of the task force, RIDOC introduced the first statewide correctional system MAT program in the country to initiate a comprehensive program to screen for OUD, to offer the full suite of medications for the treatment of OUD, to initiate or continue MAT during incarceration, and to facilitate post-release linkages to SUD treatment after release.

Text Box 12.1 provides definitions of common criminal justice terms.

Why Are There Barriers to Treatment in Correctional Settings?

A series of policy choices over the past 50 years has resulted in the United States incarcerating significantly more people than other developed countries despite having a similar rate in 1970.[1] The criminalization of behavior connected to SUDs along racial lines and the imposition of mandatory minimum sentences have had substantial impacts.[1-3] A fragmented system of re-entry and barriers around finding work, treatment, and eligibility for public assistance benefits have additionally contributed to high recidivism rates in the United States.[4-6] The punitive reaction of the United States to the increase of drug use during the 1970s and 1980s was not mirrored by other nations, where SUDs were treated as a disease and treatment was provided as a replacement for or in addition to incarceration.[7]

The United States comprises approximately 5% of the world's population and yet it accounts for almost a quarter of the world's prison population, with a rate of 716 individuals in prison per 100,000 population.[8] The prison population rate in the United States is two to 10 times the rate in other developed countries.[8] There are clear racial disparities in incarceration; African Americans are incarcerated at a rate 5.1 times that of Caucasians and are more likely to receive longer sentences for the same crimes.[9] Explanations for this inequity range from the impacts of implicit bias sentencing by judges to systemic failures of the justice system to assign suitable public defenders to each person accused of a crime.[10]

There is also a disproportionately higher number of individuals with SUDs in correctional facilities than in the community. One in five of the 2.3 million people incarcerated in the United States is locked up due to a drug offense, and 58% of prisoners in state facilities and 63% of sentenced inmates met *Diagnostic and Statistical Manual of Mental Disorders*, fourth edition (DSM-IV) criteria for drug dependence or abuse (compared to approximately 5% of the general population).[11-13] In 2005, nearly a quarter of inmates in state facilities reported using opiates.[11] In Rhode Island, approximately 53% of those admitted to the RIDOC have an SUD, and 25% have an OUD.[14] In 2014 and 2015, 21% of all fatal overdose victims in Rhode Island had been incarcerated in the two years prior to death, and in 2015, 37% of fentanyl-involved overdose decedents in Rhode Island had recently been released from prison or jail.[15] Individuals who have been previously incarcerated have a significantly higher risk of dying from overdose,[16] particularly in the first two weeks after release,[17] when they are at a higher risk of an unintentional fatal overdose,[18] as they are likely to continue to experience cravings while incarcerated and after gaining access to opioids in the community are at considerable risk for relapse and overdose.[19] This made SUD prevention, treatment, and recovery a priority public health issue not just for RIDOC but for governmental public health and its partners in the state. The use of MAT was seen as a key strategy for addressing OUD in correctional settings and during the transition back into the community.

The Role of MAT in Correctional Settings

For those in recovery from certain SUDs, MAT is often an option.[20] Today, there are three medicines approved by the US Food and Drug Administration

(FDA) that are suitable for treating OUD. As the opioid epidemic continues in the United States, with 33,000 deaths reported in 2015, policymakers, physicians, and providers will need to put aside stigma and biases and deploy MAT as an evidence-based treatment, especially within correctional facilities.[21]

Formulated in Germany before World War II, methadone's potential as a drug that could help those with OUD was first investigated in 1949 at the Lexington Federal Narcotics Farm.[22] Methadone was administered over a period of seven to 10 days, with a decreasing dose each day, mirroring the tapering efforts that currently occur in some treatment centers and correctional facilities.[22] Two physicians conducted research into this new drug after noticing that those who used heroin chronically were able to function without withdrawal or intoxication when appropriately dosed with methadone.[23] When the "war on drugs" was waged in later years, these initial studies of methadone and its clinical use in addiction treatment were on the front lines. Notably, one of the earliest studies was conducted at the Rikers Island Prison Complex in New York, where the researchers knew the potential for methadone to transform care for an incarcerated population with OUD.[24] As methadone treatment expanded in the 1970s and 1980s, it was subject to many of the same critiques as MAT is today, including the idea of "replacing one addiction with another" and concerns about diversion and abuse of the medication.[25]

Methadone was tightly regulated, and physicians required a better OUD treatment for patients who were more transient or more receptive to office-based care in a primary care medical home versus a specialty clinic. After a 30-year path to approval from the FDA, buprenorphine and buprenorphine/ naltrexone were approved to be prescribed for OUD.[26] When a demand gap developed between those who needed buprenorphine and those doctors willing to prescribe it, the US Congress passed the Drug Addiction Treatment Act of 2000 (DATA 2000), which allowed physicians to complete a continuing medical education course on appropriation use of and clinical indications for MAT therapies and to receive a waiver to prescribe buprenorphine to those with an OUD. While this program was successful, there continues to be a prescribing gap for a number of reasons, including demand for treatment, physician reluctance to obtain the waiver, and the limited number of patients a physician can treat under the waiver program.[27]

The rise and fall of MAT availability in correctional facilities does not correlate with its increase across the nation. The increase of methadone treatment in the 1970s and 1980s did not reach prisons in a meaningful or widespread way. Access to methadone has not improved over time, with only 12% of facilities offering continuing methadone maintenance if an individual was already engaging with treatment before becoming involved with the criminal justice system. [28] Historically, there have been small-scale efforts to provide

MAT within prisons, but wide adoption has not occurred despite the alarming impact of SUD generally, and OUD more specifically, in cities and states as a result of the opioid epidemic.[25] Contrary to treatment guidelines, people on MAT are often immediately withdrawn from MAT on incarceration, reducing their chances for successful treatment and recovery and increasing their risk of overdose death on release.

While public health and corrections collaboration is described by some as a "nontraditional partnership," the public health focus on correctional facilities as sites for public health interventions is not new. What is recent, however, is the scale and spread of OUD along with other SUDs in the current incarnated population, making intervention in correctional facilities a significant strategy for public health agencies for several reasons. First, the concentration of those with an OUD is extraordinarily high in correctional facilities: up to 25% in one national survey.[29] Second, the ability to engage in complete wraparound services within a correctional environment is excellent because classes can be mandated, attendance can be tracked, and medication adherence can be confirmed. Finally, those released from a correctional facility are at particularly high risk for death by overdose on release, and MAT prior to release has been shown to reduce this risk.[30,31] Essentially, the goal for public health officials is to develop a wide-reaching program that ensures that when individuals are released they are significantly less likely to use illicit drugs and overdose. These programs should offer at least two of the medications approved by the FDA for an OUD and provide wraparound services including counseling, group therapy, and trauma-informed care.

Examples of Programs Using MAT in Corrections

Unfortunately, programs that provide comprehensive supports for OUD in correctional settings exist in very few places nationwide. This is primarily due to stigma about individuals in corrections, misunderstandings about "drug replacement" therapy as an effective strategy, limited resources to support treatment and recovery programs, and other barriers. Two notable examples described below are the KEEP program at Rikers Island, New York, and the comprehensive program at the RIDOC.

KEEP Program, Rikers Island

Informed by Dole and Nyswander's 1969 study at Rikers Island, the KEEP (Key Extended Entry Program) program is the nation's longest-running correctional MAT program, having started in 1987.[32] Prior to the creation of this system, individuals with an OUD at Rikers would be withdrawn from opiods using a steadily decreasing dose of methadone. This operation carries lessons on how MAT programs can start in correctional facilities, and why, after implementation, they become popular with wardens and correctional officers. With the start of KEEP, those at Rikers on misdemenor charges were given a new option: initiating or continuing methadone with the promise of a referral to a participating comminity program on release. When introduced, it was the only program in the United States to provide methadone maintenance and one of only three programs worldwide.[32]

What enabled public health and corrections officials at Rikers to start this program? A combination of factors, some similar to those we face now. First, the increase in incarceration during the 1980s as a result of the war on drugs necessitated programs shown to reduce recidivism to prevent overcrowding. Next, the co-occurring AIDS epidemic required solutions to reduce intravenous drug use in at-risk populations. Additionally, the methadone withdrawal program at Rikers had operated smoothly, and administrators within the city's correctional department were willing to take a risk on this new program based on prior successful implementation.

Encouraging positive results were quickly observed. About 3,000 individuals received methadone maintenance through the KEEP program each year. When released, this group was more likely to follow up with treatment programs and, as a result, less likely to use heroin or commit property offenses. This occurred despite initial struggles with funding and staffing at Rikers. Over time, support for the program increased as corrections staff anecdotally observed that those given methadone were less irritable and combative, and within a few years the program was viewed as an integral part of administration at the jail for the purposes of OUD treatment and HIV prevention.

RIDOC

RIDOC has been providing limited methadone treatment since 1971 with the assistance of CODAC Behavioral Health, Rhode Island's largest and only nonprofit treatment and recovery services provider, with locations throughout Rhode Island. Prior to 2016 it was standard practice to withdraw people committed to the facility from prescribed methadone after seven days. People on other forms of opiates were only provided symptom-targeted medication. As mentioned above, in August 2015, Governor Raimondo issued Executive Order 15-14 to establish an Overdose Prevention and Intervention Task Force and an Expert Team to develop Rhode Island's Strategic Plan on Addiction and Overdose. A major component of this plan is to increase screening, assessment, and continuation or initiation of MAT for clinically appropriate individuals passing through the RIDOC.

To implement a comprehensive program with all FDA-approved MAT medications, RIDOC used community experience and knowledge through CODAC Behavioral Health. CODAC is licensed as a provider of both buprenorphine and methadone and has extensive experience providing these medications using safe, affordable, and diversion-resistant methods. Under the system of treatment withdrawal and forced abstinence, people lose their tolerance for opioids and continue to feel cravings and, once gaining access to opioids in the community, are at considerable risk for relapse and overdose. Additionally, once re-exposed to illicit opioids, the likelihood of engaging in treatment decreases significantly.[19]

In 2016, RIDOC and CODAC introduced the first correctional system MAT program in the country to initiate a comprehensive program to (1) screen for OUD, using the Texas Christian University Drug Screen[34] (TCU), (2) offer all three FDA-approved medications for the treatment of OUD, (3) initiate or continue MAT during incarceration (up to two years), both pre-trial and post-sentencing, and (4) facilitate linkages to SUD treatment after release. The medication provided is determined clinically, based primarily on past experiences, patient preference, and logistical considerations. As result of this RIDOC program, expanded MAT therapy with linkage to treatment in the community that is associated with a significant drop in statewide overdose deaths after release is now a reality. There was a statewide reduction in mortality of 12%, with a 60.5% mortality reduction for those with a history of incarceration.[14]

In Rhode Island more than 15,000 men and women cycle through the RIDOC each year, with an average daily population of 2,800.[33] Under the expanded comprehensive program, MAT is offered to three populations at RIDOC:

1. MAT is continued for individuals who enter RIDOC while on MAT in the community.
2. MAT induction is offered for new commitments at RIDOC with an OUD who are not on MAT on commitment. New commitments are referred to the MAT program through screening with the TCU tool[34] or the commitment nurse. As part of routine clinical processing on entry to the RIDOC, individuals are screened using the TCU tool. This screening tool is administered on a tablet, and the process takes five to 20 minutes. Individuals who score higher than a 2 on the TCU screen or are screened by the commitment nurse as having an OUD are referred to the MAT program.
3. Sentenced individuals who are within six months of release to the community are referred through self-referral, adult counselors working in

each facility, or medical staff. Screening and assessment typically are completed within seven days for individuals who are currently not on MAT.

For all three populations, a CODAC clinician conducts an in-depth assessment according to American Society of Addiction Medicine criteria. If appropriate for MAT, individuals meet with a prescriber who will provide education on MAT options and work with the individual to create a treatment plan. Treatment via MAT and a specific medicine (methadone, buprenorphine, or naltrexone) is chosen based on clinical history, patient preference, substance use history, and practical concerns (including the availability of certain types of treatment in the community after release). After a treatment plan is developed, each individual must consent to the treatment plan and agree to attend counseling sessions and not to misuse or share the medications. After a treatment plan is developed, agreed on, and in place, treatment begins. Before release, individuals will also be linked to community MAT programs as necessary. For patients who have received naltrexone, an intramuscular dose is provided before release. For patients who have been prescribed buprenorphine, a one-month prescription is provided on release. All patients leave with a confirmed outpatient follow-up appointment in the community to continue treatment.

On average, 250 individuals receive MAT daily, with 125 individuals released to the community per month (Table 12.2). In the first 18 months of the program, approximately 2,400 people committed were treated. Of those,

TABLE 12.2. Characteristics of Individuals Incarcerated in Rhode Island from January 1 to June 30, 2016, and from January 1 to June 30, 2017

CHARACTERISTIC	JANUARY I–JUNE 30, 2016	JANUARY I–JUNE 30, 2017
Admission for incarceration (#)	4,822	4,512
Release from incarceration (#)	4,005	3,426
Mean # of inmates receiving MAT monthly	80 (SD = 18)[a]	303 (SD = 39)
# of inmates receiving a specific MAT drug monthly, mean		
Buprenorphine	4 (SD = 3)	119 (SD = 15)
Methadone	74 (SD = 16)	180 (SD = 25)
Naltrexone	2 (SD = 1)	4 (SD = 1)
# of naloxone kits dispensed at release from incarceration	72	35

[a] Some medications for treatment of addiction were in use at RIDOC in specialized circumstances. Treatment with an opioid agonist is standard of care for pregnant women with OUD. Pregnant women with OUD incarcerated at RIDOC are typically treated with methadone and less frequently with buprenorphine. A pilot study providing naltrexone by injection had been ongoing since December 2015 prior to the start of the MAT program at RIDOC.

55% were continued on MAT, 40% were new inductions to MAT at commitment, and 5% were new inductions before release. Approximately 55% are prescribed methadone, 43% are prescribed buprenorphine, and 2% are prescribed naltrexone. When individuals consent to comprehensive MAT services, they agree to participate in comprehensive wraparound services including individual and group counseling and discharge planning for coordination and smooth transition to community-based care. Enrollment in the MAT program at RIDOC automatically admits the individual as a patient of CODAC. Once released to the community, patients can continue treatment at any of the CODAC opioid treatment program sites across the state or can be transferred to another clinic or provider. In all circumstances, CODAC will provide dosing immediately following release so that treatment is not interrupted.

Summary

Rhode Island's program brings together lessons of the past as well as the current need to address OUD in new and innovative ways today. The MAT program is demonstrating successful results. Continued public health and corrections collaboration lay the groundwork for additional innovations in program implementation, including the RIDOC's focus on health equity and the social determinants of health. For years advocates had envisioned a criminal justice system that did not perpetuate the crises of SUD and overdose and instead helped address them thought treatment and recovery supports. We also envision a public health system that similarly promotes optimal health for all working within Rhode Island communities to address health challenges, including SUD and OUD.

References

1. Weiss DB, MacKenzie DL. A global perspective on incarceration: How an international focus can help the United States reconsider its incarceration rates. *Victims Offenders*. 2010; 5(3):268–282.
2. Western B, Pettit B. Incarceration & social inequality. *Daedalus*. 2010; 139(3):8–19.
3. Alexander M. The new Jim Crow. *Ohio State J Crim Law*. 2011; 9:7.
4. Wilson DB, Mitchell O, MacKenzie DL. A systematic review of drug court effects on recidivism. *J Exp Criminol*. 2006; 2(4):459–487.
5. Pager D. *Marked: Race, Crime, and Finding Work in an Era of Mass Incarceration*. Chicago: University of Chicago Press; 2008.
6. Petersilia J. When prisoners return to communities: Political, economic, and social consequences. *Fed Probation*. 2000; 65:3.
7. Lopez G. France had a big heroin epidemic in the 1980s and '90s; here's how the country fixed it. 2018. https://www.vox.com/policy-and-politics/2018/4/17/17246484/opioid-epidemic-buprenorphine-france. Accessed January 9, 2019.

8. Walmsley R. World prison population list. Home Office London. 2003. https://www. csdp.org/research/r234.pdf. Accessed January 9, 2018.

9. Walker S, Spohn C, DeLone M. *The Color of Justice: Race, Ethnicity, and Crime in America.* Boston: Cengage Learning; 2012.

10. Spohn C. Thirty years of sentencing reform: The quest for a racially neutral sentencing process. *J Crim Justice.* 2000; 3:427–501.

11. Bronson J, Stroop J, Zimmer S, Berzofsky M. Drug use, dependence, and abuse among state prisoners and jail inmates, 2007–2009. 2017. Washington, DC: US Department of Justice, Office of Juvenile Justice and Delinquency Prevention.

12. Carson EA, Sobel W. Prisoners in 2014. Bureau of Justice Statistics. http://bjs.ojp. usdoj.gov/index.cfm. Accessed February 23, 2019.

13. Prison Policy Initiative. Mass incarceration: The whole pie 2018. https://www. prisonpolicy.org/reports/pie2018.html. Accessed January 9, 2019.

14. Green TC, Clarke J, Brinkley-Rubinstein L, et al. Postincarceration fatal overdoses after implementing medications for addiction treatment in a statewide correctional system. *JAMA Psychiatry.* 2018; 75(4):405–407.

15. Brinkley-Rubinstein L, Macmadu A, Marshall BDL, et al. Risk of fentanyl-involved overdose among those with past year incarceration: Findings from a recent outbreak in 2014 and 2015. *Drug Alcohol Depend.* 2018; 185:189–191.

16. Binswanger IA, Stern MF, Deyo RA, et al. Release from prison—A high risk of death for former inmates. *N Engl J Med.* 2007; 356(2):157–165.

17. Merrall EL, Kariminia A, Binswanger IA, et al. Meta-analysis of drug-related deaths soon after release from prison. *Addiction.* 2010; 105(9):1545–1554.

18. Krinsky CS, Lathrop SL, Brown P, Nolte KB. Drugs, detention, and death: A study of the mortality of recently released prisoners. *Am J Forensic Med Path.* 2009; 30(1):6–9.

19. Rich JD, McKenzie M, Larney S, et al. Methadone continuation versus forced with-drawal on incarceration in a combined US prison and jail: A randomised, open-label trial. *Lancet.* 2015; 386(9991):350–359.

20. Knudsen HK, Abraham AJ, Roman PM. Adoption and implementation of medications in addiction treatment programs. *J Addict Med.* 2011; 5(1):21.

21. Johnson M, Eriator I, Rodenmeyer K. Backstories on the US opioid epidemic good intentions gone bad, an industry gone rogue and watch dogs gone to sleep. *Am J Med.* 2018; 131(6):595–601.

22. Joseph H, Stancliff S, Langrod J. Methadone maintenance treatment (MMT): A re-view of historical and clinical issues. *Mount Sinai J Med.* 2000; 67(5–6):347–364.

23. Dole VP, Nyswander ME, Kreek MJ. Narcotic blockade. *Arch Int Med.* 1966; 118(4):304–309.

24. Dole VP, Robinson JW, Orraca J, et al. Methadone treatment of randomly selected criminal addicts. *N Engl J Med.* 1969; 280(25):1372–1375.

25. White WL. *Slaying the Dragon: The History of Addiction Treatment and Recovery in America.* Bloomington, IN: Chestnut Health Systems/Lighthouse Institute; 1998.

26. Campbell ND, Lovell AM. The history of the development of buprenorphine as an addiction therapeutic. *Ann N Y Acad Sci.* 2012; 1248(1):124–139.

27. Thomas CP, Doyle E, Kreiner PW, et al. Prescribing patterns of buprenorphine waivered physicians. *Drug Alcohol Depend.* 2017; 181:213–218.

28. Magura S, Lee JD, Hershberger J, et al. Buprenorphine and methadone maintenance in jail and post-release: A randomized clinical trial. *Drug Alcohol Depend.* 2009; 99(1–3):222–230.

29. Maradiaga JA, Nahvi S, Cunningham CO, Sanchez J, Fox AD. "I kicked the hard way. I got incarcerated." Withdrawal from methadone during incarceration and subsequent aversion to medication assisted treatments. *J Subst Abuse Treat.* 2016; 62:49–54.

30. Binswanger IA, Blatchford PJ, Mueller SR, Stern MF. Mortality after prison release: Opioid overdose and other causes of death, risk factors, and time trends from 1999 to 2009. *Ann Intern Med.* 2013; 159(9):592–600.

31. Marsden J, Stillwell G, Jones H, et al. Does exposure to opioid substitution treatment in prison reduce the risk of death after release? A national prospective observational study in England. *Addiction.* 2017; 112(8):1408–1418.

32. Magura S, Rosenblum A, Lewis C, Joseph H. The effectiveness of in-jail methadone maintenance. *J Drug Issues.* 1993; 23(1):75–99.

33. Rhode Island Department of Corrections. Fiscal year 2017 annual population report. http://www.doc.ri.gov/administration/planning/docs/FY17%20Annual%20Population%20Report.pdf. Accessed January 9, 2018.

34. Texas Christian University (TCU) Institute of Behavioral Research. TCU Drug Screen. https://ibr.tcu.edu/forms/tcu-drug-screen/. Accessed March 9, 2019.

III | Moving Upstream: Prevention, Partnership, and Public Health

13 | The Role of Public Health Agencies in Convening Partnerships and Collaborations to Respond to the Opioid Crisis

PHILICIA TUCKER AND MICHAEL R. FRASER

IT HAS BEEN WIDELY recognized that public health activities, especially those that involve prevention and addressing the root causes of illness and disease, are only successful when they engage not just the internal staff of a governmental public health agency but the many other external agencies and organizations with which governmental public health collaborates, including the health care delivery system, housing and education agencies, community groups, and many others.[1] Partnerships are so critical to achieving improved public health outcomes that the current US Surgeon General, Dr. Jerome Adams, has made "better health through better partnerships"[2] a significant theme of his administration. Recent frameworks to organize public health responses to the opioid epidemic have stressed the need for partnership and collaboration, including the Association of State and Territorial Health Officials (ASTHO) and the National Association of State Alcohol and Drug Abuse Directors' *Preventing Opioid Misuse in the States and Territories: A Public Health Framework for Cross-Sector Leadership*[3] and Levine and Fraser's *Elements of a Comprehensive Public Health Response to the Opioid Crisis.*[4]

While partnership and collaboration are oft-used tactics in public health, the benefits of partnership and the specific aims of such collaboration are not always clear, nor are the best tactics to use when partnering with entities that have different interests, incentives, and constituencies than governmental public health agencies. With so much focus on partnerships to address the opioid crisis at the state and local level, there is a need to describe what constitutes an effective partnership and what are useful strategies to promote effective collaboration rather than leaving such things to chance. Intentional convening of intra- and inter-agency partnerships as well as multisector approaches to collaboration are a strength of many public health agencies[5] and an essential service provided by governmental public health.[6]

The overall logic of the need for partnerships, especially around an issue as complex as the opioid crisis, is that the more assets and resources that are gathered to respond to the crisis the better—in other words, the "sum" of the response partners is greater than the impact of any one part. We agree this is the case, especially when we look at the success of state implementation of prescription drug monitoring programs (PDMP). Public health collaboration with key groups such as hospitals, health systems, medical associations, physicians and other prescribers, law enforcement, attorneys general, patient groups, and the technology industry resulted in all states having a PDMP and using it in various ways to address overprescribing among providers and prescription diversion with patients. Partnerships among law enforcement, state corrections agencies, and public health agencies have led to the expansion of treatment options for individuals who are incarcerated and reduced overdose deaths on release.[7] Public health partnerships with faith communities have led to opportunities to increase the reach of opioid use disorder and addiction treatment programs, increased availability of the overdose reversal drug naloxone, and many other public health awareness and prevention campaigns.[8] Creative collaboration with employers has led to innovative approaches to support individuals in recovery and meet the needs of employers to retain skilled and talented workers.[9] Effective partnerships among public health, substance abuse and drug and alcohol programs, social services agencies, and community leadership at the local level have led to population or community-based reductions in drug and alcohol abuse and promoted positive youth development.[10]

Partnership and collaborative activities take work, often work that is not plainly stated in position descriptions or budgeted for in agency fiscal plans. Such activities also have downsides, including loss of control by any one partner, time spent on the processes involved in shared decision making, varying commitment among partners, difficulty in engaging key leaders for the duration of partnership and collaborative activities, and difficulty sustaining the shared purpose of the partnership over the long term. Efforts to create shared vision early on and sustain mutual commitment throughout the life of the partnership are important. Describing the "win–win" aspects of partnership— that is, illustrating those things that are greater when done together and from which each partner benefits—is a helpful strategy for engaging others and sustaining their interest. The "Win-Win" project at the University of California Los Angeles Fielding School of Public Health has demonstrated the health improvement results of collaboration between public health and other sectors, including education, justice, economic development, and several others.[11,12]

This chapter presents the central role public health agencies play as leaders and/or conveners of partnership and collaboration in responding to the opioid epidemic at the state and local levels. We define "partnership" as continuum of relationships between two or more entities ranging from informal engagement around topics of interest to formal, structured memoranda of understanding or contracts that govern resource exchange, the various roles and responsibilities of the partners, and performance metrics or other accountability metrics.[1] Collaboration is similarly defined as a continuum of shared activities between two or more entities ranging from basic cooperation (shared information and mutual support), to coordination (common tasks and compatible goals), to collaboration (integration of strategies and collective purpose, to "coadunation" (unified structure; combined culture).[13] Both of these continua raise important issues about the processes to be used by partners in order to achieve shared goals in response to the opioid crisis within their jurisdictions. These include such issues as those described by Rutledge, such as:[13]

- How should we communicate among partners?
- What is our intended outcome?
- Where do we share common strategies or practices?
- How do we best communicate with each other?
- What if we disagree with each other?
- Who is responsible for what? With whose resources?
- Where is there common purpose?
- How do we make decisions together?
- What strategies do we use?
- Who is responsible for what?
- How do we hold each other accountable?

Because the answers to these questions may often be difficult to resolve, legal documents such as memoranda of understanding, memoranda of agreement, and contracts or charters can be used to govern the activity of partners and promote a shared understanding and clear purpose for partnership and collaborative efforts.

Public health has played a major role in convening partners around the opioid epidemic. This is likely the result of the nature of core public health work in the epidemiology and surveillance of the crisis, and the reality of public health practice as a "team sport"[14]—that is, improved public health outcomes are the result of active collaborations and shared resources between partners in health care, other governmental agencies, and public health's collaborative approach to problem solving. To continue to be effective public conveners, public health practitioners should follow the advice of Linden,[15] who states that leaders of effective collaborations stress the following nine factors:

1. Articulate the project's purpose in a way that excites others.
2. Get the appropriate people (partners, organizations) to the table and keep them there.

3. Help partners see their common interests in collaboration, and the benefits possible through joint efforts.
4. Generate trust and help partners design a transparent, credible process.
5. Make relationship building a priority of the collaborative work.
6. Ensure there is a senior champion for the efforts, ideally at least one from every partner.
7. Engage in collaborative problem solving and make creative use of diverse perspectives when they arise.
8. Celebrate success and share credit.
9. Provide confidence, hope and resilience.

When these factors are addressed by public health leaders, the efficacy and impact of collaborative work is increased. On an issue as important as ending the crisis of opioid misuse and preventing addiction, their application to partnership and collaborative activities is essential.

To varying degrees, the opioid crisis has affected all communities regardless of race, age, urban, rural, and/or socioeconomic status. This makes the issue of opioid misuse and addiction prevention relevant to a broad sector of community leaders and local, state, and federal policymakers. In their 2017 and 2018 ASTHO President's Challenges, Jay Butler, state health officer for Alaska, and John Wiesman, Secretary of Health in Washington State, called on their state and territorial health officer peers to take a public health approach to the prevention of substance misuse and addiction.[15,16] A key strategy of that approach was partnership and collaboration. In the following section of this chapter, we describe the roles of various partners in responding to the opioid crisis using the ASTHO President's Challenge as a guide. Figure 13.1 illustrates the many different categories of partners engaged in ending the crisis. While certainly not exhaustive of all the partnerships needed, it includes some of the key potential partners in a local or state public health response to the opioid crisis.

Attorneys General

Individuals with substance use disorder (SUD) are more likely to be incarcerated than to have the opportunity to receive treatment.[17] In 2004, more than half of those in state prisons were recorded having a drug dependence, while only 15% received treatment.[18] State attorneys general have direct authority over policies, legal matters, and the justice system within their jurisdictions.[18] Therefore, the opportunity arises for public health partnerships with attorneys general and related law and justice agencies to examine current policies and guide revisions to them. The National Attorneys General Training and Research Institute (NAGTRI) sought to work with the law enforcement and public health officials in encouraging the two communities to communicate

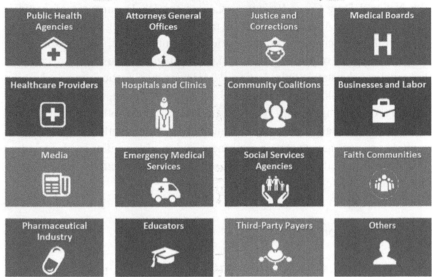

Cross-Sectoral Collaboration is Key

Public Health Agencies	Attorneys General Offices	Justice and Corrections	Medical Boards
Healthcare Providers	Hospitals and Clinics	Community Coalitions	Businesses and Labor
Media	Emergency Medical Services	Social Services Agencies	Faith Communities
Pharmaceutical Industry	Educators	Third-Party Payers	Others

FIGURE 13.1. Multiple sectors involved in prevention of substance misuse and addiction.
Source: ASTHO 2017 President's Challenge[15]

and partner together.[19] Partnering with ASTHO in 2016, NAGTRI held a symposium, *Bridging the Gaps: Reducing Prescription Drug and Opioid Abuse and Misuse Summit*, devoted to raising awareness and sharing expertise in handling the opioid epidemic to participants such as practitioners, attorneys, and public health officials.[19]

Drug courts, or special courts developed to provide alternative sentencing options such as sentencing to treatment or supervision of individuals with serious substance use or addiction disorders, are good examples of partnerships among public health, health care delivery, and the criminal justice systems with the shared goal of increasing recovery success of those with SUDs and reducing the burden on the traditional justice system.[17] These courts provide those convicted of a nonviolent misdemeanor or felony the chance to participate in local treatment with the supervision of the court rather than being immediately incarcerated.[17] Over the years, evaluation of drug courts shows various benefits to not only the participant, but also to the state. Individuals who participated in these programs were 53% less likely to be involved with criminal activity and had a 62% reduction in rearrests.[20] Drug courts are a cost-effective way of reducing incarceration, with an average savings of $5,680 to $6,208 per person.[20]

As of 2017, there were an estimated 3,100 drug courts across the United States,[20] and it is important to continue to strengthen the system and invest in potential partnerships. By offering training and technical assistance through the National Drug Court Resources Center, the US Department of Justice's Bureau of Justice Assistance assists in increasing adult drug court capacity and taking full advantage of criminal justice and public health and treatment resources. The state of Maine plans to take advantage of the use of drug courts to help address the state's opioid crisis.[21] Maine's Chief Justice proposed a pilot program that would provide increased access to treatment, sober housing, job training, counseling, family resources, and continuous follow-up for justice-involved individuals with a significant SUD.[21] Similar pilots in other states include agencies across state government and outside of it as well, including public health, Medicaid programs, departments of corrections, attorneys general offices, and others.

Justice and Corrections

In the United States, it is estimated that 90% of individuals on prescribed methadone are required to stop their treatment when incarcerated.[22] Studies estimate that those incarcerated with an SUD have a 100-fold higher risk of an overdose fatality in the first two weeks of being released from the justice system compared to the overall population.[23] In 2016, the Rhode Island Department of Corrections implemented a program that treated those incarcerated with an opioid dependence.[24] The Rhode Island Overdose Prevention and Intervention Task Force created partnerships with local opioid use disorder (OUD) resources from the criminal justice system, social and behavioral health system, and health care system so that those transitioning out of the correctional system could continue their medication-assisted treatment (MAT) and have access to resources to provide greater opportunities to a healthier life.[24] After six months, there was a 12.3% decrease in opioid overdose-related deaths in Rhode Island.[7] By connecting the criminal justice system with the resources needed to prevent opioid overdoses and increase a person's chance of success outside of incarceration, Rhode Island was able to make a significant influence on a high-risk population. Other public health agencies can use the Rhode Island example to convene similar partnerships to address post-incarceration MAT and recovery supports (see Chapter 12).

State Medical Boards

State and territorial medical boards have general oversight regarding the licensure, regulation, and discipline of physicians and other health care providers.[25] Medical boards' unique role in both the licensing and regulation of medical providers makes them important partners in establishing statewide policies for health care providers and ensuring the legitimate practice of medicine in every state. Similar state boards, such as state boards of nursing or pharmacy, offer additional partnership and collaborative opportunities. State boards, in conjunction with other stakeholders such as medical associations and large hospital systems, can establish licensure standards that include mandatory continuing education units in opioid prescribing guidelines, can discipline physicians who overprescribe opioids, and may also work with the physician community to recommend voluntary standards and practices and allow professions to "police themselves" when it comes to guideline implementation and promote opioid stewardship.

In addition to punitive disciplinary action, such as suspending or revoking a physician's license to practice medicine for failing to follow practice guidelines or obtaining required education, another role of medical boards is to assess physicians' "fitness to practice," and a board can mandate referral to treatment for a physician with an SUD.[25] Programs such as the Lifeguard program operated by the Pennsylvania Medical Society Foundation (www.pamed.org) and the KSTAR physician assessment program operated by the Texas A&M University (architexas.org/k-star-physician/assessment.html), have evolved to assess and evaluate physicians' performance and whether a physician has a drug or alcohol use disorder and to support recovery and re-entry to practice, and they play a crucial role in active monitoring and assessment of physicians in recovery. These programs also offer courses on appropriate prescribing and current guidelines to support physician education before disciplinary action is mandated.

Physicians and Other Health Care Provider Communities

Health care providers, especially those who prescribe opioids, are an obvious partner for public health agencies. Prescribers have been actively involved in the development of state pain management guidelines and development of opioid "stewardship" programs within practices (both medical and dental) and health care systems. In addition to awareness raising and education of prescribers on appropriate use of opioids, public health partnerships with health care providers are essential to expanding access to MAT and addressing addiction services treatment gaps within a state or community. Many state health agencies have worked with health care providers to encourage their participation in the US Drug Enforcement Agency's buprenorphine waiver management program, a program that allows physicians and other prescribers to prescribe buprenorphine after participating in continuing education about the medication. The US Department of Health and Human Services (HHS) recently released guidelines on the use of telemedicine in the prescribing and monitoring of patients on MAT.[26]

Unfortunately, only 47% of US counties have health providers who can prescribe buprenorphine, while 72% of rural counties do not even have a physician who can prescribe buprenorphine.[27] Several issues act as barriers for prescriber participation in the waiver program. Overall, physicians must deal with time constraints, lack of reimbursements, lack of support from other providers and partners, lack of community resources, and lack of behavioral health professionals.[28] These factors affect a provider's decision to offer MAT, and those seeking treatment may encounter long waitlists and/or poor treatment. Stigma and misunderstanding of addiction keep some health care providers from seeing patients with SUDs, believing that addiction is a personal failing rather than a chronic disease, and not wanting "those patients" in their waiting rooms.

The state of Vermont encouraged providers to participate in the waiver program along with the expansion of treatment modalities through a "hub-and-spoke" system of care (see Chapter 10). Through these and other efforts, Vermont increased the number of physicians willing to treat patients with OUD.[29] By connecting health care providers with social and behavioral services, counseling, professional advice, and other local resources, physicians were able to feel supported and more willing to get a waiver to treat patients.

Burnout among health care providers is a real barrier to health care engagement in many topics, including opioid misuse and addition. A novel approach to care, however, has been found to "bring the joy" back to practicing medicine. The University of New Mexico School of Medicine's Project ECHO (Extension for Community Healthcare Outcomes) was created to spread knowledge and improve health outcomes using a standard approach to physician engagement and education. [30] Project ECHO's "all teach, all learn" approach engages physicians in reviewing best practices, connects physicians who may be practicing in remote areas with an academic medical center or other physician expertise, and draws on the case study method that providers use in early medical education. In New Mexico, ECHO clinics supported by the state health department and other agencies included buprenorphine training, certification, and connecting to resources related to OUD, which helped to increase the number of those who could prescribe buprenorphine.[31]

Pharmacists are an often-overlooked group in the work of public health and prevention, but their role is critical in efforts to address the opioid crisis (see Chapter 8). In addition to partnering on PDMP implementation and following dispensing guidelines, pharmacists play a front-line role in dispensing naloxone and sharing health education materials and addiction prevention materials with patients. Pharmacists may also be involved in querying PDMPs and other online systems to make sure that a patient is not inadvertently co-prescribed benzodiazepine medications in conjunction with opioids, a lethal combination for many patients. They may also be able to flag suspicious or fraudulent prescriptions or identify individuals who may be diverting drugs and alert the appropriate authorities.

Hospitals and Health Care Facilities

While an obvious partner for public health agencies, the scope of public health partnership and collaboration with hospitals and clinics is often limited to access to specific health care issues or specialty care problems and conversations about how nonprofit hospitals program their "community benefit" investments. While the Patient Protection and Affordable Care Act (ACA) required nonprofit hospitals to engage in community health assessments, these are often conducted as separate activities from the assessments conducted by public health agencies, a significant missed opportunity for partnership and collaboration.[32] At a basic level, public health and hospitals should convene to discuss access issues, health assessments, and investments in community health improvement—but these are only starting issues.

Additionally, public health leaders and hospital leaders should discuss emergency department prescribing of opioids, use of state PDMP systems, and real-time surveillance of overdose deaths and equally important "close calls" in hospital settings. Hospital medical staff can set institution- or facility-specific adoption of state and national guidelines and work with their providers to implement such standards. System-wide adoption of patient pain "contracts" and other mechanisms to prevent drug diversion are additional points of collaboration between public health agencies and hospitals. Governmental public health agencies can be an especially important partner for hospital systems in a state because the health agency can act as a neutral convener for competing systems. Public health also serves as a data aggregator within a state and can share statewide data with hospitals that might otherwise have access to only their patient populations.

Community Coalitions

Community coalitions are organized, long-term partnerships used to regularly involve multiple organizations and significant leaders within the community to address a challenging situation. This allows a community to work cohesively to create objectives and goals, such as educational campaigns and prevention resources, that can be jointly agreed on to successfully respond to the opioid crisis among the population.[33] Community coalitions are a relevant way to better understand and develop ways to tackle the opioid issue because community members are most likely to share information that gives greater insight into the target population, local needs, and available prevention resources.

The US Substance Abuse and Mental Health Services Administration (SAMHSA) has provided various tools and steps to creating successful community coalitions. There are various examples of successful programs and strategies to reduce the non-medical use of prescription medication that have been evaluated and approved by SAMHSA that states can use as frameworks for their own community coalitions.[34] For example, regional work in rural/frontier Alaskan communities gathered researchers, community leaders, and local schools to work together to create a prevention strategy for parents of children in fifth through seventh grades.[34] Their goal was to reduce the access to harmful legal products, which included prescription medication, through prevention strategies that focused on parents and the home environment. Through this successful coalition, schools were able to have "family nights" that taught parents how to reduce access to harmful legal products and help prevent children from having access to products like prescription drugs in the home. Hence, states can use these models and tools to create community readiness, create common objectives, build strong relationships, and have clear outcome goals that can be implemented into their organizations.[35]

Businesses and Labor Leaders

Business and labor may not be the first sector that comes to mind when actively developing partnerships regarding the opioid crisis, but it is a very important sector as the opioid crisis has heavily impacted the US workforce. Over the past decade, the rate of those actively participating in the workforce has shown a greater drop in counties were individuals have been prescribed more opioids compared those who have been prescribed less.[36] Business and labor leaders have the opportunity to prevent abuse and misuse of opioids, especially those whose employees may have a higher risk of physical strain and thus of being prescribed opioids due to workplace injuries. According to the National Safety Council, only one-fifth of employers believed they were highly prepared to handle the threat of the opioid crisis in their workplace.[37]

Federal legislation (H.R. 5892) introduced in February 2018 by Representatives Jason Lewis (D-GA) and Matt Cartwright (D-PA) proposes the creation of a multi-agency advisory committee to guide the Secretary of Labor on practical approaches the department can adopt to reduce the impact of the opioid misuse related to the workplace.[37] Similar collaborative activities at the state and local legislative levels may also be excellent ways to create multi-sector partner groups to address the role businesses can play in supporting employees in recovery, identifying individuals who may have an

SUD and referring them to treatment, or otherwise supporting the primary prevention of opioid misuse disorder in the workplace. In June 2018, the National Business Group on Health called on its members to discuss opioid use in pain management with the health plans and pharmacy benefits managers that serve their employees.[38] The call was based on continued employer frustration with increasing rates of opioid misuse among employees, which lead to increased medical costs, abuse in the workplace, increased absenteeism, and employee overdose. Public health agencies can work with business groups and labor to identify prevention opportunities in workplace wellness programs as well as through employee assistance programs.

Media Outlets and the Press

Proactive collaboration with the media (radio, print, television, and social media outlets) is important to reach a large audience with major media markets to convey important messages, use public health education science to share prevention campaigns, increase awareness, and evoke action. In other public health contexts, media campaigns have had significant effects on health behaviors such as tobacco use and the prevention of heart disease.[39] Effective media campaigns elicit an emotional or reasoning response to individuals that persuade them to make changes in beliefs, behaviors, and social norms. The US Centers for Disease Control and Prevention (CDC)'s recent RxAwareness campaign's central message, "it only takes a little to lose a lot," is a science-based prevention campaign stressing the dangers of prescription opioids (Figure 13.2).[40] These proactive, public service approaches can have wide

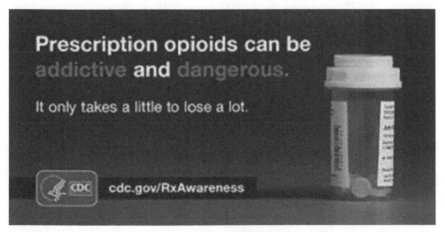

FIGURE 13.2. The CDC's RxAwareness Campaign.
Source: US Centers for Disease Control and Prevention.

reach and develop strong partnerships with media outlets for future messaging and information sharing.

Many states have state-specific media campaigns taking a more local approach to awareness raising but with the intentions of preventing opioid misuse and abuse. Vermont's "Parent Up" media campaign focuses on educating parents on preventing teen substance use through videos, resources, tools, and infographics, and position parents as the number-one influence on their teenage children.[41] Targeting the general population, Utah created the "Use Only as Directed" campaign, which was funded by the state's Commission on Criminal and Juvenile Justice. This campaign focuses on how to safely store, use, and dispose of prescription medication through various forms of media to prevent misuse and abuse of prescription pain medication (Figure 13.3). Though many campaigns pinpoint reasoning and cognitive thinking, some campaigns use more personal and emotional tools to persuade behavior change. Wisconsin's "Good Drugs Gone Bad" public service announcement uses videos targeted to teens to show the real dangers of substance use and other materials like sharing the story of a past police officer's journey of abusing prescription drugs.[41] In developing messaging, public health and prevention science suggests that it is necessary for community leaders to understand who is most at risk and what are their needs to create relevant messages that will engage the intended audience.

Emergency Medical Services

Emergency medical services (EMS) are frequently the first to respond to a 911 call regarding overdose. Partnerships with EMS responders have stressed the life-saving role of naloxone, and several states have expanded access to naloxone for all first responders in their states.[42] Proper administration of naloxone reverses the effects of an opioid overdose by blocking opioid receptor in the brain.[43] Significant public health and health care collaboration with EMS leaders has helped reduce stigma around drug use, despite some who continue to believe that the lives of individuals with SUD are not worth saving, especially after multiple saves of the same individual over time. Additional collaboration with EMS should include the EMS role in hand-off to treatment and the role EMS providers can play in early detection of overdose "hot spots" (i.e., areas where spikes in overdose may be likely due to call volume).

Another area where public health and EMS personnel have collaborated is responder safety and occupational health, especially as more and more illicit opioid overdoses involve the extremely lethal drugs fentanyl and carfentanil. Because fentanyl and carfentanil are orders of magnitude more potent than heroin, first responders are rightly concerned about their potential exposure to the substance when engaging an individual who has overdosed. Guidelines

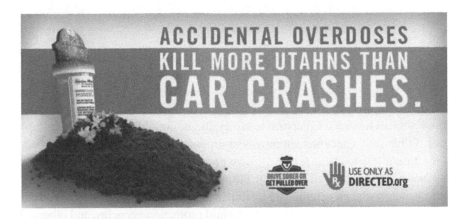

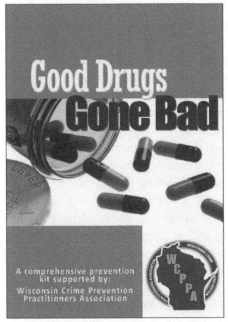

FIGURE 13.3. Examples of state-specific public awareness and educations campaign materials: Utah's "Use Only As Directed" campaign and Wisconsin's "Good Drugs Gone Bad" Campaign.

Source: https://www.upr.org/term/use-only-directed, https://tfjck.org/programs/good-drugs-gone-bad/.

for first responders have been developed in collaboration with law enforcement, health, and substance misuse and addiction agencies both federally and at the state level. These collaborations have helped reinforce trust; demonstrate that responder safety, not just overdose reversal, are priorities for public health and other state leaders; and engage EMS in response to the opioid crisis.

Social Services Agencies

Social service agencies (child welfare agencies, family services agencies, and other similar organizations) are a significant contributor to prevention, intervention, treatment, and recovery efforts for those with SUD and mental health illness. Case workers in social service agencies are critical to understanding the resources in a state to support recovery, including addiction treatment, supportive housing, education, employment supports, and food and nutrition services. In addition to client-facing services provided to individuals in need, many agencies also work with public health agencies to provide a wide range of population-based prevention and treatment services at the local, state, and federal level, such as in schools, hospitals, child protection agencies, and others.[44] Connecting those in recovery to both health-related and non–health-related social needs (e.g., housing, employment, primary and specialty health care) is necessary to sustain successful recovery from SUDs. A number of states and territories have taken coordinated approaches to the many services available to support treatment and prevention work through governor-led "blue ribbon panels," special task forces, and other high-level, multi-sector collaborations focused on both sharing data on opioid use within a state and the resources available for treatment and recovery programs.

Leaders in public health, drug and alcohol abuse/substance misuse and addiction, and the health care sectors have recently emphasized the role of adverse childhood experiences (ACEs) in contributing to potential SUDs and addiction later in life. ACEs are traumatic or stressful events (e.g., physical, emotional, or sexual abuse, parental substance abuse, other traumatic events) experienced by young children during critical stages of their development. Without developing adequate coping mechanism to deal with ACEs, a child may increase risk behaviors as a form of coping.[45] ACEs have been correlated with smoking, alcohol misuse, and illicit drug use and more specifically opioid dependence and earlier age of injection drug use.[46] Research has demonstrated a correlation between ACEs and later substance misuse and addiction in teenagers and young adults, with the more ACEs experienced the greater the correlation in substance misuse and addiction. While it is important not to jump to causal relationships without adequate study and analysis, the correlation between ACEs and substance misuse is gaining more and more understanding among social service, public health, and health care agencies.

Public health agencies can share behavioral risk surveillance data with service agencies to help identify the prevalence of ACEs in populations and design interventions and prevention programs for individuals and families in need. Recent work on developing resources and support for individual and community resiliency has been very significant in this regard, including the ASTHO 2019 President's Challenge, "Building Healthy and Resilient

Communities," and the Trust for America's Health and the Well-Being Trust's National Resilience Strategy.[45,47] The CDC has suggested various forms of ACE-prevention approaches, such as home visits, parent and family counseling, teen pregnancy support and prevention programs, substance abuse treatment, child care, and so on.[45]

The University of Washington's Communities That Care model helps community leaders and decision makers use public health strategies and programs as guides to improving their youth development.[10] Programs and resources focus on various risk and/or protective factors evolving around substance abuse, violence, school dropout, and so on, with varying interventions based on suitable age groups. Communities That Care is rooted in research that emphasizes a comprehensive approach and has tested and evaluated these programs and practices for their effectiveness. Through this approach, these practices can be integrated into current organizations to bring long-term outcomes that help to develop a healthy social environment for children at risk of behavioral issues.

Faith Communities

Communities of faith are often key leaders of social change, including supporting movements to promote social justice and support for the needy.[48] Faith leaders and their members intentionally build trusting communities with shared values and in many areas provide significant support to the homeless, the hungry, those impacted by emergencies and disasters, and those who may have extreme social needs and may have been turned away from or do not want to access government services for support. The opioid crisis is no exception when it comes to the need to partner with faith communities to help create necessary social supports, provide awareness and education programs to community members, and support recovery resources to those with SUDs and/or their families.

Faith leaders can collaborate with public health to amplify or share materials to reduce stigma, to educate community members on ways to prevent addiction, and to share information on local treatment and recovery services. HHS has developed a practical resource that covers ways the faith community can engage partners in tackling the opioid crisis. The *Opioid Epidemic Practical Toolkit: Helping Faith and Community Leaders Bring Hope and Healing to Our Communities* emphasizes the role faith communities can play in opioid crisis response and how federal resources can be used at the state and local level to support provision of SUD services by faith-based organizations.[49] Such services can include recovery and support groups, educational materials, response trainings, connecting individuals and families to local resources, youth drug prevention programs, and others.

Pharmaceutical Industry

Public health agencies have a mixed history of partnership and collaboration with the pharmaceutical industry. While pharmaceutical companies are critical to core public health interventions such as vaccinations, the industry's role in promoting and marketing opioids as safe without solid evidence that they were not addictive is currently under review and has led to several states taking legal action or contemplating legal action against opioid manufacturers and medical distributors that supplied opioids. State engagement in such litigation may complicate collaboration with companies involved in such lawsuits. However, industry can play a role in supporting educational programs for clinicians on appropriate treatment for OUD and has been actively involved in "drug takeback" events to collect unused medication and dispose of it properly, avoiding potential diversion, as evidenced by recent legislation in the state of Washington. Public health leaders should consider the way they can engage the pharmaceutical industry in ways that support their public health mission without compromising their public health ethics. This balance continues to be tricky: Many view the industry as responsible for the current crisis while also depending on it for medicines to treat addiction and many other public health programs.

Schools and Educators

Many young people spend more waking time in the classroom or at school than they do at home; as such, schools are a major opportunity for public health prevention education and intervention. SAMHSA supports states in the implementation of school-based substance abuse prevention programs.[50] These programs offer schools access to evidence-based prevention information to use with their students. SAMHSA recognizes that young people should have access to safe learning environments, but the reality is that many schools and campuses face public health problems such as substance misuse, violence, bullying, and other unsafe behavior. Educators, students, and parents/families are given access to resources that address, identify, and support youth's mental health issues to increase healthy behavior, relationships, and coping skills.[51]

College students in recovery may be faced with lack of on-campus support for recovery, leading to them having to choose between recovery or completing their studies. Collegiate recovery programs allow colleges and universities to provide recovery support, a community free of alcohol and drugs, and sometimes recovery dorms. Rutgers University in New Jersey started its recovery program in 1983 and it continues today. The program offers support, substance-free dorms, and community activities, and students have the responsibility to attend on-campus 12-step meetings weekly. These programs are cost-effective, increase health and well-being, and help decrease student dropout rates.

Third-Party Payers and Health Insurers

Third-party payers, companies that administer and manage health care benefits and expenses, have a very large role in determining patient access to and the affordability of SUD prevention and treatment. Insurer network adequacy and compliance with mental health parity laws have been the subject of intense scrutiny in many states. Advocates for those in recovery have described difficulty obtaining coverage for needed addiction treatment services, including both inpatient residential and outpatient care.[52] Providers have also indicated difficulty in working with third-party payers to obtain approval for addiction treatment medications, citing burdensome prior approval processes and or "fail-first" protocols before they are able to prescribe the medicine desired. Unfortunately, public health collaboration with third-party payers is often nonexistent, since state or territorial Medicaid programs and state insurance departments serve as the primary regulator and/or collaborator with third-party payers.

State Medicaid programs have significant roles in the financing of and access to prevention and treatment when it comes to substance misuse, especially in states where Medicaid has been expanded. In 2016, SAMHSA stated that the expansion of Medicaid helped to give coverage for SUD to over a million individuals.[53] In all states, at least one form of MAT is available for those seeking treatment, along with counseling and other recovery resources. States that have taken advantage of Medicaid expansion have seen as much as 50% of MAT being covered in their jurisdictions.[53] The use of Medicaid is critical to help decrease the burden of cost on patients, hospitals, and private providers.

Third-party payers are vital partners in the work of public health and prevention. Innovative programs to promote substance misuse and addiction prevention among their provider networks and with their members could amplify the work that public health officials conduct in their communities. Negotiating adequate reimbursement for substance abuse treatment, adjusting care limits or deductibles, and implementing other tools to prevent opioid misuse and prevention are key strategies public health agencies should discuss with third-party payers. Public health agencies can bring data and surveillance information to third-party payers and help inform third-party payers' efforts to maximize the efficient and effective care of individuals with SUD.

Additional Partners

Clearly, there are almost endless ways for public health agencies to partner with other agencies and organizations to obtain shared goals and objectives. Partners that are not mentioned specifically in this chapter but that are very important include medical examiners and coroners, the dental community, the veterinary profession, civic and other voluntary associations, clubs, and fraternal organizations, and others. The goal of this chapter was to emphasize partnership as an important strategy for addressing OUD and public health agencies' potential leadership roles in convening such partnerships in their jurisdictions. With intentional partnerships and collaborations that stress the need for win–win solutions, partnership activities can vastly amplify the limited resources available to public health agencies and expand the reach of public health programs in a state. The opioid crisis illustrates the many ways public health agencies can engage partners and collaborate to address the crisis, and ultimately end it.

References

1. US Centers for Disease Control and Prevention (CDC). Partnerships, coalitions, and collaborations. https://www.cdc.gov/oralhealth/state_programs/infrastructure/partnerships.htm. Accessed October 5, 2018.
2. US Department of Health and Human Services, Office of the Surgeon General. Biography of the Surgeon General VADM Jerome M. Adams. https://www.surgeongeneral.gov/about/biographies/bio-sg.html. Accessed October 5, 2018.
3. Association of State and Territorial Health Officials (ASTHO). Preventing opioid misuse in the states and territories: A public health framework for cross-sector leadership. https://my.astho.org/opioids/home. Accessed October 23, 2018.
4. Levine M, Fraser M. Elements of a comprehensive public health response to the opioid crisis: A guide for public health Action. *Ann Intern Med.* 2018; 169(10):712–715.
5. Association of State and Territorial Health Officials (ASTHO). About us. http://www.astho.org/About/. Accessed October 23, 2018.
6. US Centers for Disease Control and Prevention (CDC). The 10 essential public health services: An overview. 2014. https://www.cdc.gov/stltpublichealth/publichealthservices/pdf/essential-phs.pdf. Accessed October 23, 2018.
7. Green TC, Clarke J, Brinkley-Rubinstein L, et al. Postincarceration fatal overdoses after implementing medications for addiction treatment in a statewide correctional system. *JAMA Psychiatry.* 2018; 75(4):405–407.
8. Kennedy N. Faith communities and opioid crisis. Shared Justice. http://www.sharedjustice.org/most-recent/2018/8/13/the-faith-community-in-action-a-response-to-the-opioid-crisis. Accessed October 5, 2018.
9. National Safety Council. The Proactive Role Employers Can Take: Opioids in the Workplace. https://www.nsc.org/Portals/0/Documents/RxDrugOverdoseDocuments/RxKit/The-Proactive-Role-Employers-Can-Take-Opioids-in-the-Workplace.pdf. Accessed October 5, 2018.

10. Communities that Care. How It Works. https://www.communitiesthatcare.net/. Accessed February 25, 2019.

11. University of California, Fielding School of Public Health, Center for Health Advancement. Win-Win project. https://winwin.uclacha.org/. Accessed October 5, 2018.

12. University of California, Fielding School of Public Health, Center for Health Advancement. Win-Win project: Methodology. https://winwin.uclacha.org/methodology/. Accessed October 5, 2018.

13. Rutledge M. A framework and tools to strengthen strategic alliances. *OD Practitioner*. 2011; 43(2):22–27.

14. Linden R. The discipline of collaboration. In: LeBoeuf J, Hesselbein F, ed. *Leader to Leader*. 1st ed. San Francisco: Jossey-Bass; 2003:41–47.

15. Association of State and Territorial Health Officials (ASTHO). 2017 President's Challenge: Public Health Approaches to Preventing Substance Misuse and Addiction. http://www.astho.org/ASTHO-Presidents-Challenge/2017/. Accessed October 5, 2018.

16. Butler JC. 2017 ASTHO President's Challenge: Public health approaches to preventing substance misuse and addiction. *J Public Health Manag Pract*. 2017; 23(5):531–536.

17. Roberson A, Swartz M. Extended-release naltrexone and drug treatment courts: Policy and evidence for implementing an evidence-based treatment. *J Subst Abuse Treat*. 2018; 85:101–104.

18. King RS, Pasquarella J. Drug courts: A review of the evidence. Research and Advocacy for Reform. 2009. http://sentencingproject.org/wp-content/uploads/2016/01/Drug-Courts-A-Review-of-the-Evidence.pdf. Accessed September 11, 2018.

19. Manning J. Bridging the gaps to reduce prescription drug and opioid abuse and misuse. 2017. National Association of Attorneys General. www.naag.org/publications/nagtri-journal/volume-2-issue-3/bridging-the-gaps-to-reduce-prescription-drug-and-opioid-abuse-and-misuse.php. Accessed October 5, 2018.

20. US Department of Justice. Drug Courts. 2018. https://www.ncjrs.gov/pdffiles1/nij/238527.pdf. Accessed September 11, 2018.

21. Harrison J. Maine chief justice proposes expanding drug courts to address opioid crisis. *Bangor Daily News*, February 27, 2018. https://bangordailynews.com/2018/02/27/news/state/maine-chief-justice-proposes-expanding-drug-courts-to-address-opioid-crisis/. Accessed September 11, 2018.

22. Rich JD, Mckenzie M, Larney S, et al. Methadone continuation versus forced withdrawal on incarceration in a combined US prison and jail: A randomized, open-label trial. *Lancet*. 2015; 386(9991):350–359.

23. Green TC, Zaller N, Wilson PR, et al. Law enforcement attitudes toward overdose prevention and response. *Drug Alcohol Depend*. 2013; 133(2): 677–684.

24. Haskins J. Rhode Island correctional program slashes opioid overdose deaths. *The Nation's Health*. 2018; 48(3):11.

25. Federation of State Medical Boards (FSMB). About FSMB. http://www.fsmb.org/about-fsmb/. Accessed October 5, 2018.

26. Brown D. HHS encourages physicians to use telemedicine to combat opioid epidemic. *Mobile & Telehealth*, September 20, 2018.

27. White House, Office of National Drug Control Policy. The President's Commission on Combating Drug Addiction and the Opioid Crisis. 2017. https://www.whitehouse. gov/sites/whitehouse.gov/files/images/Final_Report_Draft_11-15-2017.pdf. Accessed March 17, 2019.

28. Andrilla CHA, Coulthard C, Larson EH. Barriers rural physicians face prescribing buprenorphine for opioid use disorder. *Ann Fam Med*. 2017; 15(4): 359–362.

29. Brooklyn JR, Sigmon SC. Vermont hub and spoke model of care for opioid use disorder: Cevelopment, implementation, and impact. *J Addict Med*. 2017; 11(4):286–292.

30. University of New Mexico, School of Medicine. Project ECHO: A Revolution in Medical Education and Health Care Delivery. https://echo.unm.edu/. Accessed March 17, 2019.

31. Komaromy M, Duhigg D, Metcalf A, et al. Project ECHO (Extension for Community Healthcare Outcomes): A new model for educating primary care providers about treatment of substance use disorders. *Subst Abus*. 2016; 37(1): 20–24.

32. James J. Nonprofit hospitals' community benefit requirements. *Health Affairs*. 2016. https://www.healthaffairs.org/do/10.1377/hpb20160225.954803/abs/.

33. Trudeau KJ. Development of a community readiness survey for coalitions to address prescription opioid misuse. *J Alcohol Drug Educ*. 2015; 59(3):67–97.

34. US Substance Abuse and Mental Health Services Administration (SAMHSA). Preventing prescription drug misuse: Programs and strategies. 2016. https://www. samhsa.gov/capt/sites/default/files/resources/preventing-prescription-drug-misuse-strategies.pdf. Accessed October 5, 2018.

35. US Substance Abuse and Mental Health Services Administration (SAMHSA). Components of an effective coalition. 2018. https://www.samhsa.gov/capt/tools-learning-resources/components-effective-coalition. Accessed October 5, 2018.

36. Krueger AB. Where have all the workers gone? An inquiry into the decline of the U.S. labor force participation rate. Brookings Institution. https://www.brookings. edu/wp-content/uploads/2018/02/kruegertextfa17bpea.pdf. Accessed September 12, 2018.

37. ED Workforce. Fact sheet: Ppioid legislation. https://edworkforce.house.gov/ uploadedfiles/fact_sheet_-_opioid_legislation.pdf. Accessed September 12, 2018.

38. National Business Group on Health. National business group on health recommends employers discuss opioid use for pain management with health plans and pharmacy benefit managers. https://www.businessgrouphealth.org/news/nbgh-news/press-releases/press-release-details/?ID=344. Accessed October 5, 2018.

39. Wakefield MA, Loken B, Hornik RC. Use of media campaigns to change health behaviour. *Lancet*. 2010; 376(9748):1261–1271.

40. US Centers for Disease Control and Prevention (CDC). CDC RxAwareness campaign overview. https://www.cdc.gov/rxawareness/pdf/RxAwareness-Campaign-Overview-508.pdf. Accessed October 5, 2018.

41. US Substance Abuse and Mental Health Services Administration (SAMHSA). Media campaigns to prevent prescription drug and opioids misuse. https://www.samhsa.gov/ capt/sites/default/files/capt_resource/media-campaigns-prevent-rx-drugs-opioid-misuse.pdf. Accessed September 12, 2018.

42. Zhang X, Marchand C, Sullivan B, et al. Naloxone access for emergency medical technicians: An evaluation of a training program in rural communities. *Addict Behav*. 2018; 86:79–85.

43. Jeffery RM, Dickinson L, Ng ND, et al. Naloxone administration for suspected opioid overdose: An expanded scope of practice by a basic life support collegiate-based emergency medical services agency. *J Am Coll Health*. 2017; 65(3): 212–216.

44. Scobie-Carroll A. Guest editorial: Social work students as activists in the opioid epidemic. *Field Educator*. 2017; 7(2). http://fieldeducator.simmons.edu/article/guest-editorial-social-work-students-as-activists-in-the-opioid-epidemic/. Accessed September 12, 2018.

45. Tilson E. Adverse childhood experiences (ACES): An important element of a comprehensive approach to the opioid crisis. *N C Med J*. 2018; 79(3): 166–169.

46. Gaurino H, Mateu-Gelabert P, Sirikantraporn S. The role of adverse childhood experiences in initiation of substance use and sexual behaviors among opioid-using young adults. *Drug Alcohol Depend*. 2017; 171: e79.

47. Association of State and Territorial Health Officials (ASTHO). 2019 President's Challenge. http://www.astho.org/ASTHO-Presidents-Challenge/2019/. Last accessed February 25, 2019.

48. Ager J, Fiddian-Qasmiyeh E, Ager A. Local faith communities and the promotion of resilience in contexts of humanitarian crisis. *J Refug Stud*. 2015; 28(2): 202–221.

49. US Department of Health and Human Services (HHS). Opioid epidemic practical toolkit: Helping faith and community leaders bring hope and healing to our communities. https://www.hhs.gov/about/agencies/iea/partnerships/opioid-toolkit/index.html. Accessed September 12, 2018.

50. US Substance Abuse and Mental Health Services Administration (SAMSHA). School and campus health. https://www.samhsa.gov/school-campus-health. Accessed October 5, 2018.

51 US Substance Abuse and Mental Health Services Administration (SAMHSA). Information for educators, students, parents and families. https://www.samhsa.gov/school-campus-health/information. Accessed October 5, 2018.

52. Wen H, Cummings JR, Hockenberry JM, et al. State parity laws and access to treatment for substance use disorder in the United States. *JAMA Psychiatry*. 2013; 70(12):1355–1362.

53. Connolly C. Solving the opioid crisis: A critical role for Medicaid. *Healthc Financ Manage*. 2018; 72(2):22–24.

14 | Systems Thinking and the Opioid Epidemic in Georgia

**BRIGITTE MANTEUFFEL, LEIGH ALDERMAN,
JANE BRANSCOMB, AND KAREN MINYARD**

S YSTEMS THINKING IN PUBLIC health is an analytic approach that takes a broad perspective to a health issue or challenge and considers the interrelated pieces and dependencies at play within the larger context of that issue.[1,2] Systems thinking describes the interconnected factors that combine to contribute to many of the complex public health challenges practitioners face in their day-to-day work. Key to systems thinking is the idea that to truly solve a public health problem one must understand and change the way the system works to create and sustain that problem. Changing just one part of a system can have incomplete (or even adverse) effects on overall outcomes.[3] For example, improving school lunch quality may not lead to overall obesity reduction in children because the system includes other intertwined social, environmental, economic, and other factors that influence the problem, such as food choices at home, healthy food availability at the local level, opportunities to exercise safely in neighborhoods, and many others. Similarly, a systems thinking approach to the opioid epidemic involves understanding that no single solution to the problem, such as expanding access to medication-assisted treatment (MAT), will end the epidemic in its entirety. Instead, a combination of factors that address various components and structures of the system is warranted to curb opioid misuse and addiction trends at the local, state, and national levels.

Systems thinking tools, such as maps and simulation models, have been used to study and address seemingly intractable public health challenges. Examples include mental health services delivery,[4] childhood obesity prevention,[5] tobacco control,[6] and regional health system transformation.[7] The current opioid epidemic in the United States is another example of a problem that can be understood and addressed using a systems thinking approach. The epidemic is the result of a complex system comprising varied and interrelated factors. To address the opioid crisis, and to end it, requires an understanding of the system that creates opioid misuse and addiction and the strategic, concerted actions across multiple sectors that can be leveraged to lessen and prevent it.

Some of the drivers of opioid misuse and addiction include factors such as the availability and affordability of prescribed and illicit opioids, an individual's physical and psychological pain, and access to behavioral health services. However, other diverse factors, such as prior adverse childhood events (ACEs), being incarcerated, housing, employment, and one's potential genetic susceptibility to addiction, are also connected to the crisis. Each of these drivers holds a part of the system's story and part of its solution. Understanding how these drivers interact forges a more complete picture of the problem, the populations affected, contributing factors, and potential intervention points. The Opioid Systems Map (Figure 14.1) is a useful tool for collective study and insight toward coordinated interventions to steer the system out of the current crisis. In this chapter we use the map to explain a systems thinking approach to addressing and ending the opioid crisis.

Application of Systems Thinking to the Opioid Crisis in Georgia

A major function of the Georgia Health Policy Center (the Center) is to equip policymakers with the data and tools needed to tackle complex health challenges. A particular focus is building policymakers' capacity to use systems thinking to address issues holistically.[8] System thinking makes the actors, institutions, and sectors at work on a problem more explicit, and systems tools illustrate the relationships among them. Systems tools can also describe the potential consequences, desired and undesired, of proposed policy and program interventions. A systems approach creates a more nuanced picture of an issue, helping planners and policymakers move from silos or stovepipes to focus instead on as complete a picture as possible and the combined "physics" of the system.

In 2016, Georgia's state legislators became increasingly alert to the opioid epidemic and asked to include the topic as part of the Center's Legislative Health Policy Certificate Program's Advanced Policy Institute. The Center developed the system dynamics map to show the many interrelated factors and relationships underlying the crisis. To inform the map, systems experts worked with subject matter experts, including individuals in recovery, to learn more about the opioid crisis and its many facets. Questions used to gather insight and spark additional discussion included identifying the overarching trends with regard to opioid use, misuse, and addiction; asking individuals what they see is being done to address the epidemic and what is and is not working; and

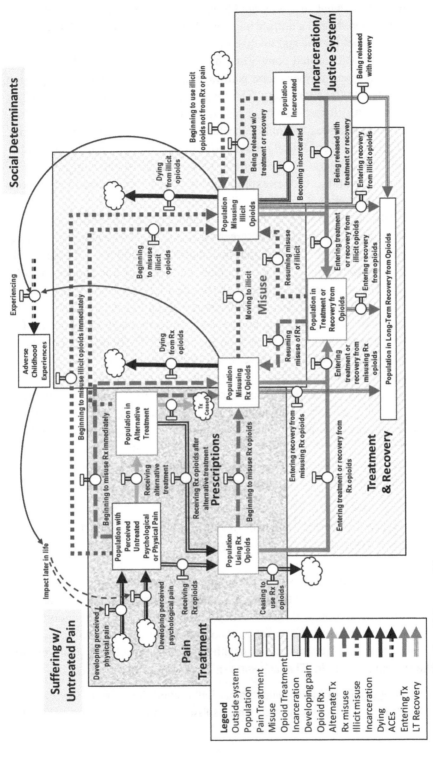

FIGURE 14.1. The Opioid Systems Map.

inquiring about what success would look like in 10 years. From this information the Center created a draft, which was then used to facilitate a larger group of experts to help refine and finalize it.

The process identified populations at risk for using opioids, those already using opioids, and former users; pathways into and out of those groups; and leverage points for intervening. The final map provides a means to visualize intervention points at different levels within the system, including both "upstream" opportunities for public health and prevention and "downstream" health care and other clinical interventions to provide treatment and/or immediate lifesaving outcomes. The map also identifies at least one reinforcing feedback loop warranting further exploration of evidence-informed interventions to break a generational cycle (described below).

In 2016, the Georgia Department of Public Health (GDPH) was awarded a three-year opioid cooperative agreement from the US Centers for Disease Control and Prevention (CDC) that included the development of a statewide opioid response plan. With input from key partners and stakeholders, GDPH developed a public health strategic map (Figure 14.2) consistent with guidance from the Association of State and Territorial Health Officials (ASTHO) for responding to prescription drug misuse, and similar to that of other states.[9] The initial GDPH strategic map defined the components of five priority areas: prevention education, data and surveillance, prescription drug monitoring program (PDMP), treatment and recovery, and control and enforcement (later revised to include a sixth area, maternal substance use). GDPH, encouraged by its funding partner to infuse a systems approach, engaged the Center to support development of the state's opioid response strategic plan. The Center incorporated systems thinking components into the state's first multi-sector strategic planning meeting design and presented the Opioid Systems Map at the meeting to inform participants' planning work.

Using the Systems Map to Better Describe Opioid Misuse, Treatment, and Recovery

The Opioid Systems Map shows groups that could be or are exposed to opioids, the relationships between these groups, and how people move from one group to another. In so doing, it makes visible the places where interventions such as certain policy decisions, practice changes, or changes in access to services, stigma, or social determinants of health can impact specific populations and the system as a whole. The map shows:

- Populations of individuals in a particular condition or state (*boxes*)
- Pathways (*arrows*) through which subsets of populations move from one condition or state to another

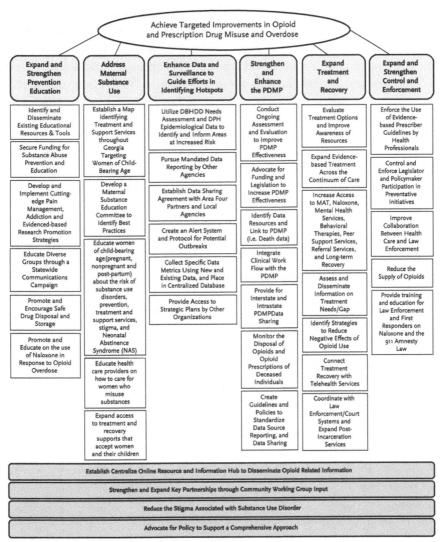

FIGURE 14.2. GDPH's Opioid and Prescription Drug Misuse and Overdose Strategic Map.

Source: Developed by Georgia Department of Public Health under the CDC Data Driven Prevention Initiative, cooperative agreement 5NU17CE924863. Reprinted by permission.

- Faucets (*circles with handles*) along each pathway indicate the process of transitioning from one group to another. These are points where interventions can be applied to speed or slow the transition.[1]

---

[1] The metaphor used to describe this in systems thinking is a bathtub, in which the water level is determined by the rate at which water flows into it through the faucet and out of it through the drain.

- Curved arrows show impacts of opioid misuse across generations.
- Clouds represent conditions that are outside the scope of the current map. Because in the real world everything is connected, system boundaries are necessarily artificial and arbitrary. For the purposes of the present map, stakeholders chose to focus attention on the parts of the system shown. As discussed below, plans are to build out more features in future iterations.

The map describes use and misuse of prescription (Rx) and nonprescription (illicit) opioids. The upper left area of the map, labeled "Suffering w/ Untreated Pain," describes pathways to accessing opioid prescriptions and alternative treatments to manage pain. Pain is defined as referring to both physical and psychological conditions that cause discomfort at a level that causes individuals to seek ways to control that discomfort (the "Population with Untreated Psychological or Physical Pain" box). There are two pathways that explain entry into this population: "Developing perceived physical pain" (arrow) and "Developing perceived psychological pain" (arrow). The clouds from which the arrows originate indicate whatever came before seeking treatment for that pain, which is outside the scope of this map. By including psychological and physical pain, the map illustrates that physical pain may have psychological components (as contributing factors or as the result of physical pain), that mental health conditions may present with pain symptoms, and that untreated mental distress/discomfort is correlated with substance misuse.

The left side of the map depicts the populations and pathways associated with pain treatment and prescriptions. The "Population with Perceived Untreated Psychological or Physical Pain" (box) may receive medical or psychological treatment for their pain (arrow: "Receiving Rx opioids") with prescription opioids ("Population Using Rx Opioids" box) or with alternative treatments (arrow: "Receiving alternative treatment"), such as other medications, physical therapy, massage, mental health services, or chiropractic care ("Population in Alternative Treatment" box). People who receive effective opioid treatment for pain may either exit or remain a member of the "Population Using Rx Opioids." Those whose pain resolves with opioid treatment would exit this box (arrow: "Ceasing to use Rx opioids"). Those who remain in this population with long-term opioid Rx could include people treated effectively for terminal cancer pain or sickle cell disease. Persons with terminal illnesses who die also exit this box (arrow: "Ceasing to use Rx opioids"). Persons whose pain is not resolved with prescription opioids could be prescribed alternative treatments and become a part of the "Population in Alternative Treatment" box.

Individuals in the "Population in Alternative Treatment" box may remain in one or more types of alternative treatment or complete treatment with resolution to their pain or distress (cloud: "Tx ceased"). However, they may be prescribed opioids if their pain is not managed effectively by alternative treatments ("Receiving Rx opioids after alternative treatment" arrow) and become part of the "Population Using Rx Opioids" box (with subsequent pathways the same as for others in that group). Those who remain in pain with alternative treatments may seek out unprescribed prescription or illicit opioids to manage their unresolved pain. They would then enter the "Population Misusing Rx Opioids" and/or the "Population Misusing Illicit Opioids" boxes.

The center section of the map, labeled "Misuse," includes the populations misusing opioids and the pathways that lead into these groups. People with untreated pain or distress ("Population with Perceived Untreated Psychological or Physical Pain" box) may self-medicate ("Beginning to misuse Rx immediately" arrow) by using prescription opioids without a prescription ("Population Misusing Rx Opioids" box; e.g., obtaining leftover pills from a medicine cabinet, family, friends, or the street) or by using heroin or illicit synthetic opioids ("Beginning to use illicit opioids immediately" arrow; "Population Misusing Illicit Opioids" box). Individuals who become dependent on and/or develop increased tolerance for their prescribed opioids may increase their dosage themselves, or seek out additional prescriptions ("Beginning to misuse Rx opioids" arrow; "Population Misusing Rx Opioids" box). Misusing prescription opioids, therefore, includes both misuse of opioids obtained with a prescription, and use of prescription opioids without a prescription. Misusing illicit opioids includes use of any nonprescription opioids, such as heroin or synthetic opioids.

The map recognizes that people without pain or a prescription can also become members of the "Population Misusing Illicit Opioids" box ("Beginning to misuse illicit opioids not from Rx or pain" arrow). For example, an individual may be encouraged to use an illicit opioid through peer pressure in school, insistence by a partner or family member, or one's own curiosity about the experience. Accidental exposure, such as to a synthetic opioid in a laboratory, in police work, as a medical examiner or medical worker, or when buying counterfeit prescription pills or other illicit drugs on the street that are made of or contaminated by synthetic opioids, while not mapped, could follow similar paths as the "Population Misusing Illicit Opioids" box (e.g., be at risk of death, develop opioid dependence, and/or need treatment for exposure to the substance). Although the risk is negligible for occupational exposure, protective measures, for example, are put in place to protect against this potential risk. Misuse of prescription opioids may lead to misuse of illicit opioids (arrow from "Population Misusing Rx Opioids" to "Population Misusing Illicit Opioids"), and the consequences of misuse of prescription and illicit opioids include death ("Dying from Rx opioids" or "Dying from illicit opioids" arrow).

The lower right corner of the map (Incarceration/Justice System) describes the relationship between opioid misuse and incarceration. The map includes a separate area for incarceration and engagement with the justice system by individuals misusing opioids to recognize and consider that relationship between justice and public health issues, and the impact of opioid misuse on the justice system. Opioid misuse may lead to incarceration ("Becoming incarcerated" arrow). Individuals misusing prescription opioids may also become involved with the justice system (not depicted on the map).

The lower third of the map depicts pathways to "Population in Treatment or Recovery from Opioids" and "Population in Long-Term Recovery from Opioids" boxes. Although recovery from opioids may involve long-term medication treatment and other supports, the map recognizes the population in long-term, stable recovery, with or without ongoing supports, to signify that this population stands outside of a relapsing cycle of opioid use, treatment, and recovery. Individuals in long-term recovery also may return to opioid use; however, this population, like any other population, could again begin opioid use through the entry points on the map, so separate arrows directly to misuse are not included.

Treatment and recovery may take several paths, which may include detoxification, medication, inpatient or outpatient treatment, self-help groups, recovery housing, or no formal treatment or supports of any kind. Populations that may enter treatment and/or recovery include those using prescription opioids, those misusing prescription opioids, or those misusing illicit opioids ("Entering treatment or recovery from Rx opioids," "Entering treatment or recovery from misusing Rx opioids," and "Entering treatment or recovery from illicit opioids" arrows) and those incarcerated with opioid use disorders ("Being released with treatment or recovery" arrow). Individuals in the "Populations Using Rx Opioids" box may develop opioid dependence and may need to be tapered from their prescriptions, including using alternative medications to manage their withdrawal. Individuals may become vulnerable to opioid misuse if this transition is not well managed ("Entering treatment or recovery from Rx opioids" arrow). The map also recognizes direct paths to long-term recovery from misuse ("Entering recovery from misusing Rx opioids" and "Entering recovery from illicit opioids" arrows) and long-term recovery achieved while incarcerated ("Being released with recovery" arrow). The arrow ("Entering recovery from opioids") from the "Population in Treatment or Recovery from Opioids" box to the "Population in Long-Term Recovery from Opioids" box shows the path to long-term recovery through treatment.

Populations who misuse opioids and are incarcerated ("Population Incarcerated" box) experience detoxification and withdrawal symptoms while incarcerated, often without treatment. On release, individuals may still be experiencing withdrawal symptoms, may have no access to treatment, may be entering recovery, or may be enrolled to receive or continue treatment services that started in the correctional facility. From the "Population in Treatment or Recovery from Opioids" box, individuals may return to misuse of prescription or illicit opioids, placing them at risk of death or incarceration, and potentially a repeating cycle of misuse and attempts at treatment and recovery.

The curved arrows on the map describe pathways for the impact of opioid misuse on secondary populations: those not using opioids themselves but impacted by the use of others. The curved arrows point to the role of opioid misuse by adults on ACEs.[10] Substance misuse by caregivers is an ACE itself but it also adds to the risk of other ACEs, including physical abuse, neglect, domestic violence, poverty, divorce, and death of a caregiver. ACEs are highly correlated with both chronic illnesses and mental health conditions, including future substance misuse, later in life.[11] As the curved arrows show at the top of the map, ACEs impact children later in life, increasing their risk of physical and mental health conditions involving pain and distress, and continuing the cycle of substance use and misuse across generations.

Using the Map to Leverage Change

How does the Opioid Systems Map help identify solutions to end the opioid crisis? In the opioid crisis, there are both immediate and long-term interventions that impact death from opioid overdose. Interventions to reduce mortality include use of naloxone for overdose reversal. Naloxone availability and use by a broad spectrum of people, including first responders, law enforcement, family members, social workers, and teachers, is a critical downstream intervention, affecting outcomes for specific populations. To reduce repeated overdose, however, additional interventions are needed so that people who experience overdose reversal do not return to the population misusing opioids. Other immediate means to reduce death include harm reduction, warm handoffs to promote access to recovery, syringe services programs, and medically supervised injection facilities that include recovery resources. The map helps illustrate these connections and needs to allow for more comprehensive solutions to the issue, for example addiction prevention interventions in addition to providing naloxone.

Upstream interventions can impact the initiation of opioid use. At the level of pain treatment, this includes changes in opioid prescribing practices. Interventions that affect this level of the system include national opioid prescribing guidelines; state PDMPs; physician and patient education; screening for substance use disorders with Screening, Brief Intervention, and Referral to Treatment (SBIRT); and the availability of and access to effective alternative treatments for pain. Access to alternative treatments may be impacted by costs, payment options, waiting lists, travel barriers, conflicts with work schedules, insurance coverage, and more. For opioids that have been prescribed but not used, reducing the amount available and where they are available (home, school, and community) reduces potential diversion and misuse. Interventions such as drug disposal locations, drug take-back programs, and medication lock boxes impact the movement of individuals into a population of misuse by changing the availability of opioids. They affect the "flow" from one group to another within the broad system.

The treatment and recovery paths on the map demonstrate the risks for return to misuse. Beginning with prescription use, changes in prescribing practices (e.g., fewer pills and shorter course of medication) reduce the need for detoxification from opioid prescriptions. Potential issues encountered in reducing opioid prescription use include provider education on detoxification protocols, patient education, and access to detoxification or opioid replacement medication. For misuse of prescription or illicit opioids, availability of trained substance use providers, access to treatment services, opioid replacement medication, managing transitions from detoxification to treatment, continuing care and support, peer support, family education and engagement (e.g., Community Reinforcement and Family Training [CRAFT], family support groups), help or warm lines, and stigma all impact initiation of treatment and recovery.

Upstream solutions address the desirability of and need for opioids. These include education about opioids to inform decisions about use. Prevention education should focus not only on children and youth but should also include those making decisions about use or continued use. These populations need education about the risks of both prescription and illicit opioids. Prevention also involves addressing conditions that may be precursors to opioid use to alleviate pain or distress. This is represented by ACEs and social determinants on the map.

Summary

There is a range of systems thinking tools and uses, including stimulating conversation and contemplation by asking carefully framed questions, using behavior-over-time graphs to look together at past trends and future desires, causal-loop diagrams, stock-and-flow maps, and computerized models. Choosing the right tool to support understanding and decision making requires a careful assessment of the users and a balance of available time and resources. The urgency and complexity of the opioid epidemic influenced the Center's use of a stock-and-flow diagram. This tool is robust enough to allow a group of stakeholders to see the system together, understand better each other's mental models, and identify priority places to intervene in the system. This type of diagram is a tool that can be developed quickly through a series of expert interviews and an expert panel work session.

While the Opioid Systems Map was developed with a sense of urgency for a specific legislative audience, it has proven to be a just-in-time tool in many other settings. Policymakers, public health officials, and project officers and funders used it to make decisions about immediate investments to address the opioid crisis with enhanced understanding of the system that influences opioid use and where those investments could be leveraged. In a few short months, legislators better understood the system, project officers and funders generated ideas about how to support grantees, and policymakers developed a state plan, all with a view of the broad and complex system that would need to be implemented by public health and other stakeholders.

An expert panel on the use of systems dynamics tools, convened by the CDC in 2014,[12] identified several guiding principles:

- The purpose for using the tool should be clearly identified and supported by the client.
- Tools should be as simple as possible, but no simpler.
- Tools should be tailored to the readiness and the level of engagement of participants, as well as the goals and the outcome of the process.
- The modeler or facilitator should have the adaptive and technical skills to use the tools.
- Tools should be used as a part of a larger change process.

The Opioid Systems Map aligns with each of these principles. The need for the map was clear. It is simple enough that a variety of audiences can use it, yet robust enough to capture many complexities of the system even while omitting some factors (represented by clouds). It can be tailored to different audiences by initially describing the key components of the system individually. Multiple team members involved in developing the map can lead groups through a process of understanding the opioid epidemic as a system; and those groups can then be part of a larger change process to address this social and public health challenge.

As the Center continues its work to address the opioid epidemic, additional systems tools are likely to be helpful. Expanding the boundaries of the system to include how money flows in the opioid epidemic and the role of industry, access and workforce supply issues, the production and distribution of licit and illicit substances, and health equity and other social determinants will be valuable to inform solutions. The opioid epidemic is not a simple problem with a ready-made solution. Rather, it is a complex system of intertwined components that need to be disentangled, understood, and addressed as part of a larger whole.

Acknowledgments

The authors acknowledge the contributions of Chris Soderquist, Pontifex Consulting, who supported facilitation and development of the initial 2016 Opioid Systems Map, and the Georgia Department of Public Health, which developed the strategic map in Figure 14.2.

References

1. Leischow SJ, Milstein B. Systems thinking and modeling for public health practice. *Am J Pub Health.* 2006; 96(3):403–405.
2. Leischow SJ, Best A, Trochim WM, et al. Systems thinking to improve the public's health. *Am J Prev Med.* 2008; 35(20):S196–S203.
3. Meadows DH. *Thinking in Systems: A Primer.* White River Junction, VT: Chelsea Green Publishing; 2008.
4. Zimmerman L, Lounsbury DW, Rosen CS, et al. Participatory system dynamics modeling: Increasing stakeholder engagement and precision to improve implementation planning in systems. *Adm Policy Ment Health.* 2016; 43(6):834–849.
5. Powell KE, Kibbe DL, Ferencik R, et al. Systems thinking and simulation modeling to inform childhood obesity policy and practice. *Public Health Rep.* 2017; 132(2 suppl):33S–38S.
6. US Department of Health and Human Services, US National Institutes of Health, National Cancer Institute. *Greater than the Sum: Systems Thinking in Tobacco Control. Tobacco Control Monograph No. 18.* April 2007. NIH Pub. No. 06-6085. Bethesda, MD.
7. Homer J, Milstein B, Hirsch GB, Fisher ES. Combined regional investments could substantially enhance health system performance and be financially affordable. *Health Aff.* 2016; 35(8):1435–1443.
8. Minyard KJ, Ferencik R, Phillips MA, Soderquist C. Using systems thinking in state health policymaking: An educational initiative. *Health Syst.* 2014; 3(2):117–123.
9. Association of State and Territorial Health Officials (ASTHO). ASTHO prescription drug strategic map. http://www.astho.org/Rx/Strategic-Map-2013-2015/Main. Accessed September 14, 2018.
10. Anda R, Butchart A, Felitti V, Brown D. Building a framework for global surveillance of the public health implications of adverse childhood experiences. *Am J Prev Med.* 2010; 39(1):93–98.
11. Anda R, Felitti V, Bremner J, et al. The enduring effects of abuse and related adverse experiences in childhood. *Eur Arch Psychiatry Clin Neurosci.* 2005; 256(3):174–186.
12. Guiding principles for use of systems thinking tools. Findings from Modeling Expert Panel Meeting: A collaborative think session, held at the US Centers for Disease Control and Prevention (CDC), Atlanta, GA, February 14–15, 2014. Georgia Health Policy Center (unpublished).

15 | A Comprehensive Approach to Addressing the Opioid Crisis

MICHAEL R. FRASER AND MARK LEVINE

A N EFFECTIVE PUBLIC HEALTH response to the opioid crisis includes understanding the many different contributors to the crisis and the need for a comprehensive versus piecemeal approach to addressing it. Several contributions in this volume highlight the need for a broad, multi-sector public health approach including Butler (see Chapter 3) who describes the need for a comprehensive set of primary, secondary, and tertiary addiction prevention strategies to be adopted within state and local jurisdictions.[1] Manteuffel and colleagues at the Georgia Health Policy Center (see Chapter 14) aptly present a systems thinking approach to understanding the epidemic that looks at the many inputs that span the "Opioid System" and contribute to the various outputs of the crisis. Several other public health researchers and practitioners have described comprehensive approaches to ending the crisis that emphasize public health's leadership role in convening multi-sector partners in health care, behavioral health, criminal justice, social service, housing, and many others to effectively treat and prevent opioid use disorder in communities.[2-7]

In 2018, we authored "Elements of a Comprehensive Public Health Response to the Opioid Crisis."[8] That article summarizes work that Levine shared with state and territorial public health, health care, and social service leaders and describes the multiple facets of Vermont's response to the opioid crisis from the vantage point of both an internal medicine physician and Vermont's Commissioner of Health. Levine's presentation, combined with research on other states' response activities gleaned from *Preventing Opioid Misuse in State and Territories: A Framework for Cross-Sector Leadership*[9] by the Association of State and Territorial Health Officials (ASTHO) and National Association of State Alcohol and Drug Abuse Directors, describes the need for a "silver buckshot"[8(p1)] approach to ending the opioid crisis. This "buckshot" approach moves beyond two or three key "silver bullet" tactics being implemented in states, including interventions such as expanding access to naloxone, expanding medication-assisted treatment (MAT) programs, and improving prescription drug monitoring programs (PDMPs) as the principal means to prevent overdose deaths and opioid misuse and addiction at the state and local levels.

We authored the "Elements" article because we believed there was a need to propel the governmental public health agency response well beyond its traditional role as data broker and convener of primarily health care partners toward a more contemporary and much-needed focus on the primary prevention of opioid misuse and addiction that forges new ground with social service agencies, employment and housing programs, law enforcement and corrections, addiction treatment providers and substance abuse prevention agencies, and many other sectors equally engaged in ending the opioid crisis. We wanted to clearly depict the broad scope of activities that needed to be accomplished within a state and across government agencies and provide a framework for organizing those activities around common themes. As we state in the "Elements" article, the outcomes of a comprehensive approach would minimally include:[8(p. 1)]

- Reducing the rate of death from unintentional overdose
- Alleviating the effect of the opioid crisis on children, families, and communities
- Reducing the supply of prescription opioids and related opportunities for diversion while developing integrated approaches to pain management
- Ensuring widespread and timely availability of MAT
- Expanding the use of evidence-based programs to prevent substance use disorder
- Offering opportunities for persons with opioid use disorder to sustain recovery and achieve their full potential.

Because so much of the work of substance misuse and addiction prevention at the state and territorial level is funded with federal dollars, the US Congress and the US Department of Health and Human Services (HHS) play incredibly important roles in guiding state and territorial activities to address substance misuse and addiction. Congressional interest in opioids has resulted in new appropriations to almost every part of HHS, including the Substance Abuse and Mental Health Services Administration (SAMHSA), the Centers for Medicare and Medicaid Services (CMS), the Centers for Disease Control and Prevention (CDC), the Health Resources and Services Administration (HRSA), the Agency for Healthcare Research and Quality (AHRQ), and others. In addition to funding, federal leadership in setting priority areas to address the crisis is equally important. As such, the recent secretaries of HHS in both the Obama and Trump administrations have developed lists of critical or priority strategies (Table 15.1) that have been and are helpful in guiding federal funding and capacity building work in the states.

These priorities place a great deal of emphasis on substance use and addiction treatment at the client level and support for investments in the reduction in the supply of opioids at the clinical/health care provider level. We posit that primary prevention, including addressing the root causes of addiction, should be expanded in future federal priority setting and should include increased investment in federal funding for states and territories to focus on the primary prevention of addiction. These activities would build on but move well beyond broad public awareness campaigns (e.g., HHS's *It Only Takes a Little to Lose a Lot* RxAwareness campaign)[10] and would include a clear push for federal, state, and local public health agencies to develop intentional and productive working relationships across sectors that have a role in ending the crisis and address the root causes of addiction at the individual and community levels.

TABLE 15.1. HHS Secretary/Presidential Administration Opioid Crisis Response Priorities, 2015 to Present

Secretary Burwell/ Obama (2015)[15]	1. Providing training and educational resources, including updated prescriber guidelines, to assist health professionals in making informed prescribing decisions. 2. Increasing use of naloxone, as well as continuing to support the development and distribution of the drug, to help reduce the number of deaths associated with prescription opioid and heroin overdose. 3. Expanding the use of MAT, which combines the use of medication with counseling and behavioral therapies to treat substance use disorders.
Secretary Tom Price/ Trump (4/2017)[16]	1. Improving access to treatment and recovery services 2. Promoting use of overdose-reversing drugs 3. Strengthening our understanding of the epidemic through better public health surveillance 4. Providing support for cutting-edge research on pain and addiction 5. Advancing better practices for pain management
Secretary Azar/ Trump (1/2019)[17]	1. Access: Better prevention, treatment, and recovery services 2. Data: Better data on the epidemic 3. Pain: Better pain management 4. Overdoses: Better targeting of naloxone 5. Research: Better research on pain and addiction

The approach we developed comprises six elements and over 60 different strategies (Table 15.2). While overwhelming to many who would prefer a shorter list of three or four items, our approach reflects the reality of the complexity of the crisis and the need for an "all-hands-on-deck" or "all-in" effort across state government. A similar call for comprehensive action has been echoed by President Trump's Commission on Combating Drug Addiction and the Opioid Crisis's 56 recommendations, most of which relate to health care and law enforcement efforts rather than the work of public health agencies.[7] Implementing each of the strategies listed in Table 15.2 involves a great deal of work. However, not implementing any one of the strategies also means that a state or territorial response could leave out entire populations, sectors, and communities for whom the crisis has devastating impacts. This is probably most true for current work in jurisdictions that do not address opioid misuse in correctional settings and approaches that focus only on the "supply side" of addiction (PDMP, prescription guidelines, limits on dispensing, alternative treatments for pain) and not the "demand side" of opioid use disorder and preventing substance use disorder in the first place.

This focus on the clinical combined with little attention to the primary prevention of addiction more broadly is what Fraser and Plescia[11] refer to as the opioid epidemic's "prevention problem": Failing to address the root causes of addiction means that the crisis will continue for the foreseeable future. A comprehensive approach must address the community-level factors that contribute to substance misuse, including what have been called "adverse community experiences"[12] and the impact of adverse events in early childhood (adverse childhood experiences [ACEs]) and the role they play in contributing to substance use and addiction (Figure 15.1).

Importantly, as a community of public health professionals and as a nation we must recognize that efforts that focus so specifically on the opioid epidemic but fail to consider substance misuse in general may be misguided. While opioid overdose deaths are clearly the most visible, tragic, and compelling aspect of the crisis, deaths from all substance misuse, including alcohol addiction, along with suicide (the other "diseases of despair"),[4] cannot be underemphasized. A focus on adverse family experiences, ACEs, and adverse community experiences and the epidemics of poor social connectivity, social isolation, and feeling undervalued by one's community on the part of youth would be a critical part of such a comprehensive approach. Solutions to these problems are all upstream and include a portfolio of proven preventive interventions including evidence-based nurse practitioner home visiting programs in early childhood, after-school curricula and activities for adolescents, and community activation along the precepts of youth and parental engagement in Iceland that involved giving youth a voice and parents stepping up to support positive youth development activities,[13] to name a few. Added to such family- and community-centered approaches must also be a

TABLE 15.2. A Comprehensive State and Territorial Approach: Elements with Key Strategies

Element 1: Leadership support

Key strategies include ensuring the following:

Engagement of gubernatorial and cross-cabinet/executive branch leadership

Support and engagement of state and territorial legislator and key legislative policy staff

Support and engagement of community leadership

Support and engagement of public and private health care delivery leadership

Support and engagement of education, corrections, housing, economic development, and social services leadership

Element 2: Partnership and collaboration

Key strategies in this element include:

Engaging cross-cabinet state and territorial agencies, departments, and commissions (e.g., attorneys general, health and human service agencies, justice and corrections, licensure boards)

Engaging substate districts, including local public health agencies

Engaging surrounding/neighbor states

Engaging public and private insurers, community health centers, urgent care centers, hospitals, integrated health care systems, and other health care delivery partners

Engaging federal funding sources and agencies

Supporting multistate collaboration and data sharing with local, state, and federal law enforcement agencies

Supporting public health collaboration with medical, veterinary, dental, and pharmacy associations and provider communities

Engaging social service agencies and community-serving private and public agencies and organizations

Engaging the media

Engaging the faith community

Engaging business leaders and chambers of commerce

Engaging community groups and coalitions

Element 3: Epidemiology and surveillance capacity

Key strategies in this element include:

Ensuring timely collection and analysis of data, including PDMP and clinical data, for public health action

Developing key indicator dashboards with real-time reporting to agency leadership and partners

Standardizing overdose reporting across the state, improving classification of opioid overdose deaths on death certificates, linking reporting systems to national efforts, and requiring overdose deaths to be reporting in existing notifiable disease systems

Maximizing the link to publicly available information and establish data sharing agreements between state agencies (e.g., public health, health care services, behavioral/mental health, education, employment, housing, and social services)

Examining variability in the incidence and prevalence of opioid use disorder by specific populations and/or in-state regions to customize response efforts

(continued)

TABLE 15.2. Continued

Element 4: Education and prevention capacity

Key prevention strategies implemented across the lifespan include the following:

Culturally appropriate education and awareness campaigns to raise awareness and address stigma associated with addiction

Evidence-based strategies to prevent ACEs by strengthening family environments for at-risk children, including evidence-based home visiting programs and positive youth development programs

School-based primary prevention programs, including peer education and leadership programs in schools and colleges

Implementation of the Drug-Free Communities program

Community mobilization, including developing and expanding community coalitions

Development and implementation of programs that address health-related social needs, including housing, education, employment support, food security

Key strategies to limit the supply of opioids (such as judicious prescribing and rational pain management) include the following:

Developing/implementing pain management core competency education for practicing clinicians and students, including dentists and other prescribers

Mandating the use of PDMPs as clinical and surveillance tools; permitting physician delegates to query PDMP systems; and providing clinicians with deidentified, specialty-specific data to help them self-monitor prescribing habits

Improving PDMP linkage to electronic health record systems/clinical providers

Permitting the sharing of PDMP data between health systems, including the US Department of Veterans Affairs and military facilities, and public health agencies

Permitting the sharing of PDMP data between states and territories

Incentivizing the use of evidence-based pharmacologic and nonpharmacologic alternatives to opioids for pain

Expanding policies that strengthen regulation of pain clinics

Developing policies that promote the implementation of prescribing guidelines and rules

Implementing/expanding policies that require electronic prescribing of opioids

Strengthening the authority of licensure boards/commissions to sanction overprescribing and/or failure to follow prescribing guidelines

Support for detailing/in-service trainings in clinical settings such as physician practices

Element 5: Treatment and recovery capacity

Key strategies to promote evidence-based efforts to diagnose and treat opioid use disorder (such as including treatment and recovery at the state and territorial level) include the following:

Treatment capacity

Supporting efforts to scale and spread of SBIRT in clinical settings, such as emergency departments and primary care practices, to identify risky substance use behavior

Increasing insurance coverage, including leveraging the Medicaid waiver process

Expanding the availability of MAT across diverse-clinical settings (addiction specialty centers, primary care, emergency departments, OB/GYN, and psychiatry) and making it widely available to all persons who require it, including justice-involved and incarcerated persons

TABLE 15.2. Continued

Developing an adequate workforce of Drug Enforcement Agency "x-waivered" physicians, nurse practitioners, and physician assistants (buprenorphine and naloxone prescribers) through strategies that incentivize provider participation in health home models (e.g., "spokes" in hub-and-spoke models)

Scaling and spreading health home models that integrate and coordinate services and support across primary care, acute care, behavioral health care, and long-term care or have added counseling services and treatment for polysubstance use and, where appropriate, co-located HIV and hepatitis screening, treatment, and recovery services

Supporting/expanding the use of peer recovery coaches in the emergency department and other hospital/large integrated delivery system settings

Establishing or expanding specialty treatment services for pregnant women and their infants

Establishing or expanding telehealth programs to increase access to care in rural/ underserved areas

Establishing or expanding diversion to treatment programs and use of drug courts by law enforcement agencies

Enforcing mental health parity laws

Expanding support for the treatment and recovery workforce

Assessing land use and other local or state ordinances that may impede construction of treatment and recovery facilities

Recovery Supports

Creating statewide networks of recovery centers with comprehensive and evidence-based services and supports

Promoting training and deployment of peer recovery coaches statewide

Promoting access to stable recovery housing

Promoting employment supports and opportunities for individuals in recovery

Element 6. Harm reduction and overdose prevention capacity

Key strategies to promote evidence-based harm reduction and overdose prevention activities include the following:

Expanding safe drug-disposal systems and sharps collection

Disseminating occupational health and safety standards for emergency/first responders

Disseminating safe storage guidelines for opioid medications to the public

Implementing evidence-based syringe services exchange programs that include referral to treatment and naloxone distribution

Implementing statewide naloxone "standing orders"

Expanding naloxone distribution programs, including training for first responders and the public on its use

Implementing the Good Samaritan law or similar protections for individuals who help those experiencing an overdose

Increasing screening and treatment for co-occurring depression, suicidal ideation, anxiety, and posttraumatic stress disorder to mitigate risk for opioid misuse

Implementing use of fentanyl test strips as a self-testing strategy to prevent overdose

Continuing to assess the efficacy and potential legal status of supervised injection facilities under specific circumstances as the evidence base emerges.

Source: Levine & Fraser, 2018[8]

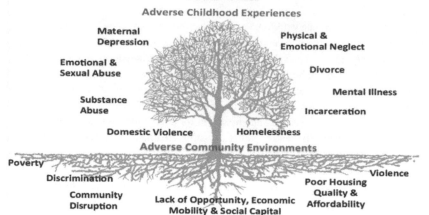

The Pair of ACEs

Adverse Childhood Experiences

Maternal
Depression

Physical &
Emotional Neglect

Emotional &
Sexual Abuse

Divorce

Mental Illness

Substance
Abuse

Incarceration

Domestic Violence   Homelessness

Adverse Community Environments

Poverty

Violence

Discrimination

Poor Housing
Quality &
Affordability

Community
Disruption

Lack of Opportunity, Economic
Mobility & Social Capital

Ellis, W., Dietz, W. (2017) A New Framework for Addressing Adverse Childhood and Community Experiences: The Building Community Resilience (BCR) Model. Academic Pediatrics. 17 (2017) pp. S86-S93. DOI information: 10.1016/j.acap.2016.12.011

FIGURE 15.1. The "Pair of Aces" Tree.

Source: Milken Institute School of Public Health, George Washington University School of Public Health. "The Pair of ACEs Tree." https://publichealth.gwu.edu/sites/default/files/downloads/Redstone-Center/Resource%20Description_Pair%20of%20ACEs%20Tree.pdf. Last accessed March 17, 2019.

focus on policy change that impacts and improves economic mobility, as lack thereof is a recurring theme in overdose deaths.

Our comprehensive approach starts with the six elements we describe but most likely should expand well beyond them. Only then will we have intervened at an appropriate number of inflection or tipping points in the crisis to turn overdose deaths and misuse trends downward. Failure to address these elements and implement the recommended strategies, and at a minimum to ensure that someone is taking the lead for each in every state and territory, will mean that we are sustaining a piecemeal response to a crisis that is impacting America in profound and unprecedented ways, including a loss of life in 2017 alone that exceeded the sum of all US causalities in the Vietnam and Iraq wars, and that is contributing to a three-year trend in declining life expectancy in the United States.[14] A commitment to this "buckshot" versus "bullet" approach can be sustained through the leadership of public health agencies but will only be successful when every entity with a role to play in the prevention of opioid use disorder, and substance misuse and addiction more broadly, fully contributes to a comprehensive and coordinated set of solutions.

References

1. Butler J. 2017 ASTHO President's Challenge: Public health approaches to prevention substance misuse and addiction. *J Pub Health Manag Prac.* 2017; 23(5):531–536.

2. Wickramatilake S, Mulvaney-Day B, Klimo MC, et al. How states are tacking the opioid crisis. *Public Health Rep.* 2017; 132(2):171–179.
3. Dasgupta N, Beletsky L, Ciccarone D. Opioid crisis: No easy fix to its social and economic determinants. *Am J Pub Health.* 2018; 108(2):182–186.
4. Trust for America's Health and the Well-Being Trust. *Pain in the Nation: The Drug, Alcohol and Suicide Crises and the Need for a National Resilience Strategy.* paininthenation.org. Accessed January 31, 2019.
5. Saloner B, McGinty E, Beletsky L, et al. A public health strategy for the opioid crisis. *Public Health Rep.* 2018; 133(Supp 1):24S–34S.
6. Murphy K, Becker M, Locke J, et al. *Finding Solutions to the Prescription Opioid and Heroin Crisis: A Road Map for States.* Washington, DC: National Governors Association Center for Best Practices, 2016. https://classic.nga.org/files/live/sites/ NGA/files/pdf/2016/1607NGAOpioidRoadMap.pdf. Accessed January 31, 2019.
7. White House, Office of National Drug Control Policy. The President's Commission on Combating Drug Addiction and the Opioid Crisis. 2017. https://www.whitehouse. gov/sites/whitehouse.gov/files/images/Final_Report_Draft_11-15-2017.pdf. Accessed March 17, 2019.
8. Levine M, Fraser M. Elements of a comprehensive public health response to the opioid crisis. *Ann Internal Med.* 2018; 169(10):712–715.
9. Association of State and Territorial Health Officials (ASTHO) and National Association of State Alcohol and Drug Abuse Directors (NASADAD). Preventing Opioid Misuse in the States and Territories: A Public Health Framework for Cross-Sector Leadership. https://my.astho.org/opioids/home. Accessed January 31, 2019.
10. RxAwareness. US Department of Health and Human Services, Centers for Disease Control and Prevention. https://www.cdc.gov/rxawareness/index.html. Accessed January 31, 2019.
11. Fraser M, Plescia M. The opioid epidemic's prevention problem. *Am J Public Health.* 2019; 109(2):215–217.
12. Pinderhughes H, Davis R, Williams M. *Adverse Community Experiences and Resilience: A Framework for Addressing and Preventing Community Trauma.* Oakland, CA: Prevention Institute; 2015.
13. Young E. How Iceland got teens to say no to drugs. *The Atlantic,* January 19, 2017.
14. Murphy S, Xu J, Kochanek K, Arias E. Mortality in the United States, 2017. National Center for Health Statistics (NCHS) Data Brief, No. 328, November 2018. https:// www.cdc.gov/nchs/data/databriefs/db328-h.pdf. Accessed January 31, 2019.
15. HHS lays out multifaceted plan to combat opioids. *Am Fam Phys.* 2015; 91(9):598.
16. US Department of Health and Human Services. Secretary Price Announces HHS Strategy for Fighting Opioid Crisis. Speech delivered at the National Rx Drug Abuse and Heroin Summit, April 19, 2017, Atlanta, GA. https://www.hhs.gov/about/leadership/secretary/speeches/2017-speeches/secretary-price-announces-hhs-strategy-for-fighting-opioid-crisis/index.html. Accessed January 31, 2019.
17. US Department of Health and Human Services. HHS 5-point strategy to combat the opioids crisis. https://www.hhs.gov/about/leadership/secretary/priorities/index.html. Accessed January 31, 2019.

16 | Five Key Strategies for an "Upstream" Approach to Preventing Opioid Misuse and Addiction

JOHN AUERBACH AND BENJAMIN F. MILLER

The Allegory of the Stream

Many in the public health community are familiar with the story of people being caught in rough waters and being pushed downstream by a strong current who are then rescued by being pulled out one by one just before drowning. Rather than asking the question, "How can we save these people coming downstream from drowning?" one of the rescuers simply asks why no one was going upstream to see why people were falling into the water in the first place. This simple question, "Why are people falling into the stream?" involves thinking about primary prevention or moving "upstream." Upstream is now a word synonymous with public health and involves addressing the root causes of diseases (keep people out of the stream) before they ever progress (fall in) and have to be cured (rescued from drowning). The allegory of the stream perfectly applies to current efforts to combat the opioid misuse and addiction crisis in the Unites States, where we are spending billions on treatment and recovery programs but very little on primary prevention activities to prevent addiction in the first place. This is not to say that attention to the downstream problem of saving lives by preventing fatal and near-fatal overdoses from opioids and other substances is not necessary. Clearly there is an urgent and important need to treat individuals with substance use disorders and support their recovery. But there is a commensurate role for public health in preventing avoidable morbidity and mortality. Our current focus on overdose prevention sets policymakers and practitioners up to continue putting all available resources into rescuing people who have already fallen into the stream without a significant investment in preventing them from falling in. As such, in addition to the lifesaving work of overdose prevention, we need to expand the work to address the problem of why people are "falling into the stream" or misusing opioids in the first place. A component of this upstream work involves adequately addressing pain—whether this be emotional pain or physical pain, our country has failed at seeing the complex connecting between our emotional health and physical health. This means being more focused on community conditions—factors that influence our health and promote healing. The continuum of this work begins with things like unemployment and continues to efforts like appropriately prescribing opioid medications to reduce the overprescribing of opioids, both of which are major factors contributing to an increases in overdose deaths.[1] Similarly, efforts to expand access to the overdose-reversing medication naloxone has been helpful. But there is other work that must be done to reduce the likelihood of opioid misuse and addiction before a prescription is ever written or a drug is ever used, and that involves addressing the social, economic, and psychological factors that impact individuals and can either increase or decrease their vulnerability to misusing substances. By reducing these factors, and building the resiliency and strength of communities, public health practitioners can make valuable contributions to preventing substance misuse and addiction.

Trust for America's Health and Well Being Trust have focused on describing the work of "moving upstream" and the needed prevention efforts in the *Pain in the Nation* series and additional educational, policy, and advocacy work.[2,3] In this work, the organizations have grouped opioid and other drug-related deaths with alcohol overdoses and injury and death from suicide because many of the upstream risk factors (opioid misuse, alcohol misuse, and suicide) are very similar, if not the same. These three, sometimes referred to as "deaths of despair," are each due in part to the way the nation views and addresses trauma, social and emotional well-being, mental illness, and substance misuse.[3(pp5-7)] Their upstream causes have a great deal to do with broad social and economic factors such as racism and other forms of discrimination, poverty, and social isolation.[4,5]

To move upstream, a comprehensive approach to the opioid crisis is needed. This approach, the organizations' National Resilience Strategy (Text Box 16.1), addresses the causes of deaths of despair by ensuring that prevention efforts are aligned along a spectrum that begins with primary prevention of trauma in early childhood by supporting families and communities in need. The National Resilience Strategy emphasizes that increased resources and attention are needed to address the primary causes of opioid misuse, alcohol misuse, and suicide. Data reinforce this need. There is evidence that addiction and mental illness in adulthood are associated with adverse childhood experiences (ACEs), such as early exposure to violence or instability in the home. ACEs also have a cumulative effect: the more experiences of ACEs in childhood, the higher the risk. Two-thirds of Americans have had at least one ACE, 40% have had two or more and more than 20% have had three or more.[6-11] Without better strategies that focus on preventing ACEs and offering effective interventions for those who are dealing with their consequences, the increases we see in drug and alcohol misuse and suicide will continue to grow and worsen.

There is a broad range of evidence-based and promising practices and programs that is available to tackle the drug, alcohol, and suicide crises. The following list offers numerous examples of these as originally highlighted in the *Pain in the Nation* report by the Trust for America's Health.[2,17] They involve reducing unhealthy behaviors, improving mental health services, and prioritizing prevention. This list may seem overwhelming to under-resourced agencies that are attempting to begin this work. The strategies described in this chapter offer a focused list of five places to begin.

Summary of Policies and Programs to Reduce Substance Misuse and Improve Well-Being

A. *Reducing Drug and Alcohol Misuse and Suicide*

   1. **Opioid response:** Much of the response to date has been focused on reacting to the acute emergencies of overdoses, insufficient treatment availability and options, and limiting the supply of opioids available for misuse. Some key efforts include:
      • **Surveillance:** to be able to track problems, and inform and target response activities, including drug use patterns, such as identifying trends in prescription drug misuse, heroin, fentanyl, and carfentanil increases in communities, and related harms such as hepatitis C and HIV
      • **Evidence-based community prevention programs** to be scaled and expanded to benefit local areas throughout the country, supporting best-practice, multi-sector partnerships that leverage the leadership, expertise, and resources within a community to support a comprehensive strategy, and expert networks to provide advice and technical assistance so effective programs are implemented for maximum impact
      • **Improving pain treatment and management practices**, including responsible prescribing of prescription opioids
      • **Increased education and training for providers,** including guidance for improving pain management and treatment
      • **Responsible prescribing of prescription opioids and prescription drug monitoring programs (PDMPs),** including continued study and use of best practices for PDMPs, and ensuring they receive sufficient support to be fully operational in every state, with a focus on using data to help inform and improve pain treatment for patients and avoiding and treating addiction
      • **Public education, safe storage, disposal, and take-back programs** to inform patients about safe use and storage and risk of dependence,

and reduce the availability of unused medicines in the community, and support tamper-resistant formulations

• **Strengthen the "public benefit" considerations of approval practices by the US Food and Drug Administration (FDA)** and support tamper-resistant and nonaddictive formulations

• **Anti-drug trafficking and stopping the supply chain of heroin, fentanyl, and other illicit, synthetic opioids** efforts must be a top priority.

• **Reducing the harms caused by overdoses and misuse** and treating substance use disorders as public health issues first, and the need for community-based, stigma-free harm reduction services that provide people the support and help they need when and where they need them by:

• **Expanding naloxone availability and Good Samaritan laws** and other policies that make the rescue drug more widely available and able to be prescribed to individuals and families at risk and community institutions (e.g., workplaces, libraries, community centers, airports/train and metro stations, universities, schools) to be able to respond to overdoses and limit liability for helping. Ensuring accessibility and affordability of naloxone is also essential.

• **Sterile syringe access** to reduce the risk and spread of HIV, hepatitis G, and vein infections.

• **Diversion strategies** to provide support and treatment to individuals with substance use disorders that focus on treating addiction as a health and not a criminal issue.

• **Treatment as prevention:** expanding the availability and quality of substance misuse services available that meet recommended, modern standards of care.

2. **Preventing excessive drinking,** which can increase risk for developing alcohol use disorders, as well as injuries, suicide, and other forms of violence and a number of chronic diseases. Some top evidence-based policies for reducing excessive drinking include:

• **Pricing, access, and availability:** increases in prices, limiting hours, and limiting the density of outlets and restaurants/stores/bars selling alcohol

• **Reducing underage drinking** through minimum legal age compliance checks, zero tolerance for underage drunk driving laws, and penalties for hosting parties with underage drinking

• **Reducing drinking and driving,** which reduces risks for crashes while also identifying individuals who may need treatment or support, through drunk driving limit laws, mandatory ignition interlocks even for first-time offenses, increases in sobriety checkpoints and increasing penalties for driving under the influence

3. **Preventing suicides** by supporting a cultural shift that focuses on providing help to individuals, especially when experiencing trauma, distress, or severe circumstances. Preventing excessive drinking, alcohol

use disorders, and opioid misuse is also an important strategy for reducing the number of suicides. In addition, leading strategies include:

- **The National Violent Death Report System** should be expanded to every state to allow for better tracking of suicide patterns and risks to develop stronger, targeted prevention strategies.
- **Statewide suicide prevention plans** that focus on building effective support systems within key institutions; training "gatekeepers" or people in positions that have significant contact with tweens, teens, and adults (e.g., educators, community and faith leaders, human resource and social service providers) to help identify those at risk; and crisis services for those in need. Special focus should be dedicated to school-based efforts and support for veterans, Native American/Alaska Natives, LGBT populations, and other higher-risk communities.
- **Suicide risk identification training for medical professionals and improving access to mental health services**
- **Limiting access to "hotspots" and lethal means for suicide.** Most suicides are carried out within a short time of having suicidal thoughts, and the risk goes down if means are not available. Thus, preventive strategies include promoting safety within communities (e.g., bridges, building access) and firearm safety policies, especially for those at risk, including safe storage, child access prevention, gun violence protective orders, and background reporting/checks for mental illness and other risks.

B.   *Improving Behavioral Health Services to Address Whole Health*

- **Expanding and modernizing behavioral health services:** With only around one in 10 people receiving the recommended treatment for mental health and substance use disorders, there is an urgent need to expand the availability of behavioral health services. The gaps are particularly acute in rural and lower-income areas. In addition, there is a need to expand the use of modern best practices for treatment in line with the research about what is most effective (including being able to provide different forms of treatment, durations, and scopes that match the needs and conditions of individual patients). Parity laws must be implemented and enforced.
- **Bolstering the behavioral workforce and expanding access to services in underserved communities:** Expanding the availability of coverage requires also increasing the behavioral health workforce, including with incentivized workforce development initiatives and expanded training and use of community health workers and peer counselor support, and models such as telehealth in many communities and other service delivery models.
- **Medication-assisted treatment (MAT)** should be available for patients as recommended or appropriate, which will require expanding the workforce trained and credentialed to support its delivery.

- **Maximize Medicare and Medicaid** to follow and support state use of best practices to treat opioid use disorder and to broadly modernize the delivery and coverage of behavioral health services. This should include continuing to support and expand integrated/aligned health care and behavioral health service models, ensuring guidelines and coverage for the scope and duration and multiple forms of recommended standards of care that meet patient needs and conditions. In addition, continued support should he provided for innovative Medicaid models that support connecting health care and social services, including Accountable Health Communities, and expanding screenings for early childhood, teen, and family risks and connections to services and supports.
- **Align and integrate behavioral health with health care,** where the "whole health" of patients is addressed, including physical and mental health needs. This will require changes that help align systems, payments, and incentives for more coordinated and integrated care. Some models include expanding training for types of professionals, referral systems, and/or co-location of services. Systems should be trauma-informed to be accessible and supportive of patients, and patients should be able to be referred to appropriate services and supports no matter where they start in the system, so there is "no wrong door" for entry to support.
- **Focusing on early identification of issues and connections to care:** There also needs to be increased focus on identifying issues early and connecting individuals and families to the care and support they need. There are numerous models and tools for screening for trauma, adverse childhood and family experiences, risk for mental illness, risk for and misuse of drugs and alcohol, and risk of suicide.
- **Coordination across health care, behavioral health, and social services** is also important, since many factors influence health, including social services. Systems must support connections to services and case management to ensure people receive the support that is needed and available.

C. *Prioritize Prevention*

Supporting Healthier Communities and Raising a Mentally and Physically Healthier Generation of Kids, with a strategy of preventing problems before they start, involves supporting evidence-based policies and programs that reduce risks for substance misuse, suicide, and other harms and that promote protective factors such as safe, secure families, homes, and communities; life and coping skills; and social-emotional development, including:

- **Multi-sector collaborative partnerships** that provide support and leadership for comprehensive approaches to problems, like the opioid, alcohol, and suicide crises, which impact the whole community.

These partnerships provide the infrastructure to leverage the expertise. resources, leadership, and capabilities of a broad range of partners (health care and hospitals, universities and schools, businesses, community and faith groups, and other organizations) across a community for stronger collective impact. These partnerships are key for being able to scale and sustain policies and programs to address the opioid, alcohol, and suicide epidemics and also to promote prevention-focused efforts on an ongoing basis.

- **Expert networks** to provide guidance on evidence-based approaches that best fit a local area's needs and technical assistance for effective implementation and evaluation of the effort
- **Early childhood strategies,** including high-quality home visiting programs, evidence-based parent education and support initiatives, high-quality child care and early childhood education, and services that support the transition from early childhood programs to elementary school
- **Modernizing the child welfare system** and need for multigenerational care, including meeting the increased needs related to the opioid epidemic, prioritizing services and support to parents and children to help keep families together and reduce the trauma of separation when possible and appropriate: supporting the ability of grandparents and other relatives to provide care for children when possible and appropriate: and comprehensive supports and case manager approaches for children in the foster care system
- **School-aged tween/teen strategies,** including prioritizing healthy positive school climates for all individuals in the school; investing in evidence-based social-emotional learning and life and coping skill programs; widespread use of modern evidence-based substance misuse prevention programs; anti-bullying programs; expanding availability for school counselors and mental health personnel and increasing school services and coordination across health, education, and social services; and school-based suicide prevention plans, including training for personnel
- **Family opportunity programs,** including income assistance programs, housing assistance, transportation, food assistance, and health care, that address core needs and promote stability
- **Economic opportunity initiatives** that promote job opportunities and training in targeted areas and improve infrastructure and community amenities and services.

The National Resilience Strategy specifies many different prevention-oriented policies to move upstream and prevent opioid misuse and addiction, along with alcohol misuse and suicide.[11] Of course it would be much easier if just one or two solutions were enough to end the crisis, but problems as complex as addiction and suicide have no easy fix. Under-resourced public health agencies and organizations should, however, consider focusing efforts on key strategies so as not to be overwhelmed by the enormity of programs and policies needed to build resilience in their communities. To assist public health practitioners in focusing their efforts, we suggest the following five major strategies:

1. Focus on children and their families.
2. Assist adults who may be at elevated risk for substance misuse.
3. Incorporate routine screening for risk factors into early childhood, school, and health care settings.
4. Support community health and social service providers that may receive referrals related to screening efforts.
5. Promote equity in broad terms and not simply in terms of health care access and health disparities.

Strategy #1: Focus on Children and Their Families

Children and adolescents who are exposed to traumatic situations or ACEs are especially vulnerable to mental health disorders. This vulnerability may be immediately apparent, or it may express itself years later. Public health practitioners should work to reduce these ACEs and/or help children and adolescents recover and heal from their impact. Such efforts may involve a range of activities, from expanding family violence prevention programs to attending to the needs of children in high-stress conditions such as home-less facilities or foster care, from supporting evidence-based curricula and social-emotional learning in schools to expanding access to home visiting, the Special Supplemental Nutrition Program for Women, Infants, and Children (WIC), and other services for low-income families (Text Box 16.2).

Public health professionals can play a key role in ensuring that the needs of children and adolescents are prioritized, particularly by targeting children who may be exposed to multiple ACEs or adolescents at highest risk for misuse. These children may well be members of the same families that public health departments are already working with because of other public health issues or health-related social needs. Action steps for public health include:

- Sharing relevant information, opportunities for skill building, and/or access to resources via existing public health services such as WIC or home visits to families
- Creating cross-agency child, adolescent, and family committees where data are shared, evidence-based and promising practices are reviewed, and action plans are developed, implemented, and evaluated for continuous improvement

- Dedicating existing staff time to partner closely with those in other sectors who work on access to such areas as early childhood education or adolescent skill-building and mentoring programs that create connections with caring adults.

Strategy #2: Assist Adults Who May Be at Elevated Risk for Substance Misuse

In addition to prioritizing efforts with children and their families, there are others for whom prevention is key: adults who experience trauma or despair. This was observed in the case of Scott County, Indiana, a rural community with an extraordinarily high number of cases of HIV in 2015, spread by widespread injection drug use and addiction. Public health professionals found that the underlying factors contributing to addiction in the county were unemployment, poverty, high dropout rates in schools, and overall hopelessness.[12]

In a 2018 article, the US Centers for Disease Control and Prevention (CDC) analyzed state-specific trends in suicide rates and assessed multiple factors contributing to suicide. While the majority of those who committed suicide had no known mental health conditions, they were likely to have experienced a recent crisis in a relationship, a difficult financial situation, or unemployment.[13] Additional research highlights the relationship between unemployment and drug overdose rates: Hollingsworth, Ruhm, and Simon[14] found that for every 1% increase in unemployment, there is a 3.6% increase in drug overdose deaths.

To address this strategy, public health officials should investigate what populations within their jurisdictions might be experiencing traumatic circumstances, such as veterans recently returned from war zones, individuals released from correctional facilities, individuals living in communities with elevated violent crime and a lack of economic opportunities, or those living in areas devastated by hurricanes or other large-scale disasters. Public health efforts to provide or promote routine screening for trauma and to offer specialized support and/or referrals for these populations can lessen the likelihood of substance misuse or harmful mental health conditions.

Strategy #3: Incorporate Routine Screening for Risk Factors into Early Childhood, School, and Health Care Settings

Public health professionals can collaborate with those in early childhood, school, and health care settings to identify and advocate for the inclusion of routine risk screening in these settings. Such screenings should identify those who already are misusing substances and those who are at high risk. For example, screening, brief interventions, and referral to treatment (SBIRT) interventions are routinely implemented in many emergency departments[15] and other clinical settings with support and assistance from the US Substance Abuse and Mental Health Services Administration (SAMHSA) and increasingly in school settings as recommended by the President's Commission on Combating Drug Addiction and the Opioid Crisis.[16] It is important to note that while screening will help detect more cases, each community must be prepared to connect the patient to treatment and recovery supports. Screening without a referral system ready to receive individuals for treatment and recovery is a disservice to the individuals and the community.

Expanding screenings for other risk factors associated with addiction are also of value. For example, patients in the Kaiser Permanente system and the Center for Community Health Improvement at the Massachusetts General Hospital are routinely screened for exposure to violence and referred appropriately when it is identified that an individual has been exposed.[17,18] Given the relationship between interpersonal violence and substance use disorder, such screening may assist in preventing further harm. Another example of related screening is provided by the Accountable Health Communities initiative of the US Centers for Medicare and Medicaid Services, which is identifying and helping patients address such issues as food insecurity, unstable housing, trauma, and other adverse experiences that may elevate the risk of substance misuse and addiction.[19]

Schools are increasingly incorporating routine screening for the potential negative impacts of trauma and root causes of addiction. The school system in Bethlehem, Pennsylvania, for example, has adopted a "trauma-informed" approach where principals and other school personnel regularly investigate if there are social and economic risk factors that may be associated with the behavior of students. If identified, school leaders reach out and attempt to assist the families involved.[20]

Strategy #4: Support Community Health and Social Service Providers Who May Receive Referrals Related to Screening Efforts

Once needs are identified, there must be somewhere to refer individuals for assistance. The public health sector has a special role in demonstrating the needs and filling the gaps for such services in the health care, community, social services, and housing sectors. Through surveys, focus groups, and other means, public health departments can prioritize the identification and assessment of needs and issues in the statewide or community health needs assessment processes and actively promote them among the public and with policymakers.

Public health officials can take the lead in convening stakeholders from multiple sectors and collaborate to move upstream. At such meetings, data gathered by health care and social service providers regarding the needs of community members could be shared to inform collaborative action.[21] There also may be relevant information from community health needs assessments and state health improvement plans. Participants in such meetings could develop collaborative efforts to fill the gaps identified, which likely will include the need for increased access to mental health or substance misuse services. The needs identified may also be related to socioeconomic factors such as access to supportive housing, as they were in Hennepin County, Minnesota,[22] or to employment resources, as they were in Scott County, Indiana.[12] Community health centers provide comprehensive, quality health care services to the patients in their communities who lack resources and access to health care. Ensuring that certain critical services such as those that address mental health and substance use are integrated onsite in these community health centers is one evidence-based solution that could add substantial value in improving clinical outcomes and help achieve cost savings.

Strategy #5: Promote Equity in Broad Terms and Not Simply in Terms of Health Care Access and Health Disparities

While substance use disorder affects individuals and families in all social and economic classes, it does not do so evenly. Those who experience racism and other forms of discrimination, poverty, and economic trauma through the loss of a job or a home are at elevated risk. When drug addiction was perceived as a condition that was disproportionately affecting the black and Latino communities, there were far fewer governmental resources to treat it than when it was perceived as impacting whites. Furthermore, studies have shown that doctors are less likely to prescribe pain medications to blacks and Latinos.[23] While discriminatory and potentially harmful to minority patients in pain, this practice ironically may partially explain why rates of opioid misuse and addiction are higher for whites. Nonetheless, there are indications that the risks of addiction are growing rapidly among the black and Latino populations. In the most recent data available (2016), both groups saw strikingly large increases in drug deaths, with blacks experiencing an increase of 39% and Latinos experiencing an increase of 24%, while the increase for whites was 19%.[24]

Public health officials can adapt their efforts to incorporate activities to eliminate racism and discrimination of all kinds. In recent years there has been increased attention to the most effective approaches to eliminate racism, including the work of philanthropies such as the Robert Wood Johnson Foundation, the California Endowment, and the W.K. Kellogg Foundation. Available resources include a summary of the lessons learned from the California Endowment's Building Healthy Communities[25] and similar efforts around the country, and the Truth, Racial Healing and Transformation Initiative funded by the W.K. Kellogg Foundation and others.[26] Notable among the state and local public health departments that have promoted effective models is the Rhode Island Public Health Department's Health Equity Zones.[27] This effort, namely a place-based strategy to promote healthy and resilient communities, is receiving national attention as the Association of State and Territorial Health Officials (ASTHO) 2019 President's Challenge (Text Box 16.3).[28]

Summary

While these five strategies are critical for state and local action, they all contribute to a sixth vital strategy: advocating for specialized funding for the

TEXT BOX 16.3 2019 ASTHO PRESIDENT'S CHALLENGE: BUILDING HEALTHY AND RESILIENT COMMUNITIES

Goals

ASTHO, the National Association of County and City Health Officials (NACCHO), and the Surgeon General's office will help governmental health officials achieve the goals of the 2019 President's Challenge by:

1. Equipping health officials to mobilize community-led, place-based collectives focused on measurable outcomes and the US Surgeon General's motto "better health through better partnerships" to build stronger communities (Figure 16.1).
2. Connecting public health officials to business leaders and policymakers who want to invest in these community-led, place-based approaches and advance economic development by reaching across sectors.

Who

Governmental public health has an important role to play in changing our mindset about how we should work with communities and who our partners should be. Together, we can implement both goals of the ASTHO President's Challenge by:

1. Supporting community-led, place-based collectives that are outcome-driven.
2. Attracting diverse investments from business leaders and policymakers who can help communities transform conditions for better living long term.

Effective community-led, place-based collectives offer a ready-made investment opportunity for business leaders and policymakers, as diverse partners are calling for community development without community displacement.

What

Health equity moved from talk to action: Mobilizing strategic investments in community-led, place-based approaches that address the socioeconomic and environmental determinants of health. This community-driven initiative aims to transform systems and policies in ways that empower local communities and limit the harms of gentrification. It also structures efforts around measurable outcomes and cross-sector outreach, raising the voice of community collectives to drive positive, meaningful change over the long term. Example models include Rhode Island's Health Equity Zones, the Fort Worth, TX's *Blue Zones Project*, and *Live Well San Diego*, among others.

Why

Strengthen community-led, place-based approaches through strategic investments that mobilize collective action to build healthy, resilient communities with better conditions for success in place.

Promote positive social connectivity uniting community members together to build social capital as a public health strategy for help with combating issues like addiction, emotional suffering, and social isolation.

Improve community resilience so communities can resist, respond to, and recover from adversity and "bounce forward" to better socioeconomic and environmental conditions, like fewer adverse childhood events.

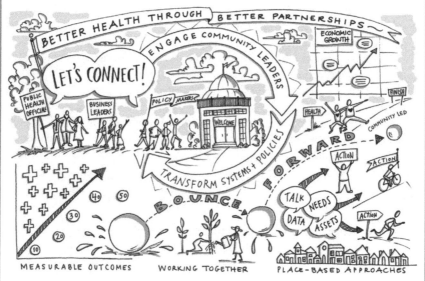

Figure 16.1 The ASTHO Challenge – Building Healthy and Resilient Communities

Source: ASTHO, 2019. Used with permission.

primary prevention of opioid use disorder, alcohol addiction, and suicide. Since the federal, state, or local funding to work upstream to address the opioid crisis is significantly lower than downstream investments, public health advocacy is needed. The case needs to be forcefully made that the opioid epidemic cannot be controlled or reversed without attention to primary prevention of addiction, and that the public health sector is uniquely qualified to promote prevention. Creating a policy agenda outlining the need for such an investment would be useful in aligning various public health entities and help collectively advocate for prevention.

One need only look at the response to HIV, another recent public health emergency, for a useful example of a comprehensive approach to an overwhelming health threat. To address the HIV/AIDS epidemic, the CDC provides state and local public health departments with sizable grants supporting primary prevention of HIV infection. The Health Resources and Services Administration (HRSA) funds the Ryan White CARE Act, which pays for a wide range of normally nonreimbursable services that are necessary for the health and well-being of those most affected by HIV, in part to make it less likely that the virus will spread. HIV/AIDS advocates fought against an inadequate federal response for years with a wide range of tactics to obtain adequate resources, but key to success was thinking creatively about the long-term needs for treatment and prevention programs.

Public health professionals can and should play a major role in preventing deaths from addiction by focusing upstream. By prioritizing children and adults at elevated risk, by giving children and families the support and skills they need to be resilient, by routinely screening and addressing the needs of those at risk, by assisting in the efforts to fill community-level service needs, and by promoting health equity, addiction can be prevented and lives can be saved. Such work can be accomplished in a limited way with existing resources. However, to mount an effective prevention campaign, increased resources for public health practitioners to support primary prevention are sorely needed.

References

1. US Centers for Disease Control and Prevention. Opioid prescribing. https://www.nber.org/aginghealth/2017no3/w23192.shtml. Accessed February 27, 2019.
2. Trust for America's Health. *Pain in the Nation Update (February 2018)*. Washington, DC.
3. Trust for America's Health. *Pain in the Nation (November 2017)*. Washington, DC.
4. Diez Roux AV. Despair as a cause of death: More complex than it first appears. *Am J Public Health*. 2017; 107(10):1566–1567.
5. Stein EM, Gennuso KP, Ugboaja DC, Remington PL. Epidemic of despair among white Americans: Trends in the leading causes of premature deaths, 1999–2015. *Am J Public Health*. 2017; 107(10):1541–1547.
6. Felitti VJ, Anada RF, Nordenberg D, et al. Relationship of childhood abuse and household dysfunction to many of the leading causes of death in adults: The Adverse Childhood Experiences (ACE) study. *Am J Prev Med*. 1998; 14(4):245–258.
7. US Centers for Disease Control and Prevention, National Center for Injury Prevention and Control, Division of Violence Prevention. https://www.cdc.gov/violenceprevention/childabuseandneglect/acestudy/index.html. Accessed February 27, 2019.

8. Middlebrooks JS, Audage NC. *The Effects of Childhood Stress on Health Across the Lifespan*. Atlanta, GA: US Centers for Disease Control and Prevention, National Center for Injury Prevention and Control; 2008.

9. US Centers for Disease Control and Prevention. Adverse childhood experiences: Looking at how ACEs affect our lives & society. https://vetoviolence.cdc.gov/apps/phl/resource_center_infographic.html. Accessed February 27, 2019.

10. Gilbert LK, Breiding MJ, Merrick MT, et al. Childhood adversity and adult chronic disease: An update from ten states and the District of Columbia, 2010. *Am J Prev Med*. 2015; 48(3):345–349.

11. U.S. Substance Abuse and Mental Health Services Administration. Adverse childhood experiences. https://www.samhsa.gov/capt/practicing-effective-prevention/prevention-behavioral-health/adverse-childhood-experiences. Accessed February 19, 2019.

12. Bruce G. Largest HIV outbreak in Indiana history: A toxic mix of drug addiction, poverty, hopelessness. *Times of Northwest Indiana*, April 18, 2015.

13. Stone DM, Simon TR, Fowler KA, et al. Vital signs: Trends in state suicide rates— United States, 1999–2016 and contributing to suicide—27 states, 2015. *MMWR*. 2018; 67(22):617–624.

14. Hollingsworth A, Ruhm CJ, Simon KI. *Macroeconomic conditions and opioid abuse, NBER Working Paper No. 23192*. 2017. https://ssrn.com/abstract=2924282. Accessed February 27, 2019.

15. Emergency Nurses Association Injury Prevention Institute/EN CARE. *Reducing Patient At-Risk Drinking: A SBIRT Implementation Toolkit for the Emergency Department Setting*. Des Plaines, IL: Emergency Nurses Association; 2008.

16. White House, Office of National Drug Control Policy. The President's Commission on Combating Drug Addiction and the Opioid Crisis. 2017. https://www.whitehouse.gov/sites/whitehouse.gov/files/images/Final_Report_Draft_11-15-2017.pdf. Accessed March 17, 2019.

17. Massachusetts General Hospital Center for Community Health Improvement. CCHI priority areas. https://www.massgeneral.org/cchi/focusareas/. Accessed February 19, 2019.

18. Permanente Medicine. Brigid McCaw, MD, discusses intimate partner violence screening for women. 2018. https://permanente.org/brigid-mccaw-md-discusses-intimate-partner-violence-screening-women/ Accessed February 19, 2019.

19. U.S. Centers for Medicare and Medicaid Services. Accountable Health Communities (AHC) model assistance and alignment tracks participant selection. https://www.cms.gov/Newsroom/MediaReleaseDatabase/Fact-sheets/2017-Fact-Sheet-items/2017-04-06.html. Accessed February 19, 2019.

20. Merlin M. United Way seeks grant to help city schools deal with trauma-exposed students. *The (Allentown, PA) Morning Call*, May 30, 2017.

21. Treatment Research Institute, Forum on Integration. Integrating appropriate services for substance use conditions in health care settings: An issue brief on lessons learned and challenges ahead. 2010. https://niatx.net/ari/uploadedfiles/presourceid770.pdf. Accessed February 27, 2019.

22. US Department of Health and Human Services, Office of the Assistant Secretary for Planning and Evaluation. Medicaid and permanent supportive housing for

chronically homeless individuals: Emerging practices from the field. 7.3. Hennepin Health. 2014. https://aspe.hhs.gov/report/medicaid-and-permanent-supportive-housing-chronically-homeless-individuals-emerging-practices-field/73-hennepin-health. Accessed February 27, 2019.

23. Hoffman KM, Trawalter S, Axt JR, Oliver MN. Racial bias in pain assessment. *Proc Natl Acad Sci USA*. 2016; 113(16):4296–4301.

24. US Centers for Disease Control and Prevention, National Center for Health Statistics. Multiple cause of death 1999–2016. https://wonder.cdc.gov/mcd.html. Accessed February 19, 2019.

25. Trust for America's Health. Advancing health equity: What we have learned from community-based health equity initiatives. https://www.tfah.org/wp-content/uploads/2018/02/advancing-health-equity-2018-convening-summary-1.pdf. Accessed February 27, 2019.

26. W.K. Kellogg Foundation. Jettisoning the belief in a hierarchy of human value. http://healourcommunities.org/. Accessed February 27, 2019.

27. Rhode Island Department of Health. Health equity zones (HEZ) initiative. http://www.health.ri.gov/programs/detail.php?pgm_id=1108. Accessed February 27, 2019.

28. Association of State and Territorial Health Officials (ASTHO). 2019 President's Challenge. http://www.astho.org/ASTHO-Presidents-Challenge/2019/. Accessed February 25, 2019.

17 | Addressing Community Trauma and Building Community Resilience to Prevent Opioid Misuse and Addiction

SHEILA SAVANNAH AND DANA FIELDS-JOHNSON,
WITH RUBEN CANTU, SANA CHEHIMI,
ALEXIS CAPTANIAN, AND KARMEN KURTZ

A S POLICYMAKERS AND THE public grapple with how to prevent opioid overdose deaths nationwide, several pioneering communities are addressing the underlying factors contributing to the opioid crisis. These communities are applying "upstream" prevention approaches rooted in effective public health practice to consider the root causes of the overdose epidemic and focus on primary prevention in addition to the more "downstream" approaches to treat addiction and prevent overdose deaths. A core element of this emerging approach is based on recognizing and addressing the role of widespread individual and community trauma and the need for solutions that build protective factors and agency within communities while supporting long-term treatment and recovery for those experiencing substance use disorders.

In this chapter, we describe how a community trauma–informed approach can be applied to address and mitigate the exposures, behaviors, and high levels of hopelessness that are fueling the opioid crisis. Further, we explore how primary prevention strategies can complement opioid treatment and long-term recovery interventions and address other conditions that co-occur in communities experiencing trauma. While our focus is on opioids, we frame the issue with a broader acknowledgment of the factors fueling a larger American epidemic of addiction. This includes recognizing that polydrug use and misuse are characteristic of emerging "diseases of despair" (suicide, drug addiction, and alcoholism) and comprehensive primary prevention offers benefits to address many chronic health conditions, including substance misuse.

Community Trauma

The current focus on substance use disorders is informed by its correlation to trauma, including adverse childhood experiences (ACEs) and has resulted in trauma-informed approaches to treatment. Similarly, there is also a growing recognition that the impact of persistent widespread trauma goes beyond the concentration of traumatized individuals within a geographic or population-based community, and manifests as community trauma. Community trauma is the result of chronic adversity in a community due to structural drivers and inequities that inflict significant harm, including displacement, economic instability and deprivation, disconnectedness, social isolation, and hopelessness. Community trauma has been directly linked to diseases of despair, including alcohol and substance abuse.[1] Overlapping factors that drive both community trauma and opioid misuse and addiction include intergenerational poverty, lack of jobs and economic opportunity such as loss of industry, substandard housing, poor-quality education, and limited or no access to key community services.

Contextual and experiential evidence gleaned from working directly with communities reveals that communities with high levels of community trauma share similar characteristics (Figure 17.1. These characteristics make it difficult for a community to develop and implement effective strategies to address opioid misuse and addiction. In the case of opioid misuse, addiction, and overdose, rural white communities with below-average income have been

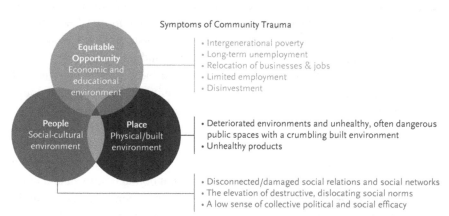

Symptoms of Community Trauma

Equitable Opportunity
Economic and educational environment

• Intergenerational poverty
• Long-term unemployment
• Relocation of businesses & jobs
• Limited employment
• Disinvestment

People
Social-cultural environment

Place
Physical/built environment

• Deteriorated environments and unhealthy, often dangerous public spaces with a crumbling built environment
• Unhealthy products

• Disconnected/damaged social relations and social networks
• The elevation of destructive, dislocating social norms
• A low sense of collective political and social efficacy

FIGURE 17.1. Symptoms of community trauma. The Prevention Institute's Adverse Community Experiences and Resilience framework (ACER) puts forth a set of symptoms of trauma at the community level. These symptoms, organized by the Prevention Institute's THRIVE framework for community environments, are present in the sociocultural environment (people), the physical/built environment (place), and the economic environment (equitable opportunity).
Source: Pinderhughes, Davis, & Williams.[3]

disproportionately impacted but there is increasing evidence that the epidemic is also spreading in urban communities of color, particularly related to the rising rates of fentanyl-related overdose deaths.[2] While these communities differ demographically, they are similarly impacted by community trauma exacerbated by structural factors such as eroding employment options, faltering schools, transportation infrastructures that reinforce social isolation, and segregation from opportunity and social mobility.

Communities facing high levels of community trauma may also exhibit lower levels of social and political efficacy, or the ability to come together to make positive changes and develop solutions for the community. A community that experiences trauma without opportunities for healing from it may not have the full capacity and efficacy to organize effectively around solutions to address threats to community health and well-being, including substance misuse and addiction.[3] This means that addressing the underlying causes and structural drivers of opioid misuse and addiction should also include strategies that support thriving communities. Countering the epidemic requires a focus on addressing and preventing community trauma so that communities themselves have the agency to identify and achieve their own solutions to the problem.

Addressing community trauma builds community resilience, which in turn strengthens a community's ability to recover from pervasive trauma and face future adversity (e.g., loss of a major industry or employer in an area, community violence, or a catastrophic weather event). By addressing community trauma and building resiliency, a community can withstand significant stressors. This interplay between community strengths and the experiences of individuals in that community is critical to understand in relation to the opioid epidemic. Individuals who have experienced personal trauma are at greater risk for drug use and addiction,[4] and community trauma exacerbates personal trauma, in part because it diminishes factors that are protective, such as social networks and supports.

Primary, Secondary, and Tertiary Prevention

As shown in Figure 17.2, there are several opportunities for prevention of substance misuse and addiction, ranging from preventing use at the earliest stages

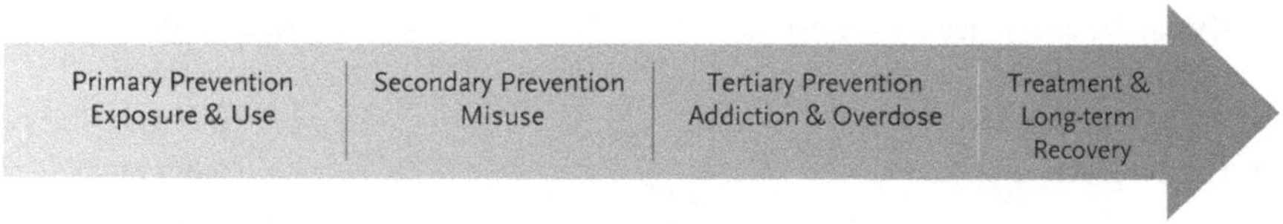

| Primary Prevention Exposure & Use | Secondary Prevention Misuse | Tertiary Prevention Addiction & Overdose | Treatment & Long-term Recovery |

FIGURE 17.2. Continuum of substance misuse and addiction prevention.
Source: Prevention Institute.

of exposure by addressing norms of medicating pain, to preventing progression to misuse and addiction, to preventing overdose deaths and treating addiction. Table 17.1 identifies the opportunities or strategies for prevention at three different levels: primary, secondary, and tertiary, much like the Association of State and Territorial Health Officials (ASTHO) 2017 and 2018 President's Challenge developed by Butler.[5] Exploring approaches along the prevention continuum helps us answer the question, "What are we preventing?" and allows us to focus on strategies that have a specific focus on contributing community factors at each level.

TABLE 17.1. Prevention Strategies and Solutions Across the Substance Use Trajectory

Prevention Strategies	Long-Term Recovery Strategies for post-treatment success:
Primary Prevention Strategies *(prevent exposure and use)* • Zoning regulations and other policies to prevent location and concentration of substance-oriented predatory businesses • Social, cultural, and peer networks and activities to increase social connection • Workplace, faith-based, school-time and out-of-school–time campaigns for stigma reduction and awareness • Healthy prosocial alternatives, including arts, culture, and recreational options for youth and families; community revitalization of parks and open spaces • Prescription drug take-back programs • Community and economic development that includes quality housing and access to transportation and ensures basic needs; workforce development, job training and placement	• Recovery-oriented systems of care (ROSCs): multi-sector groups focused on ensuring long-term recovery success • Housing and recovery support • Access to healthy and affordable foods • Transportation to reduce isolation • Peer support and networks • Trauma-informed employment opportunities • Resilience with a focus on the family unit, including family reunification • Awareness campaigns and outreach to business community and employers
Secondary Prevention Strategies *(prevent misuse and addiction)* • Improving access to treatment and clinical supports, including physical and behavioral health integration • Awareness and anti-stigma campaigns for high-risk individuals and their families • Law enforcement diversion programs and drug courts	
Tertiary Prevention Strategies *(overdose prevention)* • Rapid response teams • Naloxone distribution • Diversion programs • Bystander assistance during overdose (Good Samaritan laws) • Street outreach and education • Harm reduction strategies	

Source: Prevention Institute.

Primary prevention strategies and solutions are those that address population-level changes intended to reduce exposure and use and prevent addiction in the first place. Attention and focus on primary prevention is critical to reversing the epidemic and offers promise in understanding the overlap between solutions and strategies that prevent opioid misuse and addiction before onset and those that support long-term recovery success further along the addiction trajectory. For example, preventing exposure and use of highly addictive substances would include concentrated focus on preventing:

- Social and/or physical isolation that leads to suppressing pain, depression, and anxiety
- Unhealthy norms and lack of awareness or misinformation about addiction and addictive substances, including prescribing practices related to opioids and pain medications
- Workplace use and dependence on opioids and other substances
- High geographic concentration of unhealthy retail establishments, including pain clinics, alcohol outlets, and marijuana dispensaries
- Community deterioration, blight, economic despair, and hopelessness.

Similarly, further along the continuum, secondary prevention is an opportunity for concentrated focus on preventing or treating escalating use and misuse of substances. This point on the continuum is where intentional misuse is present, but also unintentional misuse that often results from the progressive use of pain medications requiring increased dosages over time to achieve pain relief. Its strategies are often effective once risk has advanced to use, or when an individual is "in the thick" of progressive use, with concentration on prevention of:

- Onset and advancement of complex health conditions, including undiagnosed or undertreated health and mental health conditions
- Job loss/disruption
- Criminal behaviors brought on by addiction
- Transition from prescription drugs to illegal substances and/or shared use of prescriptions and "doctor shopping"
- Barriers to accessing treatment, care, and other supports.

While a focus on tertiary prevention is often considered downstream or "after the onset of addiction," important steps can be taken to prevent exacerbation of severe impacts of substance abuse and addiction, with concentration on prevention of:

- Opioid overdoses and deaths
- Repeat emergency response and emergency room use
- Family disruption/involvement with the child welfare system and further multigenerational trauma related to substance abuse and addiction.

Current attention on medication-assisted treatment (MAT) and overdose reversal should be accompanied by an equally resourced focus on changing community environments to support long-term recovery and well-being for persons in recovery. There is a striking synergy between supports in the community environment necessary for successful long-term recovery and strategies to ensure healthy and supportive environments that benefit entire communities and prevent misuse and addiction in the first place. In particular, successful rehabilitation necessitates improving community determinants that (1) prevent relapse and/or migration to other addictive substances, (2) activate and develop untapped skills and potential for people in recovery that could support building resilience in communities, and (3) address stigma for people and families experiencing substance use disorders. Community-level strategies and solutions that may prevent onset of misuse such as quality housing and education; access to transportation; opportunities for job training and placement; meaningful employment that allows families to meet their basic needs; and social, arts, and cultural activities that promote social connection, belonging, and a sense of purpose are also critical to long-term recovery success for people already experiencing addiction.

Community Prevention Strategies and Approaches for Ending the Opioid Crisis

Stemming the tide of the opioid epidemic and preventing misuse and addiction in the first place calls for local, state, and federal strategies that advance community healing and supportive communities that promote hope and opportunity. This approach includes broadening efforts in four ways:

1. Expanding language and understanding of the crisis from addressing opioid deaths and treating addiction toward emphasizing a focus on well-being and resilience
2. Recalibrating approaches to improve community environments
3. Replacing a one-approach-for-all model with community-driven, locally tailored approaches
4. Realigning and expanding strategies that emphasize prevention and resilience as a complement to treatment and services (see the case studies in Text Boxes 17.1 and 17.2).

Expanding Our Understanding of the Crisis

We must broaden our thinking and take a wider approach to the opioid crisis that incorporates solutions beyond overdose prevention and moves upstream toward promoting well-being and resilience. A critical element in reframing efforts is acknowledging community trauma and putting into place solutions

TEXT BOX 17.1 PROMOTING COMMUNITY-LEVEL SOLUTIONS IN OHIO

The Ohio Department of Mental Health and Addiction Services is using THRIVE to assist 12 rural counties in building shared understanding of how the community environment drives opioid misuse and addiction and to support those communities in identifying solutions and strategies that change the community conditions contributing to opioid use disorder. Using THRIVE, the impacted counties have considered key community determinants of health and safety to better understand how the community environment has contributed to the opioid crisis and how it can be an actionable place for concrete solutions and strategies. THRIVE has been used to think about and advance actions to build multi-sector coalitions; to support the development of local theories of change that consider community trauma; to reduce stigma that arises when issues are seen solely as problems of individual behavior versus through a broader lens of contributing community factors; and to develop strategic plans that include upstream strategies and solutions that are linked to the underlying factors and root causes of opioid misuse and addiction. This has supported communities in prioritizing strategies that address community determinants of health such as social connection, housing, transportation, and parks and open space.

TEXT BOX 17.2 BUILDING RESILIENCE IN HUNTINGTON, WEST VIRGINIA

With double the national average of overdoses and an estimated 10% of the city's population addicted to opioids, Huntington is one of many communities that has gained national attention during the opioid crisis. The dislocation of the coal and manufacturing industries left Huntington's community members with long-term unemployment, damaged social cohesion, and deteriorated, unhealthy public spaces. City officials have focused on harm reduction and treatment efforts, including a Law Enforcement Assisted Diversion program to connect people with addiction who commit crimes to treatment and services and Quick Response Teams to assist overdose victims until they are able to access treatment. Looking to a more comprehensive approach to reverse the opioid epidemic, the city is planning and investing in strategies that account for the social, economic, and environmental factors underlying substance addiction. This includes job training and workforce development, redevelopment of vacant and dilapidated properties into spaces that drive economic growth, riverfront revitalization, enhancements in walkability, and improvements to public transit that connect people to employment and recreational opportunities.

Source: National League of Cities[7]

to encourage healing and build resilience. The strategies that have emerged to address and prevent community trauma span healing as an important starting point and include strategies among people, within communities (place and equitable opportunity), and across systems, in support of communities. Consistent across these strategies is the importance of recognizing the source of trauma (ask: "What happened to your community?"), understanding how that manifests in the community (ask: "What does it look like as symptoms or drivers?"), and then identifying actionable solutions to strengthen resilience throughout the community.

Recalibrating Approaches

Community environments (e.g., the social, physical, and economic conditions in a place or community) have tremendous influence on the stressors that people experience in their daily lives and on their risk and likelihood for opioid misuse and addiction. Our substance misuse and addiction prevention approach is based on addressing community determinants of health, which we define as the most prominent factors in communities that shape health, safety, and equity outcomes. These community determinants are relevant to all people and places, revealing how structural drivers like racism and concentrated poverty shape living conditions and experiences. Figure 17.3 provides an overview of the Prevention Institute's Tool for Health and Resilience in

Community Environments: This figure depicts THRIVE's 12 community factors that shape health, mental wellbeing, safety and equity. They are organized in three clusters representing the community environment.

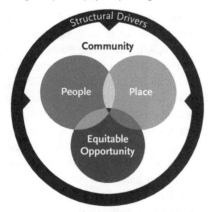

People
- Social networks & trust
- Participation & Willingness to act for the common good
- Norms & culture

Equitable Opportunity
- Education
- Living wages & local wealth

Place
- What's sold & how it's promoted
- Look, feel & safety
- Parks & open space
- Getting around
- Housing
- Air, water, soil
- Arts & cultural expression

FIGURE 17.3. Tool for Health and Resilience in Vulnerable Environments (THRIVE). THRIVE was developed in 2002 based on extensive research linking medical conditions to community resilience factors that can be strengthened for better health and safety outcomes. THRIVE affirms that the sociocultural, physical/built, and economic/educational environments at the community level (i.e., the community determinants of health) have a significant impact on health and safety outcomes and their inequitable or equitable distribution.
Source: Prevention Institute.[6]

Vulnerable Environments (THRIVE), which is a community resilience framework for understanding how structural drivers impact daily living conditions and, consequently, community outcomes for health, safety, and health equity, and how communities can implement strategies to mitigate against these structural drivers.

Replacing a One-Approach-for-All Model

There is no one-size-fits-all approach to solving the opioid epidemic. As such, there is a need for tailored solutions that consider the assets, resources, strengths, and culture of communities most impacted by opioid misuse and addiction. This is informed by community wisdom. Community wisdom is the combined knowledge, assets, intuition, and skills of community members and represents the contextual and experiential evidence that can drive community-level solutions for healing and resilience and that build the collective efficacy and agency of the community to be its own best change agent. People who have experienced addiction, those in recovery, and youth and families experiencing addiction must all be a part of defining solutions for healing, well-being, and resilience.

A community prevention approach to preventing opioid misuse and addiction ensures that all communities have a fair opportunity to achieve well-being and relies on data to identify populations and areas of geographic focus; inform strategies toward prevention, healing, and resilience; and allocate resources toward effective prevention. Community-driven and derived measures and indicators as well as existing data can be used to advance the community prevention approach to opioid misuse and abuse and build the evidence for what works and how it is making a difference in creating resilient communities.

Realigning and Expanding Strategies

Ultimately, communities must move upstream and shift from chasing the problem of opioid misuse and addiction to preventing it. Comprehensive, intensive efforts that foster solutions that address community-level determinants of health must accompany and align with strategies aimed at individual treatment and recovery. Efforts must include solutions that address housing needs, including supportive housing for individuals and families in recovery; high-quality, living-wage employment opportunities that can sustain a household; workforce development and training initiatives that build employment skills in youth and adults and provide a sense of dignity and hope; and business and economic development strategies and plans that revive the economic engines in struggling communities and regions.

Summary

Historically, substance abuse prevention work has focused on supply reduction and demand reduction with some levels of success. However, the opioid epidemic is different in many ways. It is informed by prior unsuccessful approaches that have criminalized addiction, it is more significantly linked to popularization and availability of opioids in areas with social and economic decline, and the epicenter first became apparent in a very different demographic from prior epidemics of heroin, methamphetamines, and crack cocaine. A public health approach to an epidemic of this magnitude urgently calls for us to consider all these factors in constructing a comprehensive primary prevention approach in the midst of the opioid crisis.

There is also a need to balance urgency and long-term prevention strategies to reverse the opioid epidemic in communities across the country. An effective community primary prevention and resilience approach to the epidemic considers and seeks to identify the drivers of community trauma and substance misuse and addiction and lifts up prevention strategies that promote healing and resilience and prevent misuse and addiction before they occur. The solutions critical to promote population-based well-being and resilience are also important to successful long-term treatment and recovery for people experiencing substance addiction. Thus, an expanded approach to addressing opioid misuse and addiction that includes upstream strategies to address the social, physical, and economic environment of communities can benefit everyone and is a necessary complement to solutions that prioritize treatment and recovery services along with overdose reversal. The community prevention approach is not put forth as an alternative to treatment and recovery services or approaches that address overdose prevention but instead is meant as a complement. We must do both in support of healing, resilience, equity, and safety for all.

References

1. Dasgupta N, Beletsky L, Ciccarone D. Opioid crisis: No easy fix to its social and economic determinants. *Am J Public Health.* 2018; 108(2):182–186.
2. US Centers for Disease Control and Prevention, CDC WONDER (CDC Wide-Ranging Online Data for Epidemiologic Research). https://wonder.cdc.gov. Accessed February 27, 2019.
3. Pinderhughes H, Davis R, Williams M. *Adverse Community Experiences and Resilience: A Framework for Addressing and Preventing Community Trauma.* Oakland, CA: Prevention Institute; 2016.
4. Sinha R. Chronic stress, drug use, and vulnerability to addiction. *Ann NY Acad Sci.* 2008; 1141:105–130.

5. Butler J. ASTHO President's Challenge: Public health approaches to substance misuse and addiction. *J Public Health Manag Pract.* 2017; 23(5):531–536.
6. Prevention Institute. *Tool for Health and Resilience in Vulnerable Environments (THRIVE).* Oakland, CA: Prevention Institute; 2004.
7. National League of Cities, Institute for Youth, Education, and Families. *Aligning City, County and State Resources to Address the Opioid Epidemic: Lessons Learned and Future Opportunities.* Washington, DC: National League of Cities; 2018.

18 | Early Childhood Trauma and Substance Misuse and Addiction

AN OPPORTUNITY FOR PREVENTION

MELISSA T. MERRICK, DEREK C. FORD, AND DEBRA E. HOURY

UBSTANCE USE DISORDERS (SUDS) can have devastating impacts on the health, well-being, and productivity of individuals, families, and communities across generations. Indeed, the impact of opioid misuse in the United States alone is staggering, with an estimated 399,230 deaths involving opioids from 1999 to 2017.[1] Data from the 2017 National Survey on Drug Use and Health indicate that an estimated 11.4 million people aged 12 years or older misused opioids in the past year, 769,000 of whom were adolescents aged 12 to 17 years.[2] Whereas a number of evidence-based intervention and prevention strategies have been developed to reduce and prevent substance use and misuse, many prevention efforts still lack the breadth and depth required by a comprehensive approach that spans systems, organizations, and environments, combining treatment and intervention with primary prevention efforts beginning in childhood so they can set the stage for future health and well-being. Adverse childhood experiences (ACEs), including exposure to child abuse and neglect and other violence, are well-documented risk factors for substance use, including opioid misuse and addiction, and are a viable target for preventing SUDs. This chapter provides an overview of the connections between childhood trauma and substance use and addiction, describes the impact of parental substance use on children's health and well-being, and explains the importance of comprehensive substance use prevention efforts that intentionally and thoughtfully integrate primary prevention and reduction of ACEs and other childhood trauma.

From Childhood Trauma to Substance Misuse and Addiction

Childhood experiences have a remarkable impact on health and future opportunity. They set the context for lifelong learning, behavior, and health, and provide the brain a (hopefully strong) foundation for future development. Childhood trauma, such as child abuse, neglect, and other violence and victimization, can impede the advancement of a strong foundation, affecting brain architecture and development, among other neurobiological and epigenetic impacts. While some degree of adversity and stress is a normal and predictable part of human development, exposure to frequent or prolonged adversity and trauma can result in *toxic stress*.[3] Toxic stress can disrupt optimal brain architecture and development and increase the risk for unhealthy coping behaviors such as substance misuse.[3] When toxic stress occurs continually, or is triggered by multiple sources, it can have a cumulative impact on an individual's physical and mental health for a lifetime. Indeed, the more experiences of childhood adversity, the greater the likelihood of developmental delays; engagement in risky health behaviors, including substance use; physical and mental health problems; cognitive impairment; limited life opportunities, such as high school noncompletion and unemployment; and early death.[3-9] These broad effects on health and well-being make childhood trauma an important public health issue and a vital focus for prevention efforts.

While the relationship between childhood trauma and substance use is robust, it is also complex. Not all children who experience childhood trauma will go on to use substances, and persons with no childhood trauma may still develop SUDs. However, trauma has been found to greatly increase the risk of later substance use.[10] Further, research suggests that individuals with histories of childhood trauma are more likely to report chronic pain symptoms that interfere with daily activities and are also more likely to be prescribed multiple prescription medications.[11] Similarly, according to the self-medication hypothesis of substance misuse, people who misuse substances may do so to numb the emotional pain caused by childhood trauma and toxic stress.[10] ACEs have been directly associated with substance misuse and SUDs in adulthood, including illicit drug use, with a dose–response relationship such that the more ACEs children experience, the more likely they are to have such substance use problems as adults.[4,12-14] In fact, general population surveys have estimated that 75% of individuals with SUDs have experienced trauma at some point in their lives; rates are even higher among populations seeking treatment for opioid addiction.[11]

The foundational body of research regarding ACEs has used a relatively narrow set of adversities to define ACEs, including exposure to childhood abuse (sexual, physical, and emotional), neglect (physical and emotional), and household challenges (i.e., parental incarceration, household mental illness, household substance use, parental divorce/separation, intimate partner violence) during the first 18 years of life.[4] Importantly, this definition of early adversity and childhood trauma does not represent the full scope of adversity and traumatic experiences that children are exposed to, including economic hardship, historical trauma (e.g., group trauma that extends across generations as a result of adversity, including experiences such as colonization, dislocation, and racism), bullying, peer victimization, spanking, and exposure to community violence.[15-17] Despite its frequently limited definition, ACEs provide important information about what was happening in children's lives during their childhood.

ACEs have been found to be associated with over 40 health and well-being outcomes. As early adversity increases, the risk for chronic diseases,[4,5] sexually transmitted diseases,[4] depression,[18] intimate partner violence,[19] suicide attempts,[20] smoking,[4,21] alcohol abuse,[22] sexual risk-taking,[23] and youth violence [24] also increases. Compared to someone with no ACEs, someone with six or more ACEs has nearly three times the odds of being a smoker as an adult. Similarly, someone with four or more ACEs has five times the odds of becoming addicted to alcohol and is 60% more likely to become obese. Individuals with four or more ACEs have approximately 10 times the odds of injecting drugs later in life compared to those who have had no ACEs.[4] Exposure to ACEs can also limit life opportunities, including educational attainment and employment,[6] which have far-reaching impacts beyond a single time period, person, or generation. These wide-ranging health and social consequences of ACEs underscore the importance of preventing ACEs, as early adversity and childhood trauma can set the trajectory for exposure to additional risk factors for substance use and misuse (e.g., peer victimization, sexual violence, and job and relationship problems), which can compound substance use and misuse risk over time.

Childhood trauma and violence are widespread, harmful, and costly public health concerns that have impacts on substance misuse, including opioid misuse and addiction.[25] ACEs are common and have no boundaries with regard to age, gender, socioeconomic status, race, ethnicity, or sexual orientation.[26] A recent meta-analysis found that although ACE scores of 4 or more had associations with each of 23 health outcomes, the associations between ACEs and problematic drug use were among the strongest.[27] A case-control study demonstrated that prevalence of child abuse and neglect was higher among a sample of individuals with opioid use disorder compared to a matched community sample.[28] Among those seeking medication-assisted treatment (MAT) for opioid use disorder, the prevalence of childhood trauma was high.[29,30] Similarly, among a psychiatric inpatient sample, those who misused opioids had increased odds of having childhood trauma histories that included childhood sexual and physical abuse.[31] With regard to specific ACE types, sexual abuse and parental separation (for women) and physical and emotional abuse (for men) appear to be particularly highly correlated with opioid abuse.[28] Further, in an adolescent sample, ACEs were associated with an increased risk for nonmedical use of prescription pain relievers,[32] and among adults who sought treatment for opioid use disorder, ACEs were associated with younger age of opioid initiation, injection drug use, and lifetime overdose, the three key indicators of an individual's trajectory toward opioid use disorder.[30]

Several system-level factors have contributed to the current opioid overdose epidemic, including opioid prescribing practices[33,34] and gaps between treatment need and delivery capacity of MAT services for opioid use disorder.[35] Yet, to truly advance prevention, we must also identify other structural, social, and environmental factors that contribute to prescription opioid misuse. Since early onset of prescription opioid misuse is especially predictive of subsequent opioid use disorder[36] and child abuse history has been associated with slower recovery times, less retention in treatment programs, and less recovery overall,[37–39] factors that emerge early in life and on which health systems and community organizations can effectively intervene hold promise for preventing opioid misuse. Therefore, primary prevention approaches that integrate childhood trauma theory and solutions can improve adult relationships, careers, health, and other aspects of a meaningful life.

Impacts of Parental Substance Misuse on Children and Families

In addition to the path from childhood trauma to substance misuse and addiction, it is important to understand that exposure to parental substance misuse can be traumatic for children in and of itself and can set children on their own path toward substance misuse and reduced health and life potential. Research has demonstrated that children of substance-abusing parents are more likely to experience child abuse and neglect than children in non–substance-abusing households.[40–43] We also know that substance misuse is a risk factor itself for future trauma.[10] Individuals who misuse opioids, for example, experience multiple negative consequences, including loss of employment, poor physical and mental health, suicidal behavior, and disrupted family and social relationships.[11] These impacts are not conferred only onto these individuals themselves, but also onto their children and families. As such, growing up in a home with substance misuse can translate into growing up in a home with an unemployed parent with untreated mental illness and addiction, and potentially being emotionally, if not physically, separated from a parent. Indeed, substance use has an astounding impact on the child welfare system. A recent report found that substance abuse was a contributing factor in over one-third of all foster care placements nationally.[11] The additional trauma of being taken into care may create another generation that, without appropriate trauma-informed intervention and treatment, will experience increased susceptability to additional health and well-being problems (e.g., chronic diseases, health risk behaviors including substance misuse, high school noncompletion, unemployment).

For these reasons and many others, the need to address trauma is increasingly regarded as an urgent and critical component of effective behavioral health care and an integral part of the recovery process. When children's positive experiences (e.g., social connectedness, supportive parents and mentors) outweigh their negative experiences, they may be more likely to have positive outcomes later in life.[44] As a field, we tend to know less about protective factors and how they prevent or mitigate adverse experiences. However, evidence-based policies, social norms, and programmatic strategies and approaches that create neighborhoods and communities where every child has safe, stable, nurturing relationships and environments could help prevent risk for opioid misuse and addiction and can help reverse the damage conferred by toxic stress.

Multi-Generation, Trauma-Informed Approaches to Prevention and Treatment

Unfortunately, exposure to potentially traumatic events is a common experience for children and adults in American communities, and it is especially common in the lives of people with SUDs. The impacts of childhood trauma and substance misuse are vast and can impact not only those dealing with addiction during their own lifetimes but also their children and families across generations. Strategies that focus on building safe, stable, nurturing relationships and environments early in the life of a child are cited as among the most influential means of preventing ACEs and reducing their damaging effects.[45–47] As such, primary prevention efforts that seek to prevent exposure to trauma, and secondary and tertiary prevention efforts that promote resilience in groups put at risk by exposure to adversity, are all needed.[11] Primary prevention programs can help to ensure that the next generation does not go on to misuse substances which is particularly important in communities devastated by addiction.[11] Trauma-informed treatment approaches can help people with addiction recover and return to productive, healthy lives.[11] With empirical evidence linking ACEs with many types of substance misuse, and the mounting discourse for comprehensive approaches to opioid misuse prevention, the importance of partnering across disciplines to adopt strategies to simultaneously work toward decreasing and preventing both ACEs and substance misuse has never been clearer. Further, these strategies must be implemented early in the life course, continue across the lifespan, and engage families, including parents/caregivers and children, as well as the communities where they live.

Policy and Systems-Based Prevention Strategies

Preventing childhood adversity, such as child abuse and neglect, requires strategies that build resilience in children and families, support parents to develop effective coping and positive parenting skills, and increase access to and use of comprehensive health services. Decision makers at all organizational levels can play key roles in developing and enacting policies that help children and families thrive. Therefore, raising awareness and commitment for safe, stable, nurturing relationships and environments such that children and families can reach their maximal health and life potential is warranted. Making policymakers aware of the range of impacts that early adversity can have on children can inform their policy work and program creation. The Center on the Developing Child at Harvard University, for example, offers three general principles for policymakers to consider: enhancing responsive relationships, strengthening core life skills, and reducing sources of stress.[48] These principles target protective characteristics across the social ecology at each of the individual, family, and community levels that are associated with health.[49,50] Such protective factors are important because they increase a family's ability to effectively cope and adapt to hardship and change.[47]

As an example of trauma-informed policy-based prevention efforts, Tennessee, a state hard hit by the opioid epidemic, has launched an ACE-based initiative to revise all child-serving state programs (e.g., education, health, law enforcement) to focus on the prevention of childhood trauma. The effort is expected to avoid significant costs to children and families, taxpayers, and the broader community. Specifically, it costs an estimated $200,000 annually to house a juvenile in custody and approximately $40,000 to $50,000 annually to house an adult in custody due to addiction.[11] However, programs to prevent childhood adversity are more cost-effective to offset or decrease the economic and health burdens associated with child maltreatment.[51]

Economic hardship negatively impacts children because it can cause high parental stress and increase the likelihood of children experiencing abuse or neglect. Nearly one-quarter of US children live below the federal poverty level, and in almost every state economic hardship has been documented as a common ACE.[52,53] Efforts to strengthen families' economic security may help reduce parental stress and establish greater household stability, two factors that can help protect children from additional adversity.[46,54] Policies such as the provision of adequate livable wages, full pass-through child support payments, and earned income tax credits are potential mechanisms for reducing ACEs.[46,55-57]

Assessing for ACEs and mental health conditions, questioning patients about medication misuse, and adjusting treatment decisions accordingly, including considering whether opioid therapy is the optimal treatment option, are important steps for safer and more effective pain management and prevention of opioid use disorder.[30] When prescribing opioids for the treatment of chronic pain, the *CDC Guideline for Prescribing Opioids for Chronic Pain* recommends that providers assess for anxiety, posttraumatic stress disorder, and depression; increase monitoring to lessen the risk for opioid use disorder; and ensure that treatment for mental health conditions is optimized, consulting with behavioral health specialists when needed.[58]

In 2017, Indiana lawmakers established an opioid addiction recovery pilot program to assist expectant mothers with an opioid addiction. The program provides treatment in a residential care facility and home visitation services following discharge from the facility. Moreover, 19 states have either created or funded drug treatment programs specifically for pregnant women, and 17 states and the District of Columbia provide pregnant women with priority access to state-funded drug treatment programs.[59]

Comprehensive Public Health Prevention Strategies

Essentials for Childhood: Assuring Safe, Stable, Nurturing Relationships and Environments for All Children is the US Centers for Disease Control and Prevention (CDC)'s vision and framework for comprehensive child abuse and neglect prevention.[45] *Essentials for Childhood* seeks to (1) raise awareness of the impact of child maltreatment and to increase commitment to the strengthening of protective factors that prevent the public health problem of child abuse and neglect, (2) promote the use of data to inform prevention actions, and (3) create the context for healthy children and families through norms change, programs, and policies. To facilitate a context that is supportive of children and families reaching their maximal health and life potential, CDC recently released *Preventing Child Abuse and Neglect: A Technical Package for Policy, Norm, and Programmatic Activities*.[46] This resource provides materials that can be used to prevent child abuse and neglect and includes strategies based on the best available evidence, including strengthening economic supports to families, changing social norms to support parents and positive parenting, providing quality care and education early in life, enhancing parenting skills to promote healthy child development, and intervening to lessen harms and prevent future risk. It also includes specific approaches and examples of programs, policies, or practices for each strategy along with descriptions of the evidence (Text Box 18.1). These strategies can support healthy growth and child development, modify other risk and protective factors for child abuse and neglect,

Safe, stable, nurturing relationships and environments are important for preventing child maltreatment.

Young children experience their world through their relationships with parents and other caregivers. Safe, stable, nurturing relationships and environments between children and their caregivers provide a buffer against the effects of potential stressors such as CM [child maltreatment] and are fundamental to healthy brain development. They also shape the development of children's physical, emotional, social, behavioral, and intellectual capacities, which ultimately affect their health as adults. As a result, promoting safe, stable, nurturing relationships and environments can have a positive impact on a broad range of health problems and on the development of skills that will help children reach their full potential.

Safety, stability, and nurturing are three critical qualities of relationships that make a difference for children as they grow and develop. They can be defined as follows:

- **Safety:** The extent to which a child is free from fear and secure from physical or psychological harm within their social and physical environment.
- **Stability:** The degree of predictability and consistency in a child's social, emotional, and physical environment.
- **Nurturing:** The extent to which a parent or caregiver is available and able to sensitively and consistently respond to and meet the needs of their child.

Safe, stable, nurturing relationships and environments are important to promote. There is reason to believe they can help to:

- Reduce the occurrence of CM and other adverse childhood experiences
- Reduce the negative effects of CM and other adverse childhood experiences
- Influence many physical, cognitive, and emotional outcomes throughout a child's life
- Reduce health disparities
- Have a cumulative impact on health[45,p.7]

For more information on the importance of safe, stable, nurturing relationships and environments:

www.cdc.gov/ViolencePrevention/pdf/CM_Strategic Direction--Long-a.pdf and reduce childhood victimization, thereby also interrupting the trajectories from early adversity to health risk behaviors such as opioid misuse.

Summary

The United States is experiencing a devastating opioid overdose epidemic. Efforts to ensure safe, stable, nurturing relationships and environments for all children are critical for preventing child abuse, neglect, and other early adversities. During adolescence, there are important opportunities to teach youth skills and to provide training and support to parents to help reduce the risk for youth substance abuse and other outcomes from ACEs. For patients with chronic pain, there are opportunities to enhance treatment effectiveness by improving how risks for opioid misuse, including exposure to ACEs, are assessed and by consulting with behavioral health specialists to improve the safety and effectiveness of pain management.[30,58] For individuals requiring treatment for an opioid use disorder, providers can refine their treatment protocols by understanding and addressing the consequences of childhood adversities by integrating trauma-informed care in their practice. These are just a few examples of how deliberate attention to ACEs can be incorporated into prevention activities across the lifespan. CDC's resources like the technical package and *Essentials for Childhood* can help communities make use of the best available evidence for preventing child abuse and neglect and intervening with evidence-based treatments when abuse occurs.[4] By working to reduce the prevalence and consequences of ACEs and more effectively prevent prescription opioid misuse, these strategies have the potential to protect the next generation of children from growing up in a home negatively impacted by prescription opioid misuse and from misusing substances themselves.

References

1. Scholl L, Seth P, Kariisa M, et al. Drug and opioid-involved overdose deaths—United States, 2013–2017. *MMWR Morb Mortal Wkly Rep.* 2019; 67:1419–1427.
2. Bose J, Hedden SL, Lipari RN, Park-Lee E. *Key Substance Use and Mental Health Indicators in the United States: Results from the 2017 National Survey on Drug Use and Health.* Rockville, MD: US Substance Abuse and Mental Health Services Administration; 2018.
3. Shonkoff JP. Capitalizing on advances in science to reduce the health consequences of early childhood adversity. *JAMA Pediatr.* 2016; 170(10):1003–1007.
4. Felitti VJ, Anda RF, Nordenberg D, et al. Relationship of childhood abuse and household dysfunction to many of the leading causes of death in adults: The Adverse Childhood Experiences (ACE) Study. *Am J Prev Med.* 1998; 14(4):245–258.

5. Gilbert LK, Breiding MJ, Merrick MT, et al. Childhood adversity and adult chronic disease: An update from ten states and the District of Columbia, 2010. *Am J Prev Med.* 2015; 48(3):345–349.
6. Metzler M, Merrick MT, Klevens J, et al. Adverse childhood experiences and life opportunities: Shifting the narrative. *Child Youth Serv Rev.* 2017; 72:141–149.
7. Brown DW, Anda RF, Tiemeier H, et al. Adverse childhood experiences and the risk of premature mortality. *Am J Prev Med.* 2009; 37(5):389–396.
8. Font SA, Maguire-Jack K. Pathways from childhood abuse and other adversities to adult health risks: The role of adult socioeconomic conditions. *Child Abuse Negl.* 2016; 51:390–399.
9. Merrick MT, Ports KA, Ford DC, et al. Unpacking the impact of adverse childhood experiences on adult mental health. *Child Abuse Negl.* 2017; 69:10–19.
10. National Child Traumatic Stress Network. *Understanding the Links between Adolescent Trauma and Substance Abuse: A Toolkit for Providers.* 2nd ed. 2008. https://www.nctsn.org/sites/default/files/resources//understanding_the_links_between_adolescent_trauma_and_substance_abuse.pdf. Accessed August 30, 2018.
11. Campaign for Trauma-Informed Policy and Practice. Trauma-Informed Approaches Need to be Part of a Comprehensive Strategy for Addressing the Opioid Epidemic. 2017. http://ctipp.org/Portals/0/xBlog/uploads/2017/7/17/CTIPP_OPB_No1.pdf. Accessed August 30, 2018.
12. Choi NG, DiNitto DM, Marti CN, Choi BY. Association of adverse childhood experiences with lifetime mental and substance use disorders among men and women aged 50+ years. *Int Psychogeriatr.* 2017; 29(3):359–372.
13. Dube SR, Felitti VJ, Dong M, et al. Childhood abuse, neglect, and household dysfunction and the risk of illicit drug use: The Adverse Childhood Experiences Study. *Pediatrics.* 2003; 111(3):564–572.
14. Wade R, Cronholm PF, Fein JA, et al. Household and community-level adverse childhood experiences and adult health outcomes in a diverse urban population. *Child Abuse Negl.* 2016; 52:135–145.
15. Afifi TO, Ford D, Gershoff ET, et al. Spanking and adult mental health impairment: The case for the designation of spanking as an adverse childhood experience. *Child Abuse Negl.* 2017; 71:24–31.
16. Cronholm PF, Forke CM, Wade R, et al. Adverse childhood experiences: Expanding the concept of adversity. *Am J Prev Med.* 2015; 49(3):354–361.
17. Finkelhor D, Shattuck A, Turner H, Hamby S. Improving the Adverse Childhood Experiences Study scale. *JAMA Pediatr.* 2013; 167(1):70–75.
18. Chapman DP, Whitfield CL, Felitti VJ, et al. Adverse childhood experiences and the risk of depressive disorders in adulthood. *J Affect Disord.* 2004; 82(2):217–225.
19. Whitfield CL, Anda RF, Dube SR, Felitti VJ. Violent childhood experiences and the risk of intimate partner violence in adults: Assessment in a large health maintenance organization. *J Interpers Violence.* 2003; 18(2):166–185.
20. Dube SR, Anda RF, Felitti VJ, et al. Childhood abuse, household dysfunction, and the risk of attempted suicide throughout the life span: Findings from the Adverse Childhood Experiences Study. *JAMA.* 2001;286(24):3089–3096.

21. Ford ES, Anda RF, Edwards VJ, et al. Adverse childhood experiences and smoking status in five states. *Prev Med.* 2011; 53(3):188–193.

22. Dube SR, Anda RF, Felitti VJ, et al. Adverse childhood experiences and personal alcohol abuse as an adult. *Addict Behav.* 2002; 27(5):713–725.

23. Hillis SD, Anda RF, Felitti VJ, Marchbanks PA. Adverse childhood experiences and sexual risk behaviors in women: A retrospective cohort study. *Fam Plann Perspect.* 2001; 33(5):206–211.

24. Fox BH, Perez N, Cass E, et al. Trauma changes everything: Examining the relationship between adverse childhood experiences and serious, violent and chronic juvenile offenders. *Child Abuse Negl.* 2015; 46:163–173.

25. Merrick MT, Ford DC, Haegerich TM, Simon T. Adverse childhood experiences increase risk for prescription opioid misuse. *J Prim Prev.* [under review].

26. Merrick MT, Ford DC, Ports KA, Guinn AS. Prevalence of adverse childhood experiences from the Behavioral Risk Factor Surveillance System in 23 states. *JAMA Pediatr.* 2018; 172(11):1038–1044.

27. Hughes K, Bellis MA, Hardcastle KA, et al. The effect of multiple adverse childhood experiences on health: A systematic review and meta-analysis. *Lancet Publ Health.* 2017; 2(8):e356–e366.

28. Conroy E, Degenhardt L, Mattick RP, Nelson EC. Child maltreatment as a risk factor for opioid dependence: Comparison of family characteristics and type and severity of child maltreatment with a matched control group. *Child Abuse Negl.* 2009; 33(6):343–352.

29. Sansone RA, Whitecar P, Wiederman MW. The prevalence of childhood trauma among those seeking buprenorphine treatment. *J Addict Dis.* 2009; 28(1):64–67.

30. Stein MD, Conti MT, Kenney S, et al. Adverse childhood experience effects on opioid use initiation, injection drug use, and overdose among persons with opioid use disorder. *Drug Alcohol Depend.* 2017; 179:325–329.

31. Heffernan K, Cloitre M, Tardiff K, et al. Childhood trauma as a correlate of lifetime opiate use in psychiatric patients. *Addict Behav.* 2000; 25(5):797–803.

32. Forster M, Gower AL, Borowsky IW, McMorris BJ. Associations between adverse childhood experiences, student-teacher relationships, and non-medical use of prescription medications among adolescents. *Addict Behav.* 2017; 68:30–34.

33. US Centers for Disease Control and Prevention. Vital signs: Overdoses of prescription opioid pain relievers—United States, 1999—2008. *MMWR Morb Mortal Wkly Rep.* 2011; 60(43):1487–1492.

34. US Centers for Disease Control and Prevention (CDC). CDC Wide-ranging online data for epidemiologic research (CDC-WONDER). https://wonder.cdc.gov. Accessed October 5, 2017.

35. Jones CM, Campopiano M, Baldwin G, McCance-Katz E. National and state treatment need and capacity for opioid agonist medication-assisted treatment. *Am J Public Health.* 2015; 105(8):e55–e63.

36. McCabe SE, West BT, Morales M, et al. Does early onset of non-medical use of prescription drugs predict subsequent prescription drug abuse and dependence? Results from a national study. *Addiction.* 2007; 102(12):1920–1930.

37. Branstetter SA, Bower EH, Kamien J, Amass L. A history of sexual, emotional, or physical abuse predicts adjustment during opioid maintenance treatment. *J Subst Abuse Treat.* 2008; 34(2):208–214.

38. Kumar N, Stowe ZN, Han X, Mancino MJ. Impact of early childhood trauma on retention and phase advancement in an outpatient buprenorphine treatment program. *Am J Addict.* 2016; 25(7):542–548.

39. Sacks JY, McKendrick K, Banks S. The impact of early trauma and abuse on residential substance abuse treatment outcomes for women. *J Subst Abuse Treat.* 2008; 34(1):90–100.

40. De Bellis MD, Broussard ER, Herring DJ, et al. Psychiatric co-morbidity in caregivers and children involved in maltreatment: A pilot research study with policy implications. *Child Abuse Negl.* 2001; 25(7):923–944.

41. Dube SR, Anda RF, Felitti VJ, et al. Growing up with parental alcohol abuse: Exposure to childhood abuse, neglect, and household dysfunction. *Child Abuse Negl.* 2001; 25(12):1627–1640.

42. Chaffin M, Kelleher K, Hollenberg J. Onset of physical abuse and neglect: Psychiatric, substance abuse, and social risk factors from prospective community data. *Child Abuse Negl.* 1996; 20(3):191–203.

43. Kelleher K, Chaffin M, Hollenberg J, Fischer E. Alcohol and drug disorders among physically abusive and neglectful parents in a community-based sample. *Am J Public Health.* 1994; 84(10):1586–1590.

44. Schofield TJ, Lee RD, Merrick MT. Safe, stable, nurturing relationships as a moderator of intergenerational continuity of child maltreatment: A meta-analysis. *J Adolesc Health.* 2013; 53(4, Supp):S32–S38.

45. US Centers for Disease Control and Prevention (CDC), National Center for Injury Prevention and Control. *Essentials for Childhood: Steps to Create Safe, Stable, Nurturing Relationships and Environments.* Atlanta, GA: CDC; 2014.

46. Fortson BL, Klevens J, Merrick MT, et al. *Preventing Child Abuse and Neglect: A Technical Package for Policy, Norm, and Programmatic Activities.* National Center for Injury Prevention and Control, U.S. Centers for Disease Control and Prevention. 2016. https://www.cdc.gov/violenceprevention/pdf/can-prevention-technical-package.pdf. Accessed October 5, 2017.

47. Bellazaire A. *Preventing and Mitigating the Effects of Adverse Childhood Experiences.* Denver, CO: National Conference of State Legislatures; 2018.

48. Cohen SD. *Three Principles to Improve Outcomes for Children and Families. Science to Policy and Practice.* Cambridge, MA: Center on the Developing Child at Harvard University; 2017.

49. Banyard V, Hamby S, Grych J. Health effects of adverse childhood events: Identifying promising protective factors at the intersection of mental and physical well-being. *Child Abuse Negl.* 2017; 65:88–98.

50. US Centers for Disease Control and Prevention. Child Abuse and Neglect: Risk and Protective Factors. 2016. https://www.cdc.gov/violenceprevention/childabuseandneglect/riskprotectivefactors.html. Accessed September 5, 2018.

51. Fang X, Brown DS, Florence C, Mercy JA. The economic burden of child maltreatment in the United States and implications for prevention. *Child Abuse Negl.* 2012; 36(2):156–165.

52. Sacks V, Murphey D, Moore K. *Adverse Childhood Experiences: National and State-Level Prevalence*. Bethesda, MD: Child Trends; 2014.

53. National Center for Children in Poverty. Child Poverty. http://www.nccp.org/topics/childpoverty.html. 2018. Accessed September 5, 2018.

54. Rodriguez CM, Green AJ. Parenting stress and anger expression as predictors of child abuse potential. *Child Abuse Negl.* 1997; 21(4):367–377.

55. Raissian KM, Bullinger LR. Money matters: Does the minimum wage affect child maltreatment rates? *Child Youth Serv Rev.* 2017; 72:60–70.

56. Cancian M, Yang M-Y, Slack KS. The effect of additional child support income on the risk of child maltreatment. *Soc Serv Rev.* 2013; 87(3):417–437.

57. Klevens J, Schmidt B, Luo F, et al. Effect of the earned income tax credit on hospital admissions for pediatric abusive head trauma, 1995–2013. *Public Health Rep.* 2017; 132(4):505–511.

58. Dowell D, Haegerich TM, Chou R. CDC guideline for prescribing opioids for chronic pain—United States, 2016. *JAMA.* 2016; 315(15):1624–1645.

59. Guttmacher Institute. Substance Use During Pregnancy. 2018. https://www.guttmacher.org/state-policy/explore/substance-use-during-pregnancy. Accessed September 5, 2018.

19 | Public Health and the Criminal Justice System

PARTNERSHIPS TO PROMOTE HEALTH AND PREVENT ADDICTION

GARY TENNIS, KENNETH J. MARTZ, AND JAC A. CHARLIER

PPROXIMATELY TWO-THIRDS OF AMERICA'S incarcerated population suffers with untreated or undertreated substance use disorders (SUDs),[1,2] and many of those individuals committed several crimes related to drug use and addiction on a daily basis prior to being incarcerated. To end the opioid epidemic in the United States we not only need to bolster our health care and public health response to SUD, we need to engage the criminal justice system as a specific touchpoint for public health intervention in communities and states across the country. These interventions will require sustained investment in both the public health and the *treatment capacity* available to the criminal justice sector to provide much needed behavioral and health services; this will require and advocacy for changes that better connect the work of public health and prevention agencies with the work of criminal justice as early as possible in the justice continuum, and preferably in the community. Our principal argument in examining the opportunities for public health and criminal justice collaboration is that people with opioid-use disorder and other SUDs should not have to wait until an encounter with the justice system to access drug treatment but if they become justice-involved, it is imperative that the criminal justice system serve as a belated but necessary public health and health care intervention supportive of treatment, medications as needed for supporting addiction treatment, recovery, and prevention of addiction (Text Box 19.1).

Background to the Current Criminal Justice Approach to SUD Prevention and Treatment

During the Vietnam War era, some veterans returned home to the United States with an addiction to heroin. Not surprisingly, this led to contact with

Several principles are important to consider when looking at opportunities for public health and criminal justice organizations to collaborate in ending the opioid crisis. Each of these is briefly described below.

Early and Persistent Intervention

Treatment for substance misuse and addiction should take place at the earliest possible stage in the criminal justice system (just as it should be addressed at the earliest possible stage in the health care system). If intervention and clinically appropriate treatment have not occurred or have not been successful, there should be repeated efforts to intervene and treat at every stage (including comprehensive coordination of evidence-based practices) until recovery is attained.

Treatment Based on Individualized Clinical Assessment

Historically, criminal justice stakeholders often have adopted a "one-size-fits-all" approach to treatment. But the treatment of SUDs, like the treatment of any other disease, must be tailored to an individual's specific clinical needs, based on an individualized professional assessment. The modality of treatment and the length of care should be driven by an individual's clinical needs, not the severity of his or her criminal offense.

Target the Highest-Need Populations and, for Criminal Justice, the Highest Risk

Criminal justice diversion-to-treatment programs include criteria that exclude more serious offenses or exclude individuals with longer criminal records may keep out the very people who are most likely to receive the greatest impact from being treated for SUD. Research suggests that the greatest impacts on crime reduction and improvements in well-being are achieved by focusing on those most in need of treatment.[19]

Leveraging Criminal Justice Consequences to Get Better Outcomes and Save Lives

Due to the stigma and resulting shame-driven denial around substance misuse and addiction, many individuals avoid treatment until faced with the growing and undeniable adverse consequences of their disease-related behavior. These consequences include spouses or partners threatening to leave, employers threatening termination, or facing criminal justice consequences due to crimes they have committed. However, any individual in the criminal justice system is facing jail because he or she allegedly committed a crime (e.g., theft, forgery, assault), not because it is a crime to be substance dependent. Diverting to treatment rather than the more conventional use of incarceration for the underlying crimes is a caring, humane, and lifesaving policy and not a criminalization of a disease.

Supporting Recovery

Restoring recovering criminal justice offenders to the full rights of citizenship, including the right to pursue meaningful and fulfilling work, powerfully supports their recovery. This reduces relapse and criminal recidivism, thereby improving the public's health and increasing public safety. Health-promoting, patient-centered strategies, combined with activities that address social and economic needs, should be part of efforts that take a public health approach to recovery and integration of previous incarcerated individuals with SUD back into their community.

law enforcement, including arrest, jail, and even conviction with incarceration. This took place prior to the start of America's era of mass incarceration, and at the time the public viewed the use of incarceration for people with a substance-use disorder, and especially of those that were also veterans, as an undesirable approach. In response, in 1971 the White House, through the Special Action Office for Drug Abuse Prevention, developed the initial Treatment Alternatives to Street Crimes (TASC) program model, which focused on linking criminal justice and treatment, in order to interrupt the relationship between drugs and property crime. The next year in 1972,the US Law Enforcement Assistance Administration (LEAA) (the predecessor to the US Department of Justice's Bureau of Justice Assistance), funded the first TASC program site in Delaware; it soon showed that two very different systems could work together with two shared goals: reducing crime and reducing drug use. This was followed the following year, 1973, by funding for TASC sites by the National Institute of Drug Abuse (NIDA).[3] At its inception, TASC supported a variety of pilot projects to bridge the criminal justice and the community-based drug treatment system. Today, TASC (now also known as "Treatment Accountability for Safe Communities") programs are twice as effective at reducing recidivism and relapse as non-TASC programs.[4,5] TASC is not a specialized program like drug courts, nor does it "sit" at only one justice intercept like prosecutorial or parole diversion. Instead, TASC is a highly adaptable, systems approach that is used in a wide variety of justice settings from police to parole to connection with behavioral health, housing, and other social services. Through the use of specialized case management performed in accordance with the original TASC model, communication, collaboration, and accountability between justice and treatment systems bring about proven results in reducing drug use and engaging people in drug treatment.

Providing clinically appropriate drug and alcohol treatment to criminal justice–involved individuals with substance-use disorders significantly reduces crime.[6] Ensuring the right treatment at the right time and in the right place for those who need it is far more effective in making communities safer than simply subjecting justice involved people with substance-use disorders to serial episodes of incarceration. Prosecutors and police officers generally recognize this today: The refrain "we can't arrest our way out of this problem" is now commonplace, especially in the midst of the current historic opioid epidemic. The TASC approach informs a number of contemporary efforts to address the opioid crisis described in the following sections of this chapter.

Deflection (also known as Police-Assisted Interventions)

Experienced police officers often learn who in their communities are suffering from SUDs through their day-to-day activities. Over the decades, police officers (some in recovery themselves) have informally engaged in police-assisted interventions to drug treatment. The change is that today, a growing number of police departments are now formally training their officers to positively engage those individuals and to help connect them with the SUD treatment and other services they need.[7,8] These officers learn how to build trust and a positive connection with the suffering members of their community, to encourage them, and to build the justified hope that recovery is possible. Police officers learn how to connect these individuals with appropriate treatment professionals who can conduct a clinical assessment and get them to the treatment that is right for them.

Public health officials have a strong case to make for law enforcement engagement in new approaches to preventing and treating SUD. As with other criminal justice interventions and referrals to treatment, promoting access to treatment and sustaining recovery programs is as much a smart crime-fighting strategy (an individual with a SUD may commit several crimes a day, often related to substance use issues) as it is an effective public health strategy. The Police, Treatment, and Community Collaborative (PTACC) has identified five pathways by which police may connect people with treatment.[9] This newly emerging field of pre-arrest diversion is largely being driven by the opioid epidemic and goes by a variety of terms, including deflection and first responder diversion. The change this represents for both the criminal justice system and the behavioral health system is transformational. Deflection can occur in a number of different ways and may include the following four (out of five) known pathways.

Officer Intervention Pathway: Diversion from Arrest for Criminal Offenses

Diverting individuals with SUD from arrest to treatment and other needed social services is a growing approach nationwide. The earliest example of such a program, is Seattle's Law Enforcement Assisted Diversion (LEAD) program. Currently, there are approximately 25 LEAD sites in the United States.[10] In the LEAD program, those arrested for minor offenses who appear to have a substance-use disorder are taken to treatment (and their criminal charges are held in abeyance) instead of going through the usual criminal justice process.

The person must then complete, for example, a treatment assessment or even several treatment sessions to avoid any further justice processing. A critique of some iterations of the LEAD program is that some officers report a lack of any consequences for individuals who immediately leave the program and return to the street. Due to the nature of addiction, both continued education about addiction and how SUD treatment works might help with understanding why this appears to be the case, as well as ensuring that there are actual consequences for non-participation with SUD treatment. Especially in cases where new crimes are to be avoided and an individual's own life might be at stake, leveraging future justice processing are usually warranted for LEAD participants who walk away from treatment. This may require use of a signed release by the participant, in order to comport with federal, and possibly state, confidentiality requirements.

Self-Referral Pathway

A more passive approach is publicizing and implementing a program that allows people in need of SUD treatment to access it through their local police station. No arrest is made for seeking help and even possession of small amounts of controlled substances for personal use or drug paraphernalia at the time a person is requesting treatment does not lead to arrest. Instead, the police officer directly connects the individuals with volunteers (these may be certified recovery specialists) who in turn connect the person with the appropriate SUD assessment and treatment services through a warm handoff process. A challenge with the self-referral pathway is whether or not individuals in communities or population groups that mistrust law enforcement would consider walking into a police station to ask for assistance about something that is illegal (drug use, drug paraphernalia) and not expect to be arrested. Most self-referral sites today are in majority-white communities, where the idea of possibly going to police for help is not as great a barrier. However, especially in communities of color, it remains to be seen how well self-referral will work and how it might need to be adjusted, or just avoided in favor of other strategies to connect individuals to treatment without risk of arrest.

Active Outreach Pathway

Some police departments go even further by proactively and directly reaching out to specific individuals with SUD, including the homeless and individuals with co-occurring mental illness. No specific event or activity (criminal or otherwise) by the individual is needed to initiate this pathway. Particularly in the context of community policing, as previously stated, experienced officers are usually well aware who is in need of SUD treatment, and by engaging these individuals with dignity and caring, police officers, most often accompanied or supported by a recovery specialist, peer, or SUD counselor, can be remarkably effective in making a lifesaving connection that others will not or cannot do.

As previously discussed, Active Outreach is actually not a new activity for police officers. Over the past century or more we know that police officers have engaged, unofficially and informally in such interventions. Formalizing and expanding these procedures, with training and an expectation of implementation, is promising development.

Naloxone Plus Pathway

A development uniquely arising out of and tailored to the opioid epidemic is the implementation of the "Naloxone Plus" pathway where law enforcement, often in conjunction with a recovery specialist, peer, or SUD counselor rapidly follows up with opioid overdose survivors shortly after naloxone administration, in order to offer treatment. The team will persist with attempts to engage the individual for prolonged periods of time well beyond the initial or early contact. The most common version of this is the Quick Response Team (QRT) developed in the Cinncinatti, Ohio region; this approach can now be found in over 50 sites and continues to rapidly expand across the nation.[11]

Engagement of Non–Law Enforcement Resources on the Policing Team

Having certified recovery specialists, peers, and SUD counselors, accompany officers and work together as an intervention team brings more addiction, treatment, and recovery expertise to the actual work—and in real time—with the person in need of services. One of many examples is the Bensalem Police Assisting in Recovery (BPAIR) in Bensalem, Pennsylvania.[12] The BPAIR program has built a strong interdisciplinary team with the county drug and alcohol agency to prioritize assessment and treatment for program participants and with a local treatment program with established expertise in treating more deteriorated patients. The strong partnership of the police department, the county drug and alcohol agency, and a treatment provider with the capacity to deal with criminal justice–involved patients makes the program more sustainable and more effective. Other resources can be engaged as well. Law enforcement officers faced with ever-increasingly complex work demands and expectations, can turn to these partners entities that are better suited and resourced to address what are essentially public health issues. Police intervention programs have creatively engaged other community partners as well to get the work done. For example, to further resource BPAIR, the police chief in Bensalem has partnered with a local taxicab company that has volunteered to provide participants free and immediate transportation to treatment.

Diversion at Booking for Minor Offenses

In jurisdictions where police departments opt not to engage in police-assisted interventions, there is another option: universal SUD screening at the time of booking and full assessment where there is a positive screen. Where police do engage in police-assisted interventions, diversion at booking can also be a "second chance" mechanism for arrestees to reconsider their initial choices to decline SUD treatment. Booking, or preliminary arraignment, generally takes place within a few hours of arrest, usually at the police station. A magistrate makes a preliminary determination about what charges are to be filed (these must be backed up by actual evidence presented at a preliminary hearing, which is usually held within a week or two of arrest), and a preliminary determination of bail is set. Most individuals are released on bail and provided a court date for a preliminary hearing.

Universal screening and assessment procedures are easiest to do in those jurisdictions that have established a centralized booking station for an entire jurisdiction (city, county, etc.). In such areas, a certified drug and alcohol clinician conducts an initial screening of each individual immediately prior to the actual preliminary arraignment. This clinician also keeps track of the availability of detoxification and SUD treatment openings in the area. Detox is preparation for treatment, not treatment itself, so usually a treatment bed must also be found for the arrestee to be transferred immediately upon completion of detox (which can be a three- to five-day process).[13]

Where the arrestee is determined to need and agrees to engage in SUD treatment, charges may be held in abeyance. Depending on the seriousness of the charged offenses, past criminal record, the wishes of the crime victims, and other factors, charges are simply not filed at all so long as the individual successfully engages in and completes SUD treatment. This form of officer intervention was developed by the Civil Citation Network in Florida.[14] This is not a citation in lieu of arrest but treatment in lieu of arrest with an administrative charge (not a criminal violation) that is processed without further action if the person engages in and completes treatment.

In many instances, an individual may choose not to take the treatment option. In such an instance, the individual would undergo normal criminal justice processing for the underlying offense in the same manner as if no SUD issues were present. To prevent manipulation of the treatment option approach for those who take that route, it is essential that a release be signed allowing notification to law enforcement should individuals terminate their treatment unilaterally or otherwise fail to adhere to their treatment plan and go against the advice of their treatment providers. These releases can be drafted in a manner consistent with current federal and state confidentiality regulations. When law enforcement is notified that the individual has chosen not to follow through with the decision to engage in treatment, the case is then handled as it would be for anyone else charged with the offense.

Research has demonstrated that SUDs cloud and distort the thinking. Additionally, due to the deeply ingrained and widespread stigma surrounding this disease, the afflicted are commonly in denial that they need treatment. Finally, those not in denial are typically hopeless, feeling that recovery is impossible at least for them (i.e., an individual may believe "maybe others can get better, but I'm a hopeless case"). All of these factors explain why an arrestee might make the seemingly irrational decision not to choose treatment instead of conventional criminal processing. For this reason, it is critical that the treatment option be offered again and again. For those who do not take advantage of the treatment option at the time of booking, proceeding with criminal charges means that lifesaving treatment can be offered at later points in the criminal justice process. These later points are discussed below.

Pretrial Diversion to Treatment for Cases Too Serious for Charges to Be Dropped at Booking: The Role of Drug Courts

Many cases will not be appropriate to divert at the time of booking due to the seriousness of the charge, the criminal record of the defendant, or both. These cases therefore will enter into more formal judicial processing. In this context, the best practice for diversion of the high-risk and high-need population to treatment is drug treatment court. The National Association of Drug Court Professionals (NADCP) is comprised of over 27,000 drug court judges, prosecutors, defense attorneys, probation and parole officials, pretrial service officials, treatment professionals, and, more recently, police officials as part of the team.[15] NADCP has developed a comprehensive guide for the establishment and operation of drug courts, *Adult Drug Court: Best Practice Standards, Volumes I and II.*[16] Moreover, NADCP, through its three divisions (National Drug Court Institute, National Center for DWI Courts, and Justice for Vets), offers in-depth technical assistance to courts across the nation as they work to develop drug courts for the first time where they currently are not in place, and seek to expand current drug courts to reach other populations (e.g., Veterans' Courts, DWI Courts, Mental Health Courts, Family Courts, Re-Entry Courts). NADCP also supports current drug courts in their ongoing work to engage in continuous quality improvement.

Since their genesis in Miami, Florida, in 1989, over 3,000 drug court programs (and the number is growing rapidly) have been established across all 50 states, four US territories, and over twenty other nations.[17] Drug court programs are extremely effective, reducing criminal recidivism (75% success rate for drug court graduates vs. 30% for those who are incarcerated), increasing public safety and public health, and lowering criminal justice and health care costs ($27 savings for every $1 invested).[16] As Supreme Court justices from all 50 states have agreed, drug courts are "the most effective strategy for reducing drug abuse and criminal recidivism."[15] In the following section, universal principles used by drug courts are described, including the provision of clinically appropriate SUD treatment, mental health treatment, and other social services as needed, with careful case management, usually under the supervision of a drug court judge. In instances where criminal justice sanctions would normally apply, these sanctions are either withdrawn or mitigated so long as the individual successfully completes the treatment and other requirements of the program.

Charges Dropped for Successful Completion of Drug Court Program

Depending on the seriousness of the case, an individual's criminal record, and the orientation of the criminal justice stakeholders (especially the state's sentencing commission and its courts and prosecutors), completion of the drug court program can result in the withdrawal of criminal charges for the case. Withdrawal of charges has the major benefit of allowing individuals to move forward with their life unhindered in their vocation and other life pursuits by the significant handicap of having a criminal record. Withdrawal of charges can occur immediately upon completion of the drug court program. In other instances, criminal justice authorities require that completion of the program must be followed by a specified arrest-free period of time before charges are dropped.

Incarceration Avoided by Successful Completion of Drug Court Program

In cases too serious for charges to be dropped, and even in cases where incarceration might ordinarily be called for under the prevailing sentencing guidelines and practices, beginning SUD treatment before trial can still have significant benefits for the accused, the criminal justice system, and public health, including:

Better public health outcome due to the individual's experience of personal crisis in the period following arrest and charging. Individuals facing new criminal charges are likely to be more acutely experiencing the "unmanageability" of their disease. This can lead to a client letting go of denial and becoming more receptive to undertaking the rigors of treatment.
Increased motivation because more is at stake. In these instances, the charged individual will have the additional motivation of a pending sentencing; recovering ex-offenders routinely report that the motivation of avoiding incarceration made the critical difference. This motivation is especially important if the SUD treatment provider is using a trauma-informed care approach. When painful trauma is opened up (often for the first time in the patient's life), having external reasons to persist through the difficult emotional work can be lifesaving.
Better-informed sentencing. The sentencing court will have more knowledge about the individual's future prospects. For example, if the individual is successfully engaging in treatment, the judge knows there is a greater likelihood that the recovering individual will undertake a law-abiding, productive life of recovery. The substance-dependent defendant who refuses or

is not yet ready to take advantage of the treatment opportunity, on the other hand, presents a greater risk of criminal recidivism.[18]

Less use of incarceration. Sentencing judges and prosecutors will be much more inclined to reduce what ordinarily would be a sentence of incarceration to a probation sentence if they know that the person before them is having success in a treatment regimen. They will generally understand that allowing the successful treatment regimen to continue is in the best interest of public safety and the health of the individual before them, ultimately reducing prison and other costs to society.

One caveat to offering treatment before a trial in more serious cases is that there truly must be an understanding by the courts and the prosecutors that if the individual positively engages in treatment before a trial, he or she should be sentenced to probation and allowed to continue the treatment regimen as a condition of probation. Sentencing someone to jail who is in the middle of a successful course of treatment can undo the value of the treatment that has been completed so far and causes further hopelessness in the individual. If the case is so serious that an individual must be sentenced to incarceration no matter what, the better approach is to begin "behind-the-walls" treatment prior to release.

Offenders Sentenced to Incarceration and Treatment "Behind the Walls"

Due to the nature of an offense, the defendant's criminal record, or both, some cases will be so serious that a court is going to sentence the defendant to jail or prison regardless of the role the defendant's SUD played in the case. The importance of providing clinically appropriate SUD treatment where clinically needed is extremely important in such cases since it is virtually certain that the SUD is a major criminogenic risk factor.[19] If the defendant's SUD and other criminogenic risk factors are not successfully addressed, the defendant is very likely to relapse and reoffend upon release.

As with community-based programs, "behind-the-walls" treatment should be evidence-based and include the right length of stay (this is based on individualized clinical assessment, but the research generally points to long-term treatment), the right counselor/patient ratios, matching the right level of treatment to risk and need, and a strong contingent of peer recovery counselors.[14] Lack of attention to these principles generally will result in poorer outcomes that are likely to compromise both public safety and public health concerns. One way to ensure that behind-the-walls treatment is provided in accordance with established clinical standards is to have the programs licensed by the state drug and alcohol treatment-licensing agency.

Treatment gains in behind-the-walls treatment in part depend on careful timing of the parole process so that treatment seamlessly continues in the community upon release. Immediately after completing behind-the-walls treatment, the individual should be paroled and transitioned into intensive community-based treatment with appropriate stepdown through the continuum as well as referrals and touchpoints in the community, for example using a program modeled after the Delaware experience.[20] This evidence-based model has been recognized by the Substance Abuse and Mental Health Services Administration (SAMHSA)'s National Registry of Evidence-Based Programs and has resulted in more than 200 papers, books, and presentations; the program was visited for implementation in more than 30 countries over several decades.[20] When treatment continuity fails to occur and the defendant completing behind-the-walls treatment is placed back into the prison community without ongoing care, the therapeutic work accomplished in the treatment program may be lost.[21]

Even worse, if the individual is released without the support of needed community-based treatment matched to individualized clinical need, the risk of relapse is substantial, as is the risk of overdose, because the individual's tolerance will be much lower than when he or she went into prison.[21] This is a life-and-death issue: For those with opioid use disorders, the overdose rate without proper stepdown treatment is many times greater than compared to the general population, higher even than the rate of homicide upon release to the community.[22]

Ongoing Recovery Support and the Criminal Justice System

Recovery supports for ex-offenders, such as ongoing SUD treatment, a supportive recovery community, meaningful work, stable housing, physical and emotional self-care, and caring, healthy relationships with others, are critical. Clinically sound, evidence-based SUD treatment addresses all these issues and works in helping patients build strong ties with a local recovery support community. The recovering community has a long and historic presence with recovery support programs (12-step programs being the most prominent) that have saved millions of lives. We are now entering a new era as our nation is in the midst of a "recovery revolution" in which millions of recovering individuals are forming an even more robust recovery support network to supplement and strengthen clinically appropriate treatment (usually heavily staffed with recovering clinicians). The challenge, both within and outside of the criminal justice system, will be to continue to empower the recovery community in its work providing a comprehensive array of services that will help newly recovering individuals sustain recovery over time and become a permanent addition to the 23 million Americans living in recovery.[23]

Pardons and Other Post-Release Recovery Supports

Having a criminal record today is like going through life with the proverbial "scarlet letter." A criminal record can be an obstacle to important recovery supports for an individual, such as being able to find meaningful employment, accessing public housing resources, or simply being a parent volunteer on a child's field trip. There are three approaches, not mutually exclusive, that a state can take to address this problem:

1. The automatic expungement of minor offenses after a period of crime-free years
2. "Ban-the-box" prohibitions against requiring job applicants to state on their application whether or not they have been arrested before they are determined to be the best candidate for the job
3. Streamlined and accessible pardons procedures.

In Pennsylvania, former Lieutenant Governor Mike Stack, who statutorily also served as the Board of Pardons chairman, launched a vigorous "Pathway to Pardons" initiative.[24] With the Pathway to Pardons team, he promoted the availability of pardons in countless community events across the state. This has resulted in a dramatic increase in pardons applications (nearly 50%). The Lieutenant Governor also implemented reforms to streamline the pardons process, resulting in an increase of over 125% in case merit reviews by the Pardons Board. This initiative has made the pardons process faster, less cumbersome, and more straightforward, so that the average layperson with a criminal record can obtain a pardon without hiring a lawyer as long as he or she qualifies. The advantage of the pardons option is that it entails an individualized review of each case and, perhaps more importantly, it completely "wipes the slate clean." When a person receives a pardon and his or her record is expunged under the law, it is as if no crime was ever committed; the pardoned individual is directed that "no" is the proper legal response when asked by a prospective employer if he or she has ever been arrested.

Of course, there are some instances where an individual's criminal record must be kept intact and available to protect the public. For example, expungement legislation should make an exception for child sex abuse convictions. But in other cases, the pardon option paves the way for meaningful employment opportunities and community participation that can serve to enhance recovery progress and create new opportunities and hope for individuals.

Summary: Public Health and Health Care Professionals Engaging and Collaborating with Law Enforcement

When state and local health officials gather together community stakeholders to address a jurisdiction's drug and alcohol problems, it is important to include police and other law enforcement agencies. The criminal justice system is a part of the solution to the opioid crisis and brings valuable perspectives to the discussion, as well as expanded opportunities to connect people to treatment. The police officer who arrests an individual with SUD for theft, who is also at risk of suffering a fatal overdose, is carrying out an important public health function when they link the arrestee to SUD treatment in the community. Furthermore, that arrest at least temporarily has a public health benefit by separating (temporarily of course) the at-risk individual from dangerous street drugs. Conversely, if an individual with opioid use disorder is released after a period of incarceration without treatment, the arrest might have an adverse public health consequence because the person, left untreated, might have lower tolerance due to incarceration-forced abstinence and therefore be at increased risk of fatal overdose when he or she relapses.

Prescription drug monitoring programs, underage drinking laws, outlawing of cigarette vending machines and other controls on selling tobacco to minors, and prescribing guidelines are all science-based public health interventions based on the assumption that reducing supply reduces use and misuse with a consequential public health benefit. The same is true for illegal drugs. When law enforcement seizes dangerous illegal drugs and arrests the traffickers, this reduces the supply of and access to those drugs, at least for a time, and this supply interruption has a public health benefit. Working to interrupt the flow of illegal drugs and the supply of alcohol to minors is part of the solution to ending addiction and substance misuse disorder in communities. To have the greatest possible impact on this epidemic we need an "all-hands-on-deck" approach to reducing both the demand and supply of opioids. Public health officials' active engagement with, and respect for, the vital role of law enforcement in public health efforts (and vice versa) will support the building of strong partnerships from which the entire community will benefit.

Adults with SUD in the criminal justice system would probably not be there if their disease had been identified and treated with clinical fidelity and community supports when they were younger. According to the National Institute of Drug Abuse, "as many as two-thirds of detained juveniles may have a substance use disorder [and] female juveniles who enter the system generally have higher SUD rates than males."[19] A study of those with opioid use disorder found that the average age of onset for marijuana and alcohol use was 14 and that 84% of participants who used other drugs at age 14 or younger went on to heroin use later in life.[25] If juveniles are provided a comprehensive plan to address all their critical needs using a public health approach that includes addressing the social determinants of health, then criminal justice system involvement may never occur.

This "upstream" approach in public health is common (i.e., preventing the disease before it becomes chronic or acute and requires medical attention), and a similar approach is warranted in the criminal justice sector. Tremendous possibilities exist for engaging criminal justice in public health discussions around prevention of adverse childhood events and ways to support the development of healthy and resilient communities. The opportunities for collaboration are limitless but do require new approaches and innovations. It is our hope that public health and law enforcement agencies will continue to establish strong ties, understand each other's interests, and stress the critical role that criminal justice officers and agencies can play in addressing, and ending, the opioid crisis.

References

1. Center on Addiction. Shoveling It Up II: The Impact of Substance Abuse on Federal, State, and Local Budgets. CASA Report 2009. https://www.centeronaddiction.org/addiction-research/reports/shoveling-ii-impact-substance-abuse-federal-state-and-local-budgets. Accessed December 11, 2018.
2. Proctor S. Substance use disorder prevalence among female state prison inmates. *Am J Drug Alcohol Ab*. 2012; 38(4):278–285.
3. Treatment Alternatives for Safe Communities (TASC). TASC History. http://www2.tasc.org/content/tasc-history. Accessed December 11, 2018.
4. Treatment Alternatives for Safe Communities (TASC). Making a Difference Across Illinois. 2018. http://www.tasc.org/TascBlog/images/documents/Publications/TASC_MaD_IL.pdf. Accessed December 11, 2018.
5. Treatment Alternatives for Safe Communities (TASC). Diversion and Alternatives to Incarceration. 2018. http://www.tasc.org/TascBlog/images/documents/Programs/Diversion-and-Alt2Inc-FactSheet.pdf. Accessed December 11, 2018.
6. Substance Abuse and Mental Health Services Administration (SAMHSA). Intervention Summary: Correctional Therapeutic Community for Substance Abusers. 2018. https://nrepp.samhsa.gov/Legacy/ViewIntervention.aspx?id=338. Accessed December 11, 2018.
7. Charlier J, Frost G, Kopac A, Olk T. Pre-arrest diversion: The long-overdue collaboration between police and treatment. *Police Chief*. 2018; 85(3):42–47.
8. Charlier J. You want to reduce drugs in your community? You might want to deflect instead of arrest. *Police Chief*. 2015; 82(9):30–31.
9. Police, Treatment and Community Collaborative (PTACC). Pre-arrest Diversion: Pathways to Community. 2017. https://ptaccollaborative.org/wp-content/uploads/2018/07/PTACC_visual.pdf. Accessed December 11, 2018.

10. LEAD National Support Bureau. Our mission: The LEAD National Support Bureau. https://www.leadbureau.org/. Accessed December 11, 2018.
11. Charlier J. Deflection and pre-arrest diversion: A newly emerging field in the United States. 2018. http://www2.centerforhealthandjustice.org/sites/www2. centerforhealthandjustice.org/files/publications/Pre-ArrestDiversion_SlideShow. pdf. Accessed December 11, 2018.
12. Bensalem Police Department. Bensalem police assisting in recovery. 2018. https:// bucks.crimewatchpa.com/bensalempd/15488/content/bpair. Accessed December 11, 2018.
13. US National Institutes of Health, National Institute on Drug Abuse (NIDA). *Principles of Drug Addiction Treatment: A Research Based Guide.* 2018. https:// d14rmgtrwzf5a.cloudfront.net/sites/default/files/675-principles-of-drug-addiction-treatment-a-research-based-guide-third-edition.pdf. Accessed December 11, 2018.
14. Civil Citation Network National. Adult pre-arrest verification tool. https:// civilcitationnetwork.com/. Accessed December 11, 2018.
15. National Association of Drug Court Professionals. Drug courts: Saving money, cutting crime, serving veterans. 2014. https://jpo.wrlc.org/handle/11204/3235. Accessed December 11, 2018.
16. National Association of Drug Court Professionals. Adult drug court: Best practice standards, Volumes I and II. 2015. https://ndcrc.org/resource/nadcp-adult-drug-court-best-practice-standards-volume-ii/. Accessed December 11, 2018.
17. US Department of Justice, National Institute of Justice. Drug courts. https://www.nij. gov/topics/courts/drug-courts/Pages/welcome.aspx. Accessed December 11, 2018.
18. US National Institutes of Health, National Institute on Drug Abuse (NIDA). Principles of drug abuse treatment for criminal justice populations: A research-based guide. https://www.drugabuse.gov/publications/principles-drug-abuse-treatment-criminal-justice-populations/principles. Accessed December 11, 2018.
19. Taxman F, Thanner M, Weisburd D. Risk, need and responsivity (RNR): It all depends. *Crime Delinq.* 2006; 52(1):28–51.
20. US Substance Abuse and Mental Health Services Administration (SAMSHA). Peer support and social inclusion. https://www.samhsa.gov/recovery/peer-support-social-inclusion. Accessed December 11, 2018.
21. Wexler H, Prendergast M. Therapeutic communities in the United States prisons: Effectiveness and challenges. *Ther Communities.* 2010; (31):157–175.
22. Ranapurwala SI, Shanahan ME, Alexandridis AA, et al. Opioid overdose mortality among former North Carolinai inmates: 2000–2015. *Am J Public Health.* 2018; 108(9):1207–1213.
23. Faces and Voices of Recovery (FAVOR). Shape the future of recovery. 2018. https:// facesandvoicesofrecovery.org/. Accessed December 11, 2018.
24. Commonwealth of Pennsylvania, Office of the Lieutenant Governor. Stack *Pathways to Pardons* set to become national model in opioid fight. https://www.media.pa.gov/ Pages/Lieutenant-Governor-Details.aspx?newsid=75. Accessed December 11, 2018.
25. Saint Vincent College Newsroom. Professor Kocian reports on opioid crisis to Pennsylvania state house judiciary committee. http://www.stvincent.edu/community-events/newsroom/2017/12/13/professor-kocian-reports-on-opioid-crisis-to-pennsylvania-state-house-judiciary-committee. Accessed December 11, 2018.

20 | Building Effective Public Health and Public Safety Collaborations to Prevent Opioid Overdose at the Local, State, and Federal Levels

JENNIFER J. CARROLL, RITA K. NOONAN, AND JESSICA WOLFF

The Overdose Response Strategy and Public Health and Public Safety Collaboration

For the past two years we have led the public health component of the Overdose Response Strategy (ORS), a public health/public safety collaboration between the Office of National Drug Control Policy (ONDCP)'s High Intensity Drug Trafficking Areas (HIDTAs) program and the US Centers for Disease Control and Prevention (CDC). The ORS is an innovative collaboration between federal and regional entities focused on reducing the number of fatal and nonfatal opioid-related overdoses. As of October 2018, the ORS encompasses 11 HIDTAs covering 24 states and the District of Columbia (Figure 20.1). The mission of the ORS is to reduce opioid overdose incidence by developing and sharing information about heroin, fentanyl, and other opioids across state and federal agencies. In addition, the ORS supports states in implementing evidence-based strategies to combat the opioid overdose epidemic, especially where those strategies are informed by local data. Teams comprising one drug intelligence officer and one public health analyst work in each of the 24 ORS states. These teams are responsible for helping to increase communication, data flow, and intelligence sharing between public safety and public health sectors within and across ORS states.

Through our work with this novel public health and public safety collaboration, we have learned that data collection and data sharing between interdisciplinary partners may produce challenges in new and unexpected ways. This is due in large part to the different values that parties place on data, the use of different vocabulary between partners, and the different tactics public

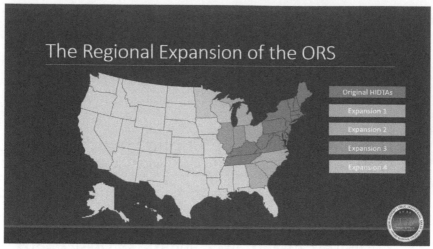

FIGURE 20.1. States participating in the HIDTA/CDC ORS as of October 2018.
Source: US Centers for Disease Control and Prevention, author created.

health and public safety use to achieve a shared goal. These challenges are described below.

Challenges for Public Health and Public Safety Collaboration

Language and Communication

Different orientations to data and to the use of data can cause confusion between partners over even the most mundane features of data science. In our work with the ORS, we have learned that the same terms may carry different meanings for persons from different professional disciplines. For example, consider the term "surveillance." Within public health, surveillance generally means "the continuous, systematic collection, analysis, and interpretation of health-related data needed for the planning, implementation, and evaluation of public health practice."[1] One common method of public health surveillance is called "sentinel surveillance," wherein certain symptoms or conditions (e.g., pneumococcus, overdose, the flu) are uniquely tracked in order to gain a better understanding of that specific epidemiology.

For public safety professionals, however, "surveillance" generally means the various measures that could be used to place a target under scrutiny. It could mean stakeouts, wiretaps, sensors, or police cameras mounted on traffic signals. By naming a particular strategy "sentinel surveillance" one might convey the use of a coordinated network of police surveillance technologies, such as closed-circuit cameras or listening devices. "Sentinel" is even the trademarked name of a line of commercial surveillance technologies available for purchase by local municipalities.[2]

This discrepancy over the term "surveillance" created confusion for us as we were discussing new data-collection technologies with public safety partners. One of those technologies, called the Overdose Detection Mapping Application (ODMAP, described in more detail below), is a tool for mapping the date, time, and approximate location of suspected overdose events. One question that quickly arose when discussing these risks and benefits of ODMAP was whether this system could be used as a tool for surveillance. We, as public health professionals, said "no," our reason being that ODMAP was a system that could not compete for accuracy or completeness with the data already being collected by existing public heath surveillance systems. Our public safety partners also said "no," because they reasoned that all of the data reported to the mapping system would be anonymized, rendering it impossible to identify or track any criminal individual or network through that system. Clearly, we and our partners were not talking about the same thing at all. Yet we all remained completely unaware of our miscommunication, feeling quite satisfied from the nods of agreement around the table that everyone was on the same page. Only later did we realize our error, as debates arose anew as to whether or not ODMAP could be promoted as a public health surveillance tool. We in public health thought this matter had already been settled; our public safety partners insisted that this question had never been raised before. We were each considering the term (and the question it implied) from a very different perspective.

Use and Disclosure of Data

From a legal standpoint, data sharing between law enforcement organizations (LEOs) and public health agencies is complicated by the fact that each sector is governed by rules and regulations that do not apply to the other. Most LEOs maintain shared data protection and distribution protocols. Most often, information held by LEOs is designated as "sensitive but unclassified" or "law enforcement sensitive" (LES). LES information is generally restricted to LEO access only. Such information is often connected to an ongoing investigation, which could be compromised if that information were released to non-LEOs.

The Health Insurance Portability and Accountability Act of 1996 (HIPAA) governs information security and data sharing by health care providers and other organizations that transmit health care data. "Covered entities," those organizations to which HIPAA rules apply, must adhere to strict regulations limiting the use and disclosure of medical records and other personal health information. HIPAA prevents hospitals and emergency services from sharing personal health information with law enforcement and other municipal agencies except under a few, narrowly defined legal circumstances.

As a result of these different regulations, public health and public safety agencies maintain different professional orientations toward each other's data and are trained to perceive different risks and benefits of data disclosure. Consider, for example, the growing practice of LEOs maintaining a list of all known individuals involved in a suspected overdose. Does an identifiable list of suspected overdose victims constitute a health record? Legally, the answer is no. LEOs are not covered entities under HIPAA and are therefore not subject to HIPAA regulations governing data protection and disclosure. However, a better question to ask of public health and public safety partnerships is this: *Should* such a list be treated as a health record, and if so, to what extent should it be maintained under those protocols to protect privacy?

In our experience, differences of opinion about the appropriate use of data rarely have much to do with legal issues. Rather, these disagreements are generally framed in terms of professional ethics, driven by each partner's appreciation for the intent of their own respective regulations. We believe that any collaboration or consensus related to data protection and disclosure between public health and public safety partners will necessarily extend beyond the restrictions set by HIPAA legislation and rules governing LES information. This is because, from a purely legal point of view, neither public health nor public safety organizations are governed by the other's rules and regulations. For this reason, it is of the upmost importance that public health and public safety partners are able to understand and respect the regulatory intent behind HIPAA and LES regulations and develop plans for cooperation that preserve the spirit of each other's professional norms and ethics in addition to respective legal constraints.

Different Approaches to the Protection of Public Welfare

In addition to maintaining different attitudes about data safety and data privacy, public health and public safety organizations also pursue fundamentally different agendas in their service to the community. Through our experience working with ORS, we have found that the explicit recognition of these differences by all parties is crucial for the development of lasting partnerships. In broad terms, public health agencies seek to improve the health and wellness of their communities through population-wide interventions designed to prevent injury, reduce susceptibility to disease, promote healthier behavior, and lower barriers to essential health care services. Public safety is also tasked with maintaining public welfare but does so by monitoring and policing public behavior, disincentivizing criminal behaviors (as opposed to incentivizing healthier or safer choices), and actively dismantling and disrupting socio-economic infrastructures or networks (i.e., the drug market) that encourage or endorse criminal activity. Finally, while public health agencies focus on population-level health, the work of our public safety partners generally centers on the individual.

It is these very differences in the functioning of public health and public safety organizations that so often make their respective activities appear to be at odds. For example, in states with strong syringe services programs, it is not uncommon to find LEOs who perceive such programs to support the very crime-promoting infrastructure they are attempting to dismantle (though it is worth noting that, per current scientific evidence, syringe service programs do *not* promote crime or substance use in their areas of operation).[3,4] Similarly, it is not uncommon to find public health professionals who perceive a local LEO policy of confiscating syringes and other supplies distributed by their program under state paraphernalia laws to be the harmful dismantling of the essential health services that they are actively trying to build. No matter how deep or how trusting public health and public safety partnerships may be, these differences could disrupt otherwise productive dialog.

Examples of Public Health and Public Safety Partnership Success

Early Warning in Ohio

When fentanyl-related overdose fatalities began to grow to alarming proportions in 2014 and 2015, the CDC and the US Drug Enforcement Administration (DEA) released nationwide alerts to inform public health agencies and first responders of this growing threat.[5,6] Unfortunately, delays in availability of data from medical examiners and coroner's offices (often six months or more depending on the level of centralization and the ability these agencies have to prioritize their own toxicology requests in state laboratories) hindered public health's ability to identify areas where fentanyl was having the most impact.

In 2015, a team of Epidemic Intelligence Service officers and staff scientists from the CDC conducted an Epidemiological Assistance (EpiAid) investigation in Ohio to identify risk factors for fentanyl-related overdose fatalities. One of the most up-to-date data sources available to this team was the record of drug seizures (i.e., police confiscations of illicit substances) containing fentanyl reported by the DEA in the National Forensic Laboratory Information System (NFLIS). The team discovered that the number of fentanyl seizures from Ohio reported in NFLIS was predictive, statistically speaking, of the volume of fentanyl-related overdose fatalities reported by medical examiners in the state.[7] In fact, the rates of fentanyl-related overdose and of fentanyl submissions to NFLIS continued to mirror one another as each waxed and waned throughout 2014 (Figure 20.2). This proved to be a particularly

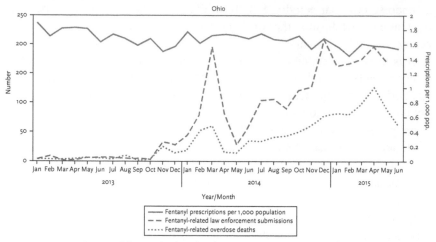

FIGURE 20.2. Rates of fentanyl-related submissions to NFLIS and fentanyl-related overdose deaths in Ohio between the first quarter of 2013 and the second quarter of 2015.[7]

fortuitous finding, as NFLIS data are generally available for review months before medical examiners and coroners in Ohio are able to release death data (as a result of backlog delays in reporting due to toxicological testing or on-going law enforcement investigation). The team determined the connection between these two indicators to be robust enough that NFLIS data could serve as a predictor of fentanyl-related overdose over time.

Soon after, a similar connection was identified between NFLIS submissions and fentanyl-related overdose deaths in Florida.[7] In light of these observations, CDC encourages state and local public health departments to continue looking to NFLIS data for early warning signs of increases in fentanyl-related fatalities.[8] Though the CDC EpiAid team cautioned local analysts to always ensure that these trends are related before jumping to conclusions, they successfully demonstrated that NFLIS and other data on drug seizures carried out by law enforcement can provide new opportunities to rapidly identify drug overdose outbreaks in ways that augment or improve existing public health surveillance systems.

Deliberate Data Sharing at RxStat in New York City

One of the primary challenges of building public health and public safety collaborations for overdose surveillance is the need to standardize different datasets collected and used by different types of agency for different purposes (e.g., police reports, medical records, surveillance data). Not only do the data need to be made comparable in some way, but public health and public safety partners must also be able to make sense of the data with a common point of view. Achieving this level of coordination can take enormous effort. Not only do partners produce different kinds of data for different purposes, but public health and public safety professionals also have limited understanding how the other operates. Differences in organizational culture and approach may prevent partners from seeing opportunities to prevent opioid overdose that are otherwise right in front of them.

Partners from the New York City Department of Health and Mental Hygiene and the New York/New Jersey HIDTA have developed an initiative to bridge these gaps in shared data and understanding. This initiative, called RxStat, convenes representatives from across public agencies with a common goal of preventing opioid overdose at the local level.[9] The diversity of stakeholders included in RxStat is a defining characteristic of the initiative. Participants from the public health sector include substance use disorder treatment providers; local hospital leadership; coordinators for New York's prescription drug monitoring program; emergency medical services providers; and representatives from correctional health, homeless services, child protective services, and social services. The public safety sector is represented by local police departments, district and regional prosecutors, drug law enforcement, the New York/New Jersey HIDTA, and local offices of probation and parole.

RxStat meetings are scheduled by a dedicated coordinator and held monthly in a large conference space provided by the hosting law enforcement agency. The agenda for these meetings is largely dedicated to stakeholders educating one another about their operations and scope of work and to the discussion of findings from existing data. Coordinated investigations are triggered by major events such as sudden, geographically clustered, surges in overdose events. Other triggers include law enforcement identification of potentially lethal drugs in the local market, or a highly publicized fatality where drug poisoning or accidental overdose is suspected. These investigations have resulted in numerous intervention strategies in New York City, including the development of new opioid prescribing guidelines for emergency departments, overdose response and naloxone training for police and other first responders, public health education campaigns to providers on Staten Island, and the identification of previously unknown points of intervention in homeless services to provide overdose prevention services and linkage to care. The designers of the RxStat in New York have produced a technical assistance manual to guide the implementation of this model in other municipalities.[9]

Overdose Response in Erie County, New York

In 2017, the Washington/Baltimore HIDTA launched ODMAP, an online tool that allows first responders to track the location of fatal and nonfatal overdoses and the administration of naloxone by police and first responders in real time. A crucial question from public health and safety officials in using ODMAP data is: How should we act on the information gleaned from this real-time reporting tool? The Erie County Department of Health (ECDOH) in New York, in cooperation with the Cheektowaga Police Department, has developed a novel use for ODMAP: directing post-overdose outreach efforts with information gathered by the ODMAP system.

In Erie County, the Community Coalition Coordinator for ECDOH daily reviews live data in ODMAP to identify nonfatal overdose events that took place in the jurisdiction in the prior 24 hours. The coordinator then contacts the Cheektowaga Police Department to obtain a public copy of the police report for any such events. The coordinator also contacts the medical examiner's office to verify the survival status of people transported to the hospital with uncertain outcomes. ECDOH then arranges a peer recovery coach and an assigned police officer to visit that individual's home. If the overdose survivor is willing to talk to the peer recovery coach, the officer leaves and the peer recovery coach offers information and assistance accessing other services, including referrals for same-day access to medication-assisted treatment (MAT) and naloxone training for the household. From September 1, 2017, to July 16, 2018, ECDOH identified 39 individuals for post-overdose outreach through ODMAP and received an additional 15 direct referrals from law enforcement. Of these, 30 (56%) had enrolled in treatment and were still receiving care after 90 days.

Lessons Learned from Public Health and Public Safety Collaboration

Public health and public safety partnerships can generate both challenges and successes. To support the future growth of these collaborations, we offer several suggestions to public health and public safety partners who are working together to realize positive change in their own communities. These include creating a shared vision, adopting best practices and innovating, and committing to a shared model of success.

Create a Shared Vision (and Document It)

For any collaboration to be successful, all parties need to agree on a shared vision, shared goals, and the best way to achieve those goals. In the ORS, public health and public safety partners collectively agreed that the main goal was the prevention of opioid overdoses. Though there were many interests among our coalition (including the primary prevention of adolescent substance use, harm reduction strategies, and so on), we mutually agreed to set the prevention of overdose fatalities as the primary goal of our partnership. The climbing death toll and the responsibility of public health and public safety professionals to prioritize the preservation of life served as marching orders. We recommend that other coalitions also focus on saving lives as a powerful motivator for action.

Having written agreements to define relationships, such as a memorandum of understanding or memorandum of agreement, is a very helpful, albeit bureaucratic, tool for maintaining productive working relationships with clarity and shared purpose. Our experience illustrates that partners should take the time necessary to define a shared vision but also to document these goals and agreements, the critical pathways toward achieving them, and the measurable outcomes to be used in evaluating success. When conversations veered toward goals or activities that were outside the previously established scope defined by our ORS, we would collectively revisit the founding documents and urge everyone to recommit to the content of the agreements.

Adopt Best Practices and Innovate

As we have described, partners may come to the table holding different views of what strategies are most intuitive or necessary for preventing overdose deaths. To stimulate a conversation about current scientific evidence on what works, CDC compiled a short, user-friendly menu of options for partners that want to address opioid overdose in their community.[10] The base of scientific evidence on what works to prevent opioid overdose is still growing. An enormous opportunity to fill in the gaps in our knowledge lies before us, provided that researchers, advocates, and public servants are willing to collaborate across sectors.

ORS has advanced two new opportunities for such innovation. First, the CDC, as a result of the ORS partnership, provided $2 million to ONDCP to support Combating Opioid Overdose Through Community-level Intervention Initiatives (COOCLI), which is now funding 13 pilot projects, led by public health/public safety partners. These initiatives are producing innovative, evidence-based, replicable solutions to the opioid epidemic in rural, suburban, and urban areas. Encouraged by these early successes, ORS intends to establish the COOCLI program as an ongoing collaboration with ONDCP. Second, on an annual basis, the ORS leverages its unique composition through cornerstone projects, mobilizing all ORS states to address shared informational needs that affect the ORS region as a whole. In 2017, the ORS implemented the "9-1-1 Good Samaritan Law" cornerstone project, which produced the single largest dataset in the United States on police experiences responding to overdose and coordinating with public health agencies. We encourage all public health and public safety collaborations to pursue opportunities for innovation and impact that their partnership makes possible.

Commit to a Shared Model of Success

In any relationship, a shared commitment to "making it work" is a critical factor for success. Establishing this commitment may be easy or difficult depending on the individuals involved; however, each stakeholder's ability to create an *institutional commitment* to the partnership, to value each other's perspective, to share credit for the work (or blame for the failure), to advocate for each other when in the company of our respective professional peers, and to establish tactics for working through difficult issues will be what makes or breaks the partnership in the long run.

Summary

Given the evolving nature of the US opioid overdose epidemic, collaboration between public health and public safety is no longer an option: It simply has to be done if we want to save lives. We believe that the ORS has demonstrated that mutual trust and understanding are foundational to successful partnerships. We hope that by attending to the concerns described in this chapter, future public health/public safety collaborations will be able to achieve successes of their own.

Disclaimer

The findings and conclusions presented in this chapter are those of the authors and do not necessarily represent the views of the US Centers for Disease Control and Prevention.

References

1. World Health Organization (WHO). Public health surveillance. 2018. http://www.who.int/topics/public_health_surveillance/en/. Accessed July 13, 2018.
2. Corbet M. SkyCop "Sentinel" surveillance program gets initial approval from the Memphis City Council. *Memphis Business Journal*, April 19, 2016.
3. Marx MA, Crape B, Brookmeyer RS, et al. Trends in crime and the introduction of a needle exchange program. *Am J Public Health.* 2000; 90(12):1933–1936.
4. Potier C, Laprévote V, Dubois-Arber F, et al. Supervised injection services: What has been demonstrated? A systematic literature review. *Drug Alcohol Depend.* 2014; 145:48–68.
5. US Centers for Disease Control and Prevention. Increases in fentanyl drug confiscations and fentanyl-related overdose fatalities. 2015. http://emergency.cdc.gov/han/han00384.asp#_edn5. Accessed February 25, 2016.

6. US Drug Enforcement Administration. DEA issues nationwide alert on fentanyl as threat to health and public safety. 2015. https://www.dea.gov/divisions/hq/2015/hq031815.shtml. Accessed August 7, 2018.
7. Peterson AB, Gladden RM, Delcher C, et al. Increases in fentanyl-related overdose deaths—Florida and Ohio, 2013–2015. *MMWR Morb Mortal Wkly Rep.* 2016;65(33):844–849.
8. US Centers for Disease Control and Prevention. Rising numbers of deaths involving fentanyl and fentanyl analogs, including carfentanil, and increased usage and mixing with non-opioids. 2018. https://emergency.cdc.gov/han/han00413.asp. Accessed August 7, 2018.
9. Heller D, Bradley O'Brien D, Harocopos A, et al. *RxStat: Technical Assistance Manual.* 2014. New York: New York City Department of Health; 2014.
10. Carroll JJ, Green TC, Noonan RK. Evidence-based strategies for prevention opioid overdose: What's working in the United States. 2018. http://www.cdc.gov/drugoverdose/pdf/pubs/2018-evidence-based-strategies.pdf. Accessed October 10, 2018.

21 | Public Health Surveillance and the Opioid Crisis

JEFFREY P. ENGEL, VALERIE N. GOODSON, MEGAN TOE,
AND MICHAEL LANDEN

PUBLIC HEALTH SURVEILLANCE IS a core activity of governmental public health agencies at the local, state, and federal level. State and local agencies have the authority to acquire health data about the population served or require reports from licensed providers of certain medically attended diseases and conditions. This authority forms the basis for fulfilling the first two of 10 essential public health services:[1]

1. Monitor health status to identify and solve community health problems
2. Diagnose and investigate health problems and health hazards in the community.

Public health surveillance is defined as the ongoing systematic collection of outcome data that are then analyzed and interpreted for the use of public health practice.[2] The roles of observation, investigation, and taking action are key for public health practitioners who often serve as first contacts with the public, medical professionals, and the systems where disease information is stored and used for follow-up and synthesis. These roles are well established in the infectious disease realm; however, as they relate to noninfectious diseases, and more specifically the current opioid epidemic, there is little standardization between states on what is being surveilled, and the definitions for some of the most important elements of the crisis, such as what constitutes an overdose death from opioids, differ (Text Box 21.1).

Without standard definitions and processes, public health practitioners may develop response protocols based on inaccurate data. As such, the opioid epidemic presents many challenges for public health surveillance, including the lack of a national behavioral health surveillance system;[3] reporting after the fact, which limits the ability for case-based follow-up; and the use of a

---

TEXT BOX 21.1 COUNCIL OF STATE AND TERRITORIAL EPIDEMIOLOGISTS' NONFATAL OPIOID OVERDOSE STANDARDIZED SURVEILLANCE CASE DEFINITION

In January 2019, the Council of State and Territorial Epidemiologists (CSTE) Executive Board approved an interim position statement on nonfatal opioid overdose standardized surveillance case definition to address the need for consistency across jurisdictions to improve national surveillance. The statement was designed to support case reporting based on public health legal authorities and traditional public health surveillance practice of case identification, follow-up investigation when possible, and identifying and combining case data across data sources. It includes (1) reporting from individual health care providers, hospitals (especially emergency departments), EMS, poison control centers, laboratories, harm reduction or comprehensive syringe service programs, and law enforcement and (2) case ascertainment or identification of potential cases by public health from administrative data (e.g., identification based on discharge diagnosis codes in hospital discharge) or from syndromic surveillance using data from emergency departments, urgent care centers, EMS, or poison control centers, where individual records are used to conduct additional case investigation in order to have data to complete and finalize case classification. The case definition for Interim-CC-19, Nonfatal Opioid Overdose Standardized Surveillance, was updated and ratified by the Council in June 2019 as 19-CC-01. The full document including data sources, ascertainment, and classification, can be found at www.cste.org.

---

variety of indicators and metrics, yielding a lack of capture of the true burden of disease.

Monitoring health status and investigating health problems define the purposes of public health surveillance, which historically developed to address communicable (infectious) diseases and environmental toxins. Event-based (and often mandated) reporting of persons afflicted by these conditions facilitates limiting exposure in the population. Hence, disease occurrence clustered in time and space can be readily investigated by a public health agency to identify the source and prevent further cases and spread of disease. Event-based surveillance, in addition to disease detection and control, also monitors population health interventions such as a mandated immunization program for school-aged children. An important consideration for this traditional form of public health surveillance is that reportability usually includes the authority to collect personal, identifiable information by the public health agency to track and monitor disease and identify contacts.

Public health surveillance of opioid use, opioid use disorder, and their consequences, including fatal and nonfatal drug overdose, is a relatively new activity for public health surveillance but has been included in decades-old public health surveillance systems and surveys. The US Substance Use and Mental Health Services Agency (SAMHSA) has administered a national survey, the National Survey on Drug Use and Health (NSDUH), since 1971 to track opioid use, opioid use disorder, and treatment for opioid use disorders. SAMHSA also funded the Drug Abuse Warning Network (DAWN) from 1974 to 2011, which focused on determining drugs causing nonfatal overdose in emergency departments. The US Centers for Disease Control and Prevention (CDC), through injury surveillance, has traditionally focused on the surveillance of poisoning and poisoning deaths. Additionally, the national network of poison control centers has aggregated reports of poisonings into several reports since 1958.

Historically, poisoning deaths had been the major focus of public health surveillance of the burden of opioid use and addiction in the 1980s and 1990s, with a focus on heroin overdose death in studies from Australia and certain locations in the United States, such as Portland, Oregon; Seattle, Washington; and New Mexico.[4-8] With the evolution of the International Statistical Classification of Diseases and Related Health Problems (ICD) system to ICD-10 in 1999, states began to review T-codes that specify drugs causing death, and it was noted that patterns of drugs causing death varied by state, emphasizing the need for state-based poisoning-death surveillance.[9] Unfortunately, having T-codes did not require specific coding of drugs causing death, as about half of the substances were nonspecific, including 27% classified only as "other and unspecified drugs, medicaments [sic] and biologic substances." In the early 2000s, reports began noting the increase of prescription opioid poisoning deaths.[10] The emergence of prescription opioids as a major cause of drug overdose death was followed by heroin, fentanyl, and other synthetic opioids. These epidemiologic trends have focused attention on the need for consistent surveillance methods, specific drug-cause coding, and timely analysis and reporting of data.

With the emergence of prescription opioids as a major cause of drug overdose death in the early 2000s, prescription drug monitoring programs (PDMPs) took hold as an important tool to track which controlled substances were dispensed, by which prescribers, and to which patients. PDMPs allow for specific tracking of prescription opioid prescribing trends at the state level as well as at the individual patient level. Linkage of PDMP data with fatal and nonfatal overdose data has become a particularly useful approach, and an increasing number of health departments have access to PDMP data for public health purposes.

Nonfatal drug overdose surveillance has emerged as an important tool alongside the development of the PDMP. Emergency department–based overdose surveillance, frequently in the form of syndromic surveillance, is being used more frequently, particularly thanks to Enhanced State Opioid Overdose Surveillance (ESOOS) funding for state and territorial programs from the CDC. A major challenge to this approach occurred with the transition to ICD-10-CM in 2015, which resulted in the need to develop new case definitions for nonfatal opioid overdose, a process that is continuing.

With the quintupling of annual opioid overdose deaths in the United States from 8,050 in 1999 to 47,600 in 2017,[11] the approach to the public health surveillance of opioid use, opioid use disorder, and their consequences, including fatal and nonfatal overdose, has substantially changed. Our current approaches can be best understood within the context of general public health surveillance and are described below.

Methods of Public Health Surveillance

Public health surveillance systems rely on both the public and the private sectors. Essentially, the system is a coordinated and legalized effort of a governmental public health agency, a health care provider or organization, and the public at large. A robust surveillance system allows the reliable and timely collection of health data that are used for public health action to reduce disease burden on society. Thus, the system requires a data source; collection of data from the source; and storage, analysis, and reporting, including data visualization and dissemination to initiate and inform public health actions to reduce disease burden. Surveillance systems for substance abuse, specifically opioids, are an important tool for public health. Table 21.1 summarizes the surveillance systems and methods discussed in this chapter.

Table 21.1 also illustrates the multiple government and nongovernment agency involvement at the federal, state, and local level and the multiple opportunities for nonstandardized methodologic approaches and data sources to be used. The systems listed vary considerably in their accuracy, completeness, and timeliness but can be complementary when used programmatically by a governmental or jurisdictional public health agency to monitor various aspects of the opioid problem in populations. DAWN is a federal program that was established by the US Drug Enforcement Administration (DEA) in 1974, transferred to the National Institute of Drug Abuse (NIDA) in 1980, and then transferred to the SAMHSA in 1992. The original system collected information from a select number of metropolitan-area hospitals to track emergency department visits associated with drug abuse. DAWN's stated goal was to identify and establish patterns of drug abuse and assess trends over time.

In 2003, SAMHSA redesigned the system to expand anonymous data collection of all drug-related medical emergencies. The updated version allowed SAMHSA to release data at shorter intervals (monthly compared to annually) and served as an early warning system for participating cities.[12] Though DAWN

TABLE 21.1. Surveillance Systems in Use or Available for Opioid Drug Abuse

SYSTEM	METHOD	DATA SOURCE	AGENCY/CENTER
DAWN	Sentinel	Hospital ED visits	SAMHSA/CBHSQ
NSDUH	Survey	Randomly selected individuals	SAMHSA/CBHSQ
HCUP-NEDS	Event-based	Hospital ED visit claims	AHRQ
NHCS	Survey	Hospital discharges	CDC/NCHS
PDMP	Event-based	Dispensed controlled substance prescriptions	State
ESOOS, SUDORS	Event-based	Hospital ED EHR, toxicology reports, death scene investigation	State, CDC/NCIPC
Poison Control	Call-based	Public, provider, other	State, territorial, and regional Poison Centers
National Overdose Deaths	Event based	Death certificate	State, CDC/NCHS

ED, emergency department; EHR, electronic health record.
Source: Authors' research.

data were not nationally representative and the work of case finding through chart reviews required additional staffing, DAWN provided a timely opportunity for action and follow-up on drug-related events. DAWN was discontinued in 2011, although some of its components were transferred from 2012 to 2017 to the CDC's National Center for Health Statistics (NCHS) National Hospital Care Survey (reviewed below); however, its usefulness as an early warning system was lost. DAWN was refunded by Congress in 2016 and is scheduled to recommence under SAMHSA's direction in 2019.

SAMHSA also conducts the National Survey on Drug Use and Health (NSDUH), a yearly survey collecting information on tobacco, alcohol, drug use, mental health, and other health-related issues. The sample includes residents of all 50 states and the District of Columbia. NSDUH data is used by policymakers, researchers, public health entities, and a variety of other agencies to make informed decisions about prevention and treatment efforts, funding, and educational materials.[13] While not timely because data are released up to two years after collection, NSDUH data provides decision makers with an opportunity to review population estimates for change over time as it relates to drug use. NSDUH has limitations as a public health surveillance system because it is a relatively small randomized sample conducted through telephone interviews. The sample size limits generalizability to small-area populations, making it less useful for rural populations.

The Healthcare Cost and Utilization Project (HCUP) sponsored by the US Agency for Healthcare Research and Quality (AHRQ) is a national database providing patient discharge data. The HCUP's Nationwide Emergency Department Sample (NEDS) provides annual national estimates of all payer hospital emergency department visits. The annual release of data comes approximately 18 months after year-end, limiting the timeliness of the information provided.[14] The strength of NEDS is the completeness of data, estimating millions of annual emergency department visits throughout the United States, including all payers and the uninsured; it provides patient demographic characteristics and information on the hospital where the patient was treated and multiple clinical and nonclinical variables for each encounter. As an administrative database based on hospital billing codes, the accuracy of the data may be compromised because billing codes optimize hospital reimbursements and may not reflect the primary reason for the hospital visit.

The National Hospital Care Survey (NHCS) is a data collection tool to track national patterns of health care services within hospital settings. The assessment tool collects personal identifiers, which allows for linkage of records to other systems such as the National Death Index. Data on patient care are collected from a sample of US-based hospitals to be used by policymakers and researchers to understand trends impacting the health care delivery system.[15] These national statistics on health care utilization are published by NCHS under a restricted-access file and are not available for up to three years after they are collected. While this system collects data on individual patients over time, access to use the data to inform decision makers about emerging threats is limited.

Though their use is not mandated in all states and territories, PDMPs are data collection systems operated at the state level by health departments, boards of pharmacy, or law enforcement agencies. PDMPs were originally developed for use by clinicians and law enforcement to monitor and evaluate prescription dispensing information. However, in response to the increase in prescription pain management using opioids, PDMPs became a useful tool to identify individuals and prescribers who may be contributing to opioid misuse and abuse. PDMPs serve as a useful surveillance tool because data are entered by dispensing pharmacies soon after filling, most updating daily. Additionally, the prescriber's DEA number is linked with each record, so querying the system can identify possible overprescription. The system also allows identification of "doctor shopping" by persons who may be misusing or diverting opioids. PDMPs are limited as a public health surveillance system because they cannot predict or confirm ingestion of the medication by the patient, have various levels of access for public health agency staff, and in some jurisdictions are linked to or even managed by law enforcement agencies.

The CDC's National Center for Injury Prevention and Control (NCIPC) has developed robust public health surveillance for the opioid epidemic using the injury prevention paradigm. ESOOS directly funds 32 states and the District of Columbia to improve the timeliness and the quality of data on drug overdose and emphasizes the public health model of surveillance data for action.[16] ESOOS incorporates the State Unintentional Drug Overdose Reporting Surveillance (SUDORS) module into the National Violent Death Reporting System (NVDRS) to report overdose mortality. SUDORS data include demographics; circumstances of death; toxicology results; data from law enforcement, death certificates, prescription drug monitoring program, emergency medical services, and death scene investigations; drug use and treatment history; and other documented circumstances and risk factors. As part of the ESOOS's aim to improve data timeliness, fatal opioid overdoses are reported within eight months of death. Funded states submit SUDORS data twice yearly. Strengths and limitations of SUDORS data depend on the data quality of death certificates, medical examiner and coroner reports, and toxicology reports. The improved timeliness, accuracy, and completeness of the data, including the ability to identify and report polysubstance use and decedent circumstances, are strengths of ESOOS for drug overdose mortality. For overdose morbidity, the non-SUDORS component of ESOOS relies on hospital emergency department and emergency medical services (EMS) data. Similar to other systems described that use emergency department data, ESOOS sources include hospital billing data, facing the constraints of timeliness and accuracy.

A promising and emerging public health surveillance system for the opioid epidemic is syndromic surveillance, where local and state jurisdictions collect electronically a line-listing of every emergency department visit at participating hospitals. Reporting may be voluntary or mandated, depending on state and local laws and ordinances. De-identified lists include several data elements, such as age, gender, ZIP code of residence, and, unique to this system, chief complaint and nurse triage notes. Within hours to days, discharge diagnoses from ICD-10 codes are added to the line-listing. The CDC's Center for Surveillance, Epidemiology and Laboratory Services (CSELS) assembles syndromic data on the National Syndromic Surveillance Program (NSSP) platform (also known as BioSense). The strength of syndromic surveillance is its timeliness because it provides near real-time analysis and the ability to track outbreaks and provide situational awareness. By relying on both diagnosis codes and natural language algorithms of the chief complaint and nurse triage notes, syndromic surveillance for overdose morbidity is increasingly used as a rapid source of information. As a national system, CDC and states are working to incorporate NSSP methods into ESOOS, and the challenges include a need for standardized definitions and validation of the method as an accurate public health surveillance system for opioid overdose. Another limitation is the anonymity of the system, preventing public health agencies from identifying patients who have overdosed to link them to addiction care or to conduct community investigations of overdose clusters.

The United States has 55 poison control centers, with each center reporting calls received regarding poison exposure within minutes. The timeliness of the system is unique and enables real-time updates for public health departments, policymakers, and the public. System weaknesses include concerns about the completeness and accuracy of the data, given that the data are based solely on the number of calls received. Some jurisdictions combine call center data with their syndromic surveillance systems for more complete data, but national validation and usefulness of this approach is lacking.

Mortality surveillance is conducted by the CDC's NCHS National Vital Statistics System (NVSS). It provides death certificate data, including overdose deaths, from state vital registrars. National mortality data are released 12 months after the end of the data year. To address the lack of timeliness, NCHS releases quarterly provisional estimates and vital statistics rapid release reports. These currently include monthly provisional counts of drug overdose deaths. An advantage of the national mortality data is their completeness and accuracy, with validated case definitions for overdose deaths; however there is a need to improve both the drug specificity and timeliness of information.

What Is Next for Public Health Surveillance and the Opioid Crisis?

The major challenge of public health surveillance of opioid misuse in populations is the lack of an historical and consistent government approach to behavioral health and substance use surveillance. The technical problems that result include the lack of standardized measures and consistent data access (e.g., PDMP) at health departments throughout the United States. Consensus recommendations for surveillance case definitions and indicators can ensure that public health agencies are consistently identifying comparable data and allow for a more accurate calculation and reporting of the local, state, and national impact, ultimately leading to public health action (see Text Box 21.1). Connections between opioid overdose and other conditions associated with substance use and mental illness require a broader, less siloed or stovepiped public health approach to diseases of despair.

Standard surveillance, particularly for analysis of hospitalization and emergency department data, is necessary to ensure accurate, consistent measurement across the United States. Areas of recent improvement include the expansion of

CDC's opioid overdose prevention funding programs to states, with required reporting measures, and coordination between medical examiners, coroners, and epidemiologists to improve the specificity of overdose death certificate reporting. Federal, state, and local epidemiologists need to develop guidance for ICD-10-CM drug poisoning case definitions and a standardized surveillance case definition for nonfatal opioid overdose. State health departments require sustained funding and technical assistance to implement and maintain these standardized methods for long-term reporting and ongoing data- informed intervention and policy efforts.

To address issues of drug coding specificity, recommendations to improve death certificate data call for coordinated efforts by vital registrars, medical examiners, and coroners.[17] In 2015, the Council of State and Territorial Epidemiologists (CSTE) created an epidemiologic tool to analyze the free text on death certificates, and in 2016 the group released "Recommendations and Lessons Learned for Improved Reporting of Drug Overdose Deaths on Death Certificates." The CDC's NCHS needs to accelerate progress with state and local medicolegal death investigators and public health surveillance to implement recommendations for improved completeness and consistency in drug overdose investigation, toxicology testing, and death reporting. Access to key data sources is not currently uniform across states, with some state health departments having limited access to their state PDMP, and some state and local health departments not consistently receiving hospitalization and emergency department data. PDMP and hospital data are essential for a complete public health surveillance system.

A skilled epidemiology workforce is critical for public health surveillance. The need for further investment in workforce development and capacity building in health department injury and substance use expertise can provide long-term benefits to address the opioid crisis. The 2017 CSTE Epidemiology Capacity Assessment Report identified the need for 63 additional substance use epidemiologists nationally, with 93% of state public health agencies indicating that they need to improve their capacity for substance use surveillance.[18] A critical component of appropriate public health surveillance is the ability to use the data collected to inform both prevention and treatment. Improved capacity and development of state public health substance use and injury epidemiologists will enable improved "data to action" and the ability to inform evidence-based interventions for communities and individuals in need. Additionally, workforce development of behavioral health and substance use epidemiologists at public health departments, including fellowships and early and mid-career internships, are needed. Early career mentorship and ongoing technical assistance, trainings, and resource dissemination for epidemiologists at all stages of their careers, will also improve capacity.

A new opportunity for public health epidemiologists is to shift the surveillance approach to include case-based reporting as infectious disease surveillance has been funded to do. Identifying nonfatal overdose cases enables public health and care providers to intervene and provide linkage to care and harm reduction programs. By incorporating case-based reporting, consistent with the National Notifiable Disease Surveillance System format that receives sufficient funding, public health can replicate the successes used in infectious diseases to intervene in nonfatal cases. As more states are declaring drug overdose a state reportable condition, opportunities to evaluate the effectiveness of various interventions based on nonfatal opioid overdose case reporting are increasing. At the federal level, improved coordination among the various agencies and their surveillance systems can address gaps and ensure programmatic and consistent systems.

Summary

This chapter describes some of the national public health surveillance programs and initiatives for opioid use, opioid use disorder, and their consequences. Promising practices are emerging to improve data collection and the exchange of information between public health and health care to improve accuracy, completeness, and timeliness. PDMP, syndromic surveillance, and poison center call data all are capable of real-time data flows but need synthesis into standardized surveillance systems and validation of methods. Adequate, long-term funding for overdose surveillance is required to ensure the continued use and improvement of these systems. Newer technologies need to replace static datasets like the medical encounters captured only by hospital discharges. Not reviewed here are electronic case reporting and electronic laboratory reporting that use clinical decision support algorithms operating within the electronic medical record to automatically send data to public health. These systems are in use or in development for infectious disease surveillance. Electronic death reporting is improving timeliness as well, but toxicology results from postmortem samples need shorter turnaround times. Legal authority will need to accompany automated technological advances to ensure protection of patient confidentiality, minimize stigma, and not confound health reports with criminal activity.

A prepared public health workforce will be necessary to manage newer technologies and interface better with behavioral health and substance use agencies. More epidemiologists are needed in the field of behavioral health and substance use surveillance, and workforce development is particularly needed in early and mid-career public health agency epidemiology staff. The practicing epidemiologist will also need much more training in the field of information science and data exchange, particularly as systems come online that vastly improve bidirectional information flow with health care providers. Ending the crisis will most certainly require a prepared public health workforce capable of managing modern systems with common definitions to improve our response to this devastating opioid epidemic.

References

1. US Centers for Disease Control and Prevention (CDC). The 10 Essential Public Health Services. 2018. https://www.cdc.gov/publichealthgateway/publichealthservices/essentialhealthservices.html Accessed July 23, 2018.
2. Teutsch SM, Churchill, RE. *Principles and Practice of Public Health Surveillance*. 2nd ed. New York: Oxford University Press; 2000.
3. Lyerla R, Stroup DF. Toward a public health surveillance system for behavioral health. *Public Health Rep*. 2018; 133(4):360–365.
4. Fingerhut LA, Cox CS, Warner M. *International Comparative Analysis of Injury Mortality. Findings from the ICE on Injury Statistics*. Advance Data from Vital and Health Statistics, no. 303. Hyattsville, MD: NCHS; 1998.
5. Garrick TM, Sheedy BA, Abernathy J, et al. Heroin-related deaths in Sydney, Australia. How common are they? *Am J Addict*. 2000; 9(2):172–178.
6. US Centers for Disease Control and Prevention (CDC). Heroin overdose deaths—Multnomah County, Oregon, 1993–1999. *MMWR Morb Mortal Wkly Rep*. 2000; 49(28):633–636.
7. US Centers for Disease Control and Prevention (CDC). Unintentional opiate overdose deaths—King County, Washington, 1990–1999. *MMWR Morb Mortal Wkly Rep*. 2000; 49(28):636–640.
8. Landen M, Castle S, Nolte K, et al. Methodological issues in the surveillance of poisoning, illicit drug overdose, and heroin overdose deaths in New Mexico. *Am J Epidemiol*. 2003; 157(3):273–278.
9. US Centers for Disease Control and Prevention (CDC). Unintentional and undetermined poisoning deaths—11 states, 1990–2001. *MMWR Morb Mortal Wkly Rep*. 2004; 53(11):233–238.
10. Ballesteros MF, Budnitz, DS, Sanford CP. Increase in deaths due to methadone in North Carolina. *JAMA*. 2003; 290(1):40.
11. Scholl L, Seth P, Kariisa M, et al. Drug and opioid-involved overdose deaths—United States, 2013–2017. *MMWR Morb Mortal Wkly Rep*. 2019; 67:1419–1427.
12. US Substance Abuse and Mental Health Services Administration. Drug Abuse Warning Network (DAWN). https://www.samhsa.gov/data/data-we-collect/dawn-drug-abuse-warning-network. Accessed December 30, 2018.
13. US Substance Abuse and Mental Health Services Administration. National survey on drug abuse and health. https://www.samhsa.gov/data/data-we-collect/nsduh-national-survey-drug-use-and-health. Accessed December 30, 2018.
14. US Agency for Healthcare Research and Quality (AHRQ). Overview of the Nationwide Emergency Department Sample (NEDS). 2018. https://www.hcup-us.ahrq.gov/nedsoverview.jsp. Accessed January 2, 2019.

15. US Centers for Disease Control and Prevention. About the National Hospital Care Survey. 2018. https://www.cdc.gov/nchs/nhcs/index.htm. Accessed December 30, 2018.
16. US Centers for Disease Control and Prevention. Enhanced state opioid overdose surveillance. 2017. https://www.cdc.gov/drugoverdose/foa/state-opioid-mm.html. Accessed December 30, 2018.
17. Slavova S, O'Brien D, Creppage K, et al. Drug overdose deaths: Let's get specific. *Public Health Rep*. 2015; 130(4):339–342.
18. Arrazola J, Binkin N, Israel M, et al. Assessment of epidemiology capacity in state health departments—United States, 2017. *MMWR Morb Mortal Wkly Rep*. 2018; 67:935–939.

22 | The Role of Prescription Drug Monitoring Programs (PDMPs) in Addressing the Opioid Overdose Epidemic

GRANT BALDWIN, JAN L. LOSBY, WESLEY M. SARGENT, JR., JAMIE MELLS, AND SARAH BACON

History of Opioid Prescribing and the Use of PDMPs

Deaths involving prescription opioids in the United States increased in lock-step with increases in opioid prescribing beginning in the late 1990s.[1] In 2016, over 17,000 people died from prescription opioids, the most ever recorded in the United States.[2] The increase of opioid-related deaths was largely the result of proliferate use of prescription opioids to treat chronic non-cancer pain in the United States.[3,4] The number of opioid prescriptions peaked in 2012 at 289 million prescriptions, or 82.5 prescriptions per 100 persons in the United States.[5,6] From 1999 to 2010, opioid prescribing per capita measured in morphine milligram equivalents (MME) increased more than fourfold, from 180 MME to 782 MME.[7] While opioid prescribing has decreased since 2012, the rate of 512 MME per capita in 2017 is still nearly three times the amount prescribed in 1999.[8]

Moreover, opioid prescribing varies markedly across the United States. In one study, the opioid prescribing rate per 100 persons varied 2.7-fold from Alabama to Hawaii, the highest to lowest prescribing states respectively.[6] When looking at prescribing rates at the county level, differences are even more pronounced. County-level prescribing varied nearly sixfold in 2017 between highest and lowest counties.[8] Importantly, this variation in prescribing cannot be explained fully by underlying differences in demographic characteristics or the prevalence of conditions treated with opioids.[6]

PDMPs are secure, online, state-based databases that contain detailed information about controlled substance prescriptions written by clinicians and dispensed by pharmacists within a jurisdiction.[9] There are 53 operational PDMPs located in 50 states, the District of Columbia, Puerto Rico, and Guam.[10] Moreover, there are two national platforms (RxCheck from the US Department of Justice's Bureau of Justice Assistance and PMP InterConnect from the National Association of Boards of Pharmacy) that facilitate bilateral exchange of PDMP data across states. Currently 46 states and the District of Columbia are exchanging data with other states via one or both of these existing PDMP data hubs.[11,12]

Dispensers (e.g., pharmacists, dispensing clinicians) are responsible for entering the required controlled substance prescriptions into state PDMPs. States determine which drugs are monitored and required to be reported by dispensers, and it ranges nationally from Schedules II–IV to II–V.[10] Dispensers may also be required to report other drugs of concern that are not scheduled (e.g., gabapentin), and this varies from jurisdiction to jurisdiction. The central aim of a PDMP is reduce the diversion and misuse of controlled substances such as prescription opioids.[9] In addition, PDMPs are used to monitor prescribing trends by insurers and health system administrators as well as by public health practitioners responsible for population-level surveillance.[13]

In addition to informing point-of-care clinical decision making to improve patient safety and alert clinicians to a patient's use of multiple providers or multiple pharmacies, PDMPs are an asset to other professions.[9] Law enforcement officials and others in the criminal justice sector may use data collected by PDMPs when investigating unusual prescribing patterns or assessing whether someone might be operating a "pill mill."[9] Pill mills are pain management clinics where a high volume of prescription drugs is inappropriately prescribed and dispensed.[14] Law enforcement officials may also use PMDP data in drug courts and other criminal diversion programs.[13] Medical licensing boards use PMDP data to assess aberrant prescribing practices by clinicians.[9] Health systems, insurers, and public health officials use aggregated PDMP data as part of their efforts to evaluate a quality improvement initiative, an opioid stewardship program to improve opioid prescribing system-wide, or broad changes in prescribing patterns across a city, county, or state.[9] Finally, medical examiners and coroners use PDMP data when assessing the circumstances of a drug overdose death.[13]

Initially, PDMPs were set up as tools for law enforcement to monitor and enforce drug laws.[15] The first PDMP was set up in New York in 1918 as a means to address a growing drug problem.[15] At the time, heroin and cocaine were prescribed by clinicians and dispensed at pharmacies in accordance with federal and state law.[15] California established a PDMP in 1939; over the next 50 years seven more states followed suit, and these PDMPs remain in operation today: Hawaii (1943), Illinois (1961), Pennsylvania (1972), New York (1973), Rhode Island (1978), Texas (1981), and Michigan (1989).[15] These initial PDMPs were paper-based, so data often lagged weeks or months behind when the prescription was written or dispensed; they were used primarily by law enforcement officials to monitor prescribing of Schedule II controlled substances.[15] Prior to PMDPs becoming computerized systems, multi-copy (duplicate or triplicate), serialized state-issued prescribing forms were used to catalog prescribing practices.[15] In the case of triplicate forms, one copy remained with the clinician, one copy remained with the pharmacist, and one copy was sent to the state agency administering the PDMP.[15]

In 1990, Oklahoma became the first state to use electronic transmission of PDMP data.[15] The ever-expanding computer and internet revolutions made it easier and safer to securely store and share PDMP data and to better integrate those data into clinical workflow.[15] In addition to Oklahoma, six other states or territories added PDMPs in the 1990s: Massachusetts (1992), Nevada and Utah (1995), Indiana (1997), and Guam and Kentucky (1998). The number of states and territories with operational PDMPs rapidly accelerated at the beginning of the 21st century for two reasons. First, there was growing concern about nonfatal overdoses and overdose-related deaths from prescription opioids.[15] Second, federal funding for PDMPs became available.[15] In 2002, the Harold Rogers Prescription Drug Monitoring Grant Program was established by the Bureau of Justice Assistance to establish PDMPs.[15] To further support PDMP development, funding became available in 2005 through the National All Schedules Prescription Electronic Reporting Act, administered by the US Substance Abuse and Mental Health Services Administration (SAMHSA).[15] Starting in 2015, the US Centers for Disease Control and Prevention (CDC) started funding a number of states to expand and maximize the use of PDMPs through the Overdose Prevention in States Initiative. By 2018, all 50 states, Washington DC, and Guam reported functioning PDMPs.[15]

Clinical Uses and Public Health Applications of State-Based PDMPs

As states began legislating the creation of PDMPs, a substantial amount of variation developed between them, particularly because the practice of medicine is regulated at the state level. Specifically, there are differences in which state office manages the PDMP, which drugs are included in the PDMP, how timely the data are in the PDMP, who has access to PDMP data, how PDMP data can be used, whether PDMP data are integrated into clinical electronic health records (EHRs) and if data are shared with other states, and whether clinicians are required by state law to register and use the PDMP. For example, concerns about individual patient privacy, security of large data systems, and infringing on clinician discretion in the practice of medicine are drivers of these differences. This between-state variability influences the utility and value of PDMP data. Table 22.1 illustrates the differences in PDMPs across states.[10]

TABLE 22.1. Select Differences in State PDMPs, August 2018

CHARACTERISTIC	STATES OR TERRITORIES

Operating State Agency

Pharmacy Board (n = 20): AK, AZ, CO, IA, ID, KS, LA, MN, MS, MT, ND, NH, NM, NV, OH, SD, TN, TX, WV, WY

Department of Health (n = 18): AL, AR, DC, FL, GA, GU, IL, KY, MA, MO, NE, NY, OR, PA, RI, SC, VT, WA

Professional Licensing Agency (n = 6): DE, IN, MI, UT, VA, WI

Law Enforcement (n = 4): CA, HI, NJ, OK

Substance Abuse Agency (n = 4): MD, ME, NC, PR

Consumer Protection Agency (n = 1): CT

Schedules of Drugs Covered

Schedules II–V Only (n = 14): AZ, CO, FL, GA, MD, MI, MT, NC, NM, OK, PA, PR, SD, TX

Schedules II–V and Drugs of Concern* (n = 27): AL, AR, CT, DC, DE, GU, HI, ID, IL, IN, KY, LA, MA, MN, MS, ND, NE, NJ, NY, OH, TN, UT, VA, WA, WI, WV, WY

Schedule II–IV Only (n = 10): AK, CA, IA, ME, MO, NH, NV, RI, SC, VT

Schedule II–IV and Drugs of Concern* (n = 2): KS, OR

Data Collection Frequency

Point of Sale (n = 1): OK

Point of Sale/24 Hours (n = 2): NY, UT

Daily or Next Business Day (n = 45): AK, AL, AR, AZ, CO, CT, DC, DE, FL, GA, IA, ID, IL, IN, KS, KY, LA, MA, MD, ME, MI, MN, MO, MS, MT, NC, ND, NE, NH, NJ, NM, NV, OH, PA, RI, SC, SD, TN, TX, VA, VT, WA, WI, WV, WY

2 or 3 Days (n = 2): OR and PR

7 Days (n = 2): CA, HI

14Days (n = 1): GU

Mandatory Enrollment of Prescribers and Dispensers

Prescribers and Dispensers (n = 31): AK, AR, AZ, CA, CO, FL, ID, IN, KY, LA, MD, ME, MN, MS, MT, NC, ND, NH, NJ, NM, NV, OH, OR, PA, RI, TN, TX, VA, VT, WV, WY

Prescribers Only (n = 12): AL,CT, DE, GA, IA, HI, IL, MA, MI, SD, UT, WA

Dispensers Only (n = 1): GU

No Mandatory Enrollment (n = 9): DC, KS, MO, NE, NY, OK, PR, SC, WI

---

*Drugs of concern include butalbital-containing products that are not controlled. In some states this also includes ephedrine, pseudoephedrine, and phenylpropanolamine-containing products.

Source: Authors' own work and Brandeis University, Prescription Drug Monitoring Program Training and Technical Assistance Program. PDMP Maps and Tables. 2018. http://www.pdmpassist.org/content/pdmp-maps-and-tables. Accessed December 4, 2018.

PDMPs have an important role in public health both as a clinical tool and a tool for public health surveillance. As a tool to help inform clinical decisions, PDMPs' potential utility was highlighted in CDC's "Guideline for Prescribing Opioids for Chronic Pain."[16] CDC recommends that clinicians review a patient's controlled substance prescriptions using state PDMP data to determine whether the patient is receiving opioid dosages or dangerous concurrent prescriptions of opioids and benzodiazepines that may put him or her at high risk for overdose. CDC recommends that clinicians review PDMP data when starting opioid therapy for chronic pain and periodically during opioid therapy for chronic pain, ranging from every prescription to every three months.[16] Patterns of concern in the PDMP include obtaining medications from multiple providers and filling prescriptions at multiple pharmacies, especially when prescriptions are filled in quick succession or on the same day, or when filling prescriptions far from the patient's address on record. To address the concern that some patients with chronic pain may not have access to opioid medications, Green, Mann, and Bowman[17] recommend that prescribers discuss what they are seeing in the PDMP with patients rather than making a judgment that could result in the patient not receiving appropriate care.

In addition to their clinical application in managing patient care, PDMPs are also used for epidemiologic surveillance and to assist in substance abuse monitoring, evaluation, and prevention efforts. The data contained in PDMPs can be used in a manner analogous to a disease registry that supports epidemiologic analyses and interventions when an outbreak or epidemic is detected. PDMP data can serve as an early warning system to identify "hotspots" or areas with high prescribing rates. Examples may include de-identified patient, prescriber, and dispenser-specific information organized by geographic area (state, county, ZIP code, or municipality) and by time period to illuminate trends in both medical and nonmedical use of prescription drugs. For example, Project Lazarus, a comprehensive overdose prevention program in North Carolina, uses PDMP data to target intervention services and to measure community prevention efforts.[18]

Factors that Encourage or Inhibit PDMP Use by Clinicians

There are several factors that can encourage or inhibit prescriber use of PDMPs. Clinicians are more likely to use PDMPs that present data in "real time" (current or very recent data), that are used by all prescribers, and that can actively identify potential problems such as multiple prescribers or multiple prescriptions.[19] PDMPs can help identify patients who may be at higher risk for overdose (e.g., taking high opioid dosages, taking benzodiazepines with opioids) or who may be misusing prescription opioids (e.g., receiving opioid prescriptions from multiple providers). This can prompt the clinician to act to improve patient safety by initiating clinician–patient conversations about safety concerns while remaining sensitive to a patient's treatment goals and medical needs. Providers who identify aberrant prescriber history can respond accordingly and make a referral to mental health or substance abuse treatment.[17,20]

Requiring PDMP checks also has a positive effect on prescriber use of PDMPs. Buchmueller et al.[21] found stronger effects on opioid prescribing when providers are required to access the PDMP. They also found that PDMPs significantly reduced measures of misuse (e.g., opioid prescriptions from five or more providers) in Medicare Part D.[21] In contrast, they found that PDMPs without such provisions had no effect on opioid prescribing or misuse. PDMPs can also bolster provider confidence in managing access to opioid medications. For example, emergency department prescribers reported feeling more comfortable prescribing controlled substances when they received information from PDMPs because they are often unfamiliar with their patients' medical histories and unsure what other controlled substances they may be taking.[22]

Prescribers may use PDMP data at the point of care, allowing them to identify patients with multiple provider episodes or potentially overlapping benzodiazepine and opioid prescriptions that place them at risk of opioid use disorder or overdose. McAllister et al.[22] found that all prescribers who were surveyed indicated that accessing PDMP data altered their prescribing behavior in favor of more judicious use of opioids. An Indiana-based assessment of PDMPs in pharmacy practice indicates that pharmacists who always use a PDMP are more likely to refuse to dispense opioids than pharmacists who never do.[23] Baehren et al.[24] found that when PDMP data were used in an emergency department, 41% of cases had altered prescribing after the clinician reviewed PDMP data, with 61% of the patients receiving fewer or no opioid pain medications than had been originally planned and 39% receiving more opioid medication than previously planned because the physician was able to confirm the patient did not have a recent history of controlled substance use.

PDMPs have broad support from clinicians, especially PDMPs that provide easy access or use within an existing clinical workflow.[25,26] Barriers to PDMP use vary across the United States and are correlated strongly with the PDMP design; the state's health information technology infrastructure; and state regulations on prescriber registration, access, and utilization.[27] The additional time required to verify a patient's current medication history is cited in several studies as a major barrier to wider implementation and use by clinicians.[28,29] A recent survey of over 600 members of the American Association of Neurological Surgeons found that participants working in states with mandatory PDMP verification estimated that it took on average three to five minutes to check the PDMP per patient.[28] Nationally, a relatively small number of health systems have integrated PDMP data within their EHR due to the cost of linking these data systems.[30] For the vast majority of prescribers, the PDMP is accessed by logging into a separate website or portal outside of their EHR system. Investing in PDMP integration within clinical workflow can greatly reduce this barrier. In states with relatively small investments in their PDMPs, a prescriber's experience is directly affected by how the PDMP is accessed in a clinical setting.[25,27]

Knowledge and training on how to interpret PDMP data has also been a major barrier cited by clinicians for not using their state PDMP. States are taking steps to ameliorate this barrier through a variety of approaches, such as generating patient risk scores based on algorithms; integrating MME calculator software that allows providers to quickly assess a patient's daily MME; or including clinical decision tools to assist prescribers in making more informed, faster decisions about patients' treatment.[31] Limited interstate data sharing is also a barrier that has great variability across the nation.[31] A clinician's ability to query neighboring state databases is directly impacted by the data-sharing agreements that have been entered into by the adjoining states. The availability of PDMP data has also impacted the US Department of Veterans Affairs (VA) and the US Indian Health Service (IHS). A recent survey of VA physicians noted that incomplete or unavailable prescription data was a major obstacle to increasing PDMP use.[26] In 2016, the US Department of Health and Human Services issued a policy requiring IHS prescribers to query the PDMP before prescribing opioids and pharmacists to report their dispensing activity to the PDMP.[32] In addition, it directed IHS to ensure that memoranda of understanding were signed with the appropriate state offices.[32] Tribal internet connectivity is also dependent on state and federal resources, and most tribal nations have limited resources with which to develop the necessary health information technology infrastructure.

Best Practices and Successful Strategies to Promote PDMP Use

States have implemented a range of ways to improve provider access and ease of use to PDMPs. In fact, the Prescription Drug Monitoring Program Training and Technical Assistance Center (TTAC) at Brandeis University identified 67 best practices to enhance PDMPs in the following seven practice categories (see Text Box 22.1):[33]

1. Data collection and data quality
2. Data linking and analysis
3. User access and report dissemination
4. Enrollment, outreach, education, and utilization
5. PDMP promotion
6. Interorganizational coordination
7. PDMP usability, progress, and impact.

TEXT BOX 22.1 CURRENT PDMP BEST PRACTICE CHECKLIST

Below is the most recent draft of the checklist (dated January 15, 2016) that takes into account feedback from states during two webinars on PDMP best practices. Most of the items in this version were included in the 2016 TTAC state assessment.

Instructions: Under "Current Status," please indicate which of the listed practices/policies are not planned, planned, in progress. or achieved by typing an "x" in the appropriate box. Under "Priority Assessment" please indicate your disagreement or agreement with the practice or policy, then list any barriers to its adoption and its priority for adoption, if not already adopted. Mary of these practices are described in the 2012 Pew white paper on PDMP best practices, available at http://www.pdm.passist.org/pdf/COE_documents/Add_to_TTAC/Brandeis_PDMP_ Report. pdf.

Optional On this last page of this form, please indicate your suggestions for additional practices/policies not inducted in the current checklist.

State: Date:

PDMP Practice/Policy	Current Status				Priority Assessment		
	Not planned	Planned	In progress	Achieved	Disagree with practice, please give reason	Agree with practice (and reason, optional)	Barriers to adoption, if any (describe briefly)	Priority for Adoption: zero-0, low-1, medium-2, high-3

DATA COLLECTION AND DATA QUALITY							
Collect data on all schedules of controlled substances							
Adopt latest ASAP reporting standard							

Collect data on non-scheduled drugs implicated in abuse as determined by the state

Record positive identification of the person picking up prescriptions (customer ID)

Collect data on method of payment, including cash

Daily or real-time data collection

Monitor pharmacy reporting compliance

Institute effective data correction and missing data procedures

Integrate electronic prescribing and PDMP data collection

DATA LINKING AND ANALYSIS

Use a proven method to match/link the same patient's records

Conduct periodic analyses to identify at-risk patients, prescribers, and dispensers

PDMP Practice/Policy	Current Status				Priority Assessment			
	Not planned	Planned	In progress	Achieved	Disagree with practice, please give reason	Agree with practice (and reason, optional)	Barriers to adoption, if any (describe briefly)	Priority for Adoption: zero-0, low-1, medium-2, high-3
Conduct epidemiologic analyses for surveillance, early warning evaluation, prevention								
Use automated expert software and systems to expedite analyses and reports								
Record data on prescriber disciplinary status, patient lock-ins								
Link to prescriber specialty data								
USER ACCESS AND REPORT DISSEMINATION								
Provide continuous online access and automated reports to authorized users								
Customized solicited reports for different types of end-users								

User-friendly interfaces
(e.g., decision support tools,
risk scores)

Enhance patient reports with
summary data (e.g., MMEs,
MPEs)*

Prescriber self-lookup

Batch (multi-patient) reporting for
prescribers and delegates

Integrate PDMP reports with . . .
health information exchanges

EHRs

pharmacy dispensing systems

Provide PDMP data to . . .

prescribers

medical residents

dispensers

law enforcement

licensure boards

patients

Medicare

PDMP Practice/Policy	Current Status				Priority Assessment			
	Not planned	Planned	In progress	Achieved	Disagree with practice, please give reason	Agree with practice (and reason, optional)	Barriers to adoption, if any (describe briefly)	Priority for Adoption: zero-0, low-1, medium-2, high-3
Medicaid								
private third-party payers								
workers' compensation programs								
substance abuse treatment								
clinicians								
medical examiners/coroners								
drug courts								
researchers (encrypted/de-identified data)								
Send unsolicited reports and/or alerts to . . .								
prescribers								
dispensers								
law enforcement								
licensure boards								
Proactive alerts								
letters to top prescribers								

ENROLLMENT, OUTREACH, EDUCATION, UTILIZATION

Streamline/automate enrollment

Presentations and trainings for end-user groups

Online user guides and educational materials

Proactive identification and outreach to enroll high-impact users (e.g., top prescribers)

Prescriber report cards

Delegate accounts

Mandate PDMP enrollment:

prescribers

dispensers

Mandate PDMP training:

prescribers

dispensers

Mandate PDMP utilization:

prescribers

dispensers

Financial or other incentives

Letters to new prescribes

PDMP Practice/Policy	Current Status				Priority Assessment			
	Not planned	Planned	In progress	Achieved	Disagree with practice, please give reason	Agree with practice (and reason, optional)	Barriers to adoption, if any (describe briefly)	Priority for Adoption: zero-0, low-1, medium-2, high-3
PDMP PROMOTION								
Conduct presentations								
Distribute reports								
Website content:								
Annual PDMP reports								
Quarterly PDMP reports								
Data dashboards								
PDMP enhancement news								
Other reports								
INTERORGANIZATIONAL COORDINATION								
Interstate data sharing								
Collaborate with other health agencies/organizational in applying and linking PDMP data:								
Veterans Affairs								

Indian Health Service

Department of Defense

PDMP USABILITY, PROGRESS, AND IMPACT

Conduct satisfaction and utilization surveys of end-users

Conduct audits of PDMP system utilization tor appropriateness and extent of use

Track/report progress in adapting practices (checklist)

Track/report PDMP enrollment and utilization data, prescribing, and risk measures (e.g., MPEs, MMEs)*

Use PDMP data as outcome measures in evaluating program and policy changes

Analyze other outcome data (e.g., overdoses, deaths, hospitalizations, ER visits) to evaluate the PDMP's impact

*Note: Morphine Millegram Equivalents, Multiple Provider Episodes.

PDMP Practice/Policy	Current Status			Priority Assessment			
	Not planned	Planned	In progress	Achieved	Disagree with practice, please give reason	Agree with practice (and reason, optional)	Barriers to adoption, if any (describe briefly)	Priority for Adoption: zero-0, low-1, medium-2, high-3

PDMP FUNDING AND SUSTAINABILITY

Secure funding that is independent of economic downturns, conflicts of interest, and changes in PDMP policies

Enact legislation to maintain sufficient funding over time

Periodic review of PDMP performance to ensure efficient operations and identify opportunities for improvement

Promote visibility of PDMP impact to motivate funding (e.g., via annual reports and news releases)

Optional: Please list here any PDMP practices or policies not mentioned above you think should be included in the checklist, then indicate their adoption status and priority:

Practice/Policy	Current Status				Assessment of Priority for Adoption		
	Under consideration	Planned	In progress	Achieved	Reason for adoption	Barriers to adoption, if any (describe briefly)	Priority for Adoption: low-1, medium-2, or high-3

Excerpted from Tracking PDMP Enhancement: The Best Practice Checklist (March 3, 2017).[33] Reprinted with permission.

In addition, CDC promotes four best practices that may be particularly useful in improving PDMP utility: universal use, active management, timely or real-time reporting, and ease of use/ease of access.[34]

Universal Use

The utility of PDMPs as clinical tools for clinicians is contingent on clinician and delegated use of PDMPs within a state (i.e., a clinician is able to allow other medical staff to access the PDMP for clinical care). For example, state law may permit a nurse practitioner (i.e., delegate) to query a patient's PDMP report on behalf of the clinician as a part of the patient visit and care. Most states (41) have implemented polices that require providers to check a state PDMP (i.e., mandatory PDMP use) prior to prescribing certain controlled substances.[35] Dowell et al.[16] found both a reduction in opioids prescribed (8%) and prescription opioid deaths (12%) after the combined implementation of mandatory PDMP use and pain clinic laws. It is important to note that in terms of mortality comparisons, the analysis did not show an absolute reduction, but it was reduced in comparison to what would have been expected given existing trends without the law. Legislation requiring mandated use of PDMPs in four states (Kentucky, New York, Ohio, Tennessee) was associated with an increase in PDMP use and decreases in multiple provider episodes and the prescribing of specific medications.[36] Further, a reduction in the quantity of opioids and benzodiazepines dispensed was found in Ohio after that state enacted legislation requiring PDMP use (i.e., statutory requirement to check the PDMP).[37] Mandates are most associated with behavioral change when they are implemented to maximize utility and in a manner that does not overburden clinicians.[38]

Active Management

PDMPs can inform providers on prescribing trends and improve clinical practice at the point of care by sending proactive reports on individual patients at highest risk and on potentially inappropriate prescribing. Providers surveyed in Massachusetts found both hard copy and electronic proactive reports and alerts to be useful clinical tools.[39] Young et al.[40] found that providers who received proactive reports were associated with decreases in seven patient risk measures, which included the number of Schedule II opioid prescriptions, dosage units, total days' supply, total MME, and average daily MME. This study controlled for patient behavior through the use of a matched comparison group.

Timely or Real-Time Reporting

Dispensers (e.g., pharmacists) are responsible for entering prescriptions into state PDMPs. However, the submission of data to state PDMPs varies from biweekly to daily or even in real time (i.e., under five minutes).[41] Greenwood-Ericksen et al.[42] noted that it was critical for providers to have access to timely data so that PDMPs can be used as tools for detecting patients at risk for opioid misuse, opioid use disorder, and overdose. Requiring timely data reporting was one of five PDMP features associated with stronger protective effects on the relative risks of prescription opioid–related poisoning.[43] This longitudinal, observational study assessed the associations between administrative PDMP features and risks of prescription opioid–related poisoning in a nationally representative sample of privately insured adults from 2004 to 2014.

Easy to Use/Easy to Access

Promising practices to improve provider use and access to PDMPs include integrating PDMP data into EHRs and simplifying the PDMP registration process (e.g., automatic PDMP registration with license renewal). PDMP data are useful for clinical decision making only to the extent that they are readily available and easy for a prescriber to consult in the course of providing care. Integration with existing health systems data and systems allows prescribers to incorporate PMDP data into their regular decision-making process. In fact, ease of use and accessibility to PDMP data within clinical workflow is associated with increased PDMP usage.[44] Evidence suggests that the increased availability of PDMP data, via integrated EHR connections, was associated with an increase in PDMP use and a decrease in prescribed opioids. Queries at one PDMP integration pilot site in Illinois increased from an average of 6.9 per provider registered with the PDMP in 2013 to 998.2 in 2015 (145-fold increase), compared to only a slight increase in the state overall. Further, from 2013 to 2015, there was a 22% decrease in the number of prescribed opioids issued from the same PDMP integration pilot site versus a 13% increase in prescribed opioids during that period for the state overall.[44]

Impact of PDMPs on Health Outcomes

The effect of PDMPs on prescribing behavior and health outcomes remains unclear, with conflicting reports. One of the major reasons PDMPs are so difficult to study is the vast variability across states depending on PDMP functionality and features. Also, most studies have focused largely on estimating the effect of PDMPs on prescribing behaviors or health outcomes while statistically adjusting for complementary prevention programs (e.g., naloxone distribution initiatives or pill mill laws). As noted earlier, the exception to this is Dowell et al.,[16] who measured the combined effect of state pain clinic laws and PDMPs—thus looking at the additive effect on overdose rates. Despite these methodologic challenges and the variability in PDMP administrative features, there is some evidence that PDMPs reduce the amount and number of drugs prescribed, particularly opioids.[14,45–48] However, additional evidence is needed to confirm these effects.

Prior to using PDMPs, providers may already have developed practice patterns and clinical behaviors that shape their prescribing habits. Deyo et al.[49] sought to determine if prescriber registration with and use of Oregon's PDMP led to fewer high-risk opioid prescriptions or overdose events. Their research found that the numbers of patients with high-dose prescriptions, multiple prescribers, or inappropriate prescriptions decreased gradually over time in both registered and nonregistered groups. However, registered prescribers did not show greater or faster declines than nonregistrants, either in the short term or the long term after PDMP registration. Basically, cautious prescribers were more likely to check the PDMP more frequently rather than frequent use of the PDMP making prescribers more cautious. Combined with other efforts to regulate prescribing and dispensing, Florida's PDMP has been shown to reduce the number of opioid prescriptions among high-volume prescribers,[14,48] reduce diversion of prescription opioids,[50] and reduce the number of deaths involving oxycodone.[51] In New York and Tennessee, checking the PDMP helped reduce the number of patients receiving opioid prescriptions from multiple prescribers.[19]

Compared to research examining impacts on prescribing behavior, it is less common for studies to investigate the impact of PDMPs on health outcomes. For example, in a recent systematic review looking at the association between PDMPs and opioid-related overdose, Fink et al.[52] concluded that evidence is largely insufficient to draw definitive conclusions about the effect of PDMPs on overdose. Of the 17 studies meeting the authors' inclusion criteria, 10 linked PDMP implementation to reductions in fatal overdoses. Mandatory review of PDMP data by providers before writing prescriptions was the most studied program feature associated with this outcome. Other features correlating with a decrease in fatal overdoses were frequent (at least weekly) updates of PDMP data, sharing data across states, provider authorization to access PDMP data, and monitoring of noncontrolled substances.[52] As PDMPs continue to evolve, more research is needed to evaluate the effectiveness of specific features of PDMPs to inform their evolving implementation. In addition, more research is needed regarding how complementary prevention programs (e.g., medication-assisted treatment [MAT], naloxone distribution, and pill mill laws) interact with PDMPs to affect population health. Finally, robust research is needed to examine the impact of PDMPs on patient health and overall community health and substance misuse and addiction.

Challenges of PDMP Implementation and Use

While provider use of PDMPs has been associated with a reduction in prescribing of opioids and benzodiazepines,[21–24,37,49,53] barriers to PDMP data access within clinical workflow remain. There are significant barriers, including the consolidation of the health information technology market and the associated costs of both implementing and sustaining PDMP/health information technology integration and interstate interoperability.

Another barrier is the lack of universal technical standards that are used for exchanging prescription information between health information technology systems.[54] Pharmacies, PDMPs, and EHRs all "communicate" or exchange information with different standards;[44] therefore, application programming interfaces (API) are needed to "translate" and exchange the data between systems. Health information technology vendors have developed APIs that can translate between the various standards, but there are significant financial costs associated with the use of these APIs.

In addition to the costs associated with interstate PDMP data exchange, the primary legal barrier is resolving which end-user groups are allowed access to PDMP data in the states where data are being shared.[44] Cepeda et al.[55] found that patients identified as visiting multiple doctors and pharmacies (i.e., more than one prescriber with at least one day of overlap at three or more pharmacies) traveled a median of 83.8 miles to fill prescription opioids, while those identified as demonstrating greater levels of multiple doctor or pharmacy visits (i.e., at least five multiple doctor/pharmacy episodes) traveled a median of 199.5 miles to fill prescription opioids. Therefore, it is critical to resolve any barriers that prohibit the access of interstate PDMP data within clinical workflow, as patients may cross state lines to obtain opioid prescriptions. With regards to PDMP and health information technology integration, one of the primary legal barriers centers on which providers are allowed to view the PDMP data in various states.[44]

What's Next for PDMPs?

PDMPs have evolved a great deal since their creation as paper-based law enforcement and regulatory tools. States are taking steps to expand the utility and functionality of PDMPs. For example, Ohio requires all providers to enter either the International Classification of Diseases, 10th edition (ICD-10), or Current Dental Terminology diagnosis code in the state PDMP for all controlled substance prescriptions. Additionally, the Ohio PDMP integrates an MAT locator.[56] The MAT locator allows providers to quickly access the SAMHSA buprenorphine treatment locator database. The MAT locator generates a list of locations for treatment from within the state PDMP so that providers can facilitate referral to treatment for patients who have been identified and diagnosed with opioid use disorder. West Virginia recently passed legislation requiring medical providers to report instances of overdose or suspected overdose that occurred because of illicit or prescribed medications.[57] These data will be used to assist providers with clinical decision making and care, such as making referrals to treatment for opioid use disorder or other forms of wraparound services.

State PDMPs and PDMP vendors have also been developing new risk scores that are proactively sent to providers when a patient's PDMP report is requested. For example, some states set thresholds that indicate patient risk or inappropriate use.[58] In addition, some PDMP vendors use proprietary algorithms to generate a relative overdose risk score based on a patient's PDMP records.[44] A few common thresholds that trigger proactive PDMP alerts are:

The "5-5-6" multiple provider episodes for prescription opioids (five or more prescribers and five or more pharmacies in a six-month period)
Current active prescriptions totaling 50 MMEs and 90 MMEs
Overlapping active opioid and benzodiazepine prescriptions.

One particular risk score is the NARxCHECK score, which is calculated and featured prominently on one consolidated PDMP/EHR interface.[59] Providers are able to view the score and quickly determine whether to view the full PDMP report.[59] If the provider clicks on the risk score, the full PDMP report is generated within the clinical workflow.[59] Also, there are some other thresholds that states may adopt to trigger a proactive report or risk alert, such as multiple provider episodes (e.g., high number of prescribers, prescriptions filled in a short time period), MME of 90 or more, and overlapping benzodiazepine and opioid prescriptions.[58]

As PDMP data are increasingly linked with other data sources, there is increased potential to cross over the legal threshold of what is classified as (1) protected health information and subject to the Health Insurance Portability and Accountability Act (HIPAA) or (2) information obtained from a federally assisted substance use treatment program and protected by the 42 CFR, Part 2 regulation.[60] This regulation protects the confidentiality of patients who have been diagnosed with and are receiving treatment for alcohol and drug abuse. As states work to expand the amount of information providers have about their patients, additional safeguards will need to be developed to ensure that non-medical staff do not have access to data that would fall under HIPAA and be subject to legal challenges. Both the technological and the legal implications of evolving PDMPs will be important to continue to monitor into the future. Future developments that enhance interstate data sharing and ensure patient privacy protections, to increase real-time data reporting, and to provide better clinical workflow integration/integration with EHRs are all welcome additions to PDMPs of the future.

Summary

As the prescription opioid overdose epidemic evolved and expanded beginning in the late 1990s, it became increasingly important for clinicians, pharmacists, law enforcement officials, medical licensing boards, health system administrators, insurers, public health officials, and others to have near real-time access to opioid prescribing data to ensure patient safety and to inform prevention and response activities. The number of states with functional PDMPs rapidly expanded during this period; however, widespread variation continues across state PDMPs despite knowing what enables or inhibits PDMP use by prescribers and pharmacists. A number of best practices exist to maximize PDMP utility, and these need to be adopted whenever possible. While the number of prescription opioid-related overdose deaths has never been higher, new opportunities to reduce the number of prescriptions and to help clinicians and public health practitioners use PDMPs for prevention work exist. A significant first step in increasing PDMP use by clinicians is to better integrate PDMPs into clinical workflow and to encourage common best practice features and functionality across PDMPs to improve clinical and public health prevention and response efforts.

Disclaimer

The conclusions in this chapter are those of the authors and do not necessarily represent the official position of the US Centers for Disease Control and Prevention (CDC).

References

1. Paulozzi LJ, Jones CM, Mack KA, Rudd RA. Vital signs: Overdoses of prescription opioid pain relievers—United States, 1999–2008. *MMWR Morb Mortal Wkly Rep.* 2011; 60(43):1487.
2. Seth P, Scholl L, Rudd RA, Bacon S. Overdose deaths involving opioids, cocaine, and psychostimulants—United States, 2015–2016. *MMWR Morb Mortal Wkly Rep.* 2018; 67(12):349–358.
3. Boudreau D, Von Korff M, Rutter CM, et al. Trends in long-term opioid therapy for chronic non-cancer pain. *Pharmacoepidemiol Drug Saf.* 2009; 18(12):1166–1175.
4. Von Korff M, Saunders K, Ray GT, et al. De facto long-term opioid therapy for non-cancer pain. *Clin J Pain.* 2008; 24(6):521.
5. Levy B, Paulozzi L, Mack KA, Jones CM. Trends in opioid analgesic–prescribing rates by specialty, US, 2007–2012. *Am J Prev Med.* 2015; 49(3):409–413.
6. Paulozzi LJ, Mack KA, Hockenberry JM. Vital signs: Variation among states in prescribing of opioid pain relievers and benzodiazepines—United States, 2012. *MMWR Morb Mortal Wkly Rep.* 2014; 63(26):563–568.
7. Guy JG, Zhang K, Bohm MK, et al. Vital signs: Changes in opioid prescribing in the United States, 2006–2015. *MMWR Morb Mortal Wkly Rep.* 2017; 66(26):697–704.
8. Guy GP, Zhang K, Schieber LZ, Young R, Dowell D. County-level opioid prescribing in the United States, 2015–2017. *JAMA Intern Med.* [Epub ahead of print, February 11, 2019].

9. McBournie A, Lawal S, Carrow G, et al. Prescription drug monitoring programs: evidence-based practices to optimize prescriber use. Pew Charitable Trusts. 2016. https://www.pewtrusts.org/-/media/assets/2016/12/prescription_drug_monitoring_programs.pdf. Accessed December 4, 2018.

10. Brandeis University, Prescription Drug Monitoring Program Training and Technical Assistance Program. PDMP Maps and Tables. 2018. http://www.pdmpassist.org/content/pdmp-maps-and-tables. Accessed December 4, 2018.

11. US Department of Justice, Bureau of Justice Assistance. Frequently Asked Questions about the RxCheck Hub. 2018. https://coapresources.org/Content/Documents/pdmpDataSharing/RxCheckHubFAQ.pdf. Accessed December 4, 2018.

12. National Association of Boards of Pharmacy. PMP InterConnect. 2018. https://nabp.pharmacy/initiatives/pmp-interconnect/. Accessed December 4, 2018.

13. Clark T, Eadie J, Kreiner P, Strickler G. Prescription drug monitoring programs: An assessment of the evidence for best practices. Prescription Drug Monitoring Program Center of Excellence. 2012. https://www.pewtrusts.org/~/media/assets/0001/pdmp_update_1312013.pdf. Accessed March 1, 2019.

14. Rutkow L, Chang HY, Daubresse M, et al. Effect of Florida's prescription drug monitoring program and pill mill laws on opioid prescribing and use. *JAMA Intern Med*. 2015; 175(10):1642–1649.

15. Prescription Drug Monitoring Program Center of Excellence, Brandeis University. History of Prescription Drug Monitoring Programs. 2018. http://www.pdmpassist.org/pdf/PDMP_admin/TAG_History_PDMPs_final_20180314.pdf. Accessed December 4, 2018.

16. Dowell D, Zhang K, Noonan RK, Hockenberry JM. Mandatory provider review and pain clinic laws reduce the amounts of opioids prescribed and overdose death rates. *Health Aff*. 2016; 35(10):1876–1883.

17. Green TC, Mann MR, Bowman SE, et al. How does use of a prescription monitoring program change medical practice? *Pain Med*. 2012; 13(10):1314–1323.

18. Albert S, Brason FW, Sanford CK, et al. Project Lazarus: Community-based overdose prevention in rural North Carolina. *Pain Med*. 2011; 12(Supp 2):S77–S85.

19. Johnson H, Paulozzi L, Porucznik C, et al. Decline in drug overdose deaths after state policy changes—Florida, 2010–2012. *MMWR Morb Mortal Wkly Rep*. 2014; 63(26);569–574.

20. Irvine J, Hallvik S, Hildebran C, et al. Who uses a prescription drug monitoring program and how? Insights from a statewide survey of Oregon clinicians. *J Pain*. 2014; 15(7):747–755.

21. Buchmueller TC, Carey C. The effect of prescription drug monitoring programs on opioid utilization in Medicare. *Am Econ J*. 2018; 10(1):77–112.

22. McAllister MW, Aaronson P, Spillane J, et al. Impact of prescription drug-monitoring program on controlled substance prescribing in the ED. *Am J Emerg Med*. 2015; 33:781–785.

23. Norwood CW, Wright ER. Integration of prescription drug monitoring programs (PDMP) in pharmacy practice: Improving clinical decision-making and supporting a pharmacist's professional judgment. *Res Social Adm Pharmacy*. 2016; 12(2):257–266.

24. Baehren DF, Marco CA, Droz DE, et al. A statewide prescription monitoring program affects emergency department prescribing behaviors. *Ann Emerg Med*. 2010; 56(1):19–23.

25. Pugliese JA, Wintemute GJ, Henry SG. Psychosocial correlates of clinicians' prescription drug monitoring program utilization. *Am J Prev Med*. 2018; 54(5):e91–e98.

26. Radomski TR, Bixier FR, Zickmund SL, et al. Physicians' perspectives regarding prescription drug monitoring program use within the Department of Veterans Affairs: A multi-state qualitative study. *J Gen Intern Med*. 2018; 33(8):1253–1259.

27. Elder JW, DePalma G, Pines JM. Optimal implementation of prescription drug monitoring programs in the emergency department. *West J Emerg Med*. 2018; 19(2):387–391.

28. Babu MA, Nahed BV, Heary RF. Commentary: Prescription drug monitoring programs and the neurosurgeon: Impact on workflow and overall perceptions. *Neurosurgery* 2018; 83(4):e169–e176.

29. Christianson H, Driscoll E, Hull A. Alaska nurse practitioners' barriers to use of prescription drug monitoring programs. *J Am Acad Nurse Pract*. 2018; 30(1): 35–42.

30. Finklea K, Sacco LN, Bagalman E. *Prescription Drug Monitoring Programs. Report #7-5700*. Washington, DC: US Library of Congress, Congressional Research Service; 2014.

31. National Dialogue for Healthcare Innovation (NDHI). National Dialogue for Healthcare Innovation's Opioid Crisis Solutions Summit: A Roadmap for Action. 2018. https://www.hlc.org/app/uploads/download.php?dl=app/uploads/2018/06/Opioid-Roadmap-FINAL.pdf. Accessed December 6, 2018.

32. US Department of Health and Human Services, Indian Health Service. *The Indian Health Manual*. Rockville, MD: US Indian Health Service; 2016.

33. Prescription Drug Monitoring Program Training and Technical Assistance Center (PDMP TTAC) and Brandeis University Prescription Drug Monitoring Program Center of Excellence. Tracking PDMP Enhancement: The Best Practice Checklist. 2017. http://www.pdmpassist.org/pdf/2016_Best_Practice_Checklist_Report_20170228.pdf. Accessed December 6, 2018.

34. US Centers for Disease Control and Prevention. What States Need to Know about PDMPs. 2017. https://www.cdc.gov/drugoverdose/pdmp/states.html. Accessed December 6, 2018.

35. Brandeis University Prescription Drug Monitoring Program Center of Excellence. PDMP Mandatory Query by Prescribers and Dispensers. 2018. http://www.pdmpassist.org/pdf/Mandatory_Query_20180615.pdf. Accessed December 5, 2018.

36. Brandeis University Prescription Drug Monitoring Program Center of Excellence. PDMP Prescriber Use Mandates: Characteristics, Current Status, and Outcomes in Selected States. 2016. http://www.pdmpassist.org/pdf/Resources/Briefing_on_mandates_3rd_revision_A.pdf. Accessed December 6, 2018.

37. Winstanley EL, Zhang Y, Mashni R, et al. Mandatory review of a prescription drug monitoring program and impact on opioid and benzodiazepine dispensing. *Drug Alcohol Depend*. 2018; 188:169–174.

38. Haffajee RL, Jena AB, Weiner SG. Mandatory use of prescription drug monitoring programs. *JAMA*. 2015; 313(9):891–892.

39. Thomas CP, Kim M, Nikitin RV. Prescriber response to unsolicited prescription drug monitoring program reports in Massachusetts. *Pharmacoepidemiol Drug Saf.* 2014; 23(9):950–957.

40. Young LD, Kreiner PW, Panas L. Unsolicited reporting to prescribers of opioid analgesics by a state prescription drug monitoring program: An observational study with matched comparison group. *Pain Med.* 2018; 19(7):1396–1407.

41. Brandeis University Prescription Drug Monitoring Program Center of Excellence. PDMP Data Collection Frequency. 2017. http://www.pdmpassist.org/pdf/PDMP_Data_Collection_Frequency_20171001.pdf. Accessed December 6, 2018.

42. Greenwood-Ericksen MB, Poon SJ, Nelson LS. Best practices for prescription drug monitoring programs in the emergency department setting: Results of an expert panel. *Ann Emerg Med.* 2016; 67(6):755–764.e4.

43. Pauly NJ, Slavova S, Delcher C, et al. Features of prescription drug monitoring programs associated with reduced rates of prescription opioid-related poisonings. *Drug Alcohol Depend.* 2018; 184:26–32.

44. US Centers for Disease Control and Prevention. Integrating and expanding prescription drug monitoring program data: Lessons from nine states. 2017. https://www.cdc.gov/drugoverdose/pdf/PEHRIIE_Report-a.pdf. Accessed December 6, 2018.

45. Fisher J, Sanyal C, Frail D, Sketris I. The intended and unintended consequences of benzodiazepine monitoring programmes: A review of the literature. *J Clin Pharm Ther.* 2012; 37(1):7–21.

46. Simoni-Wastila L, Qian J. Influence of prescription monitoring programs on analgesic utilization by an insured retiree population. *Pharmacoepidemiol Drug Saf.* 2012; 21(12):1261–1268.

47. Haegerich TM, Paulozzi L, Manns B, Jones CJ. What we know and don't know about state and system level policy strategies to prevent prescription drug overdose. *Drug Alcohol Depend.* 2014; 145:34–47.

48. Chang H-Y, Lyapustina T, Rutkow L, et al. Impact of prescription drug monitoring programs and pill mill laws on high-risk opioid prescribers: A comparative interrupted time series analysis. *Drug Alcohol Depend.* 2016; 165:1–8.

49. Deyo RA, Hallvik SE, Hildebran C, et al. Association of prescription drug monitoring program use with opioid prescribing and health outcomes: A comparison of program users and nonusers. *J Pain.* 2018; 19(2):166–177.

50. Surratt HL, O'Grady C, Kurtz SP, et al. Reductions in prescription opioid diversion following recent legislative interventions in Florida. *Pharmacoepidemiol Drug Safety.* 2014; 23(3):314–320.

51. Delcher C, Wagenaar AC, Goldberger BA, et al. Abrupt decline in oxycodone-caused mortality after implementation of Florida's prescription drug monitoring program. *Drug Alcohol Depend.* 2015; 150:63–68.

52. Fink DS, Schleimer JP, Sarvet A, et al. Association between prescription drug monitoring programs and nonfatal and fatal drug overdoses. *Ann Intern Med.* 2018; 168(11):783–790.

53. Bao Y, Pan Y, Taylor A, et al. Prescription drug monitoring programs are associated with sustained reductions in opioid prescribing by physicians. *Health Aff.* 2016; 35(6):1045–1051.

54. US Department of Health and Human Services (HHS), Office of the National Coordinator for Health Information Technology. Standards and Interoperability Framework S&I Framework: Prescription Drug Monitoring Program & HIT Integration Implementation Guide. 2014. https://oncprojectracking.healthit.gov/wiki/display/TechLabSC/PDMP+Home?preview=/16123422/16319238/PDMP%20IG%206.21.2016.docx. Accessed December 6, 2018.

55. Cepeda MS, Fife D, Yuan Y, Mastrogiovanni G. Distance traveled and frequency of interstate opioid dispensing in opioid shoppers and nonshoppers. *J Pain.* 2013; 14(10):1158–1161.

56. Ohio Automated Rx Reporting System. Ohio PDMP Aware User Support Manual. 2017. https://ohiopmp.gov/Documents/General/PHARMACIES_PRESCRIBERS/OARRS%20User%20Manual.pdf. Accessed December 6, 2018.

57. West Virginia Uniform Controlled Substance Act: Article 9 Controlled Substances Monitoring. 2018. http://www.wvlegislature.gov/Bill_Text_HTML/2017_SESSIONS/RS/amendments/SB333%20HJUD%20AM%204-3%20NEW.htm. Accessed December 6, 2018.

58. Brandeis University Prescription Drug Monitoring Program Center of Excellence. Guidance on PDMP Best Practices: Options for Unsolicited Reporting. 2016. http://www.pdmpassist.org/pdf/PDMP_admin/Update%20to%20%20Guidance%20on%20Unsolicited%20Reporting%20final.pdf. Accessed December 6, 2018.

59. Huizenga JE, Breneman BC, Patel VR, et al. NARxCHECK score as a predictor of unintentional overdose death. 2016. https://apprisshealth.com/wp-content/uploads/sites/2/2017/02/NARxCHECK-Score-as-a-Predictor.pdf. Accessed December 6, 2018.

60. US Government Publishing Office. 42 CFR 2—Confidentiality of Alcohol and Drug Abuse Patient Records. https://www.gpo.gov/fdsys/granule/CFR-2010-title42-vol1/CFR-2010-title42-vol1-part2. Accessed December 6, 2018.

23 | Prescribing Guidelines and Opioid Stewardship

MARK BICKET AND CALEB ALEXANDER

IVEN THE CENTRAL ROLE that the overuse of prescription opioids has played in the opioid epidemic, prescribing guidelines and opioid stewardship are critical strategies to reduce opioid-related addiction, injury, and death. Prescribing guidelines are important because, when they are constructed well and instituted effectively, they are an important driver of prescriber behavior, and thus improve the safe and effective use of opioids in clinical practice. The concept of opioid stewardship, on the other hand, refers to the design of clinical and public health policies and procedures to maximize the risk/benefit balance of opioids at both an individual and a population level. Prescribing guidelines represent one important approach to fostering opioid stewardship, although there are many others, including public health surveillance, sound organizational policies, and patient and family engagement.

Guidelines provide an efficient means of disseminating best practices to prescribers, patients, and others in a position to influence clinical care, such as policymakers and payers. Rigorously developed guidelines offer a valuable synthesis of the field and thus serve as an important resource for individuals and organizations looking for an authoritative examination of the evidence base supporting the use of opioids in clinical practice. By improving access to evidence, guidelines promote care that is better aligned with such information. For example, opioid guidelines have encouraged the use of nonpharmacologic and non-opioid pharmacologic therapies prior to the initiation of an opioid in many settings.[1] Similarly, based on growing evidence that the dose and duration of early prescriptions is associated with the likelihood of conversion to chronic opioid use,[1-3] these formal recommendations have decreased the number of opioids prescribed on "first fills." While clinicians and patients are often considered the primary end users of guidelines, they ultimately shape practice at many levels, including through payment models, standards and accountability for health systems, and quality measures for prescribers and institutions.

While numerous guidelines during the past two decades have addressed the management of individuals in pain or the use of opioids in clinical practice, arguably none has been more carefully developed, nor as influential in shaping clinical practice, as the US Centers for Disease Control and Prevention's (CDC) "Guideline for Prescribing Opioids for Chronic Pain" in 2016.[1] Developed using standardized and high-quality methods along with input from federal, public, and expert stakeholders, the Guideline outlines 12 key recommendations oriented to primary care physicians and others who manage pain and consider opioid prescriptions as a treatment for chronic pain (Text Box 23.1).

In addition, recommendations cover when to initiate or continue opioids, how to select opioids and appropriate follow-up intervals, and how to monitor for potential harms. The CDC has provided a checklist and many additional tools to help clinicians implement these recommendations. The Guideline was released at a time of heightened awareness and concern regarding the epidemic, and its comprehensiveness and rigor, combined with the CDC's credibility and national reach, have helped foster the dissemination and implementation of the Guideline throughout numerous local, regional, and national public health and health care delivery systems, and this has accelerated a national decline in opioid prescribing.[4]

Given the enormity of the opioid epidemic, and the central role that prescription opioids have played in its genesis, many other guidelines have also been developed. While none is likely to have been as impactful as the CDC's, these are nevertheless noteworthy, as they reflect a wide breadth of clinical settings and also demonstrate how the evidence base and in turn clinical practice guidelines have evolved over time (Text Box 23.2).

For example, in 2012 the American College of Emergency Physicians published a clinical policy on prescribing opioids for adults in the emergency department, based on systematic review and expert opinion, concluding that opioids are not routinely recommended as a treatment for an acute exacerbation of chronic non-cancer pain in the emergency department.[5] In contrast, in 2018 the US Departments of Veterans Affairs and Defense released clinical practice guidelines, based on systematic review, that substantially overlaped with the Guideline.[6] Other opioid prescribing guidelines exist for both highly prevalent (e.g., low back pain, surgery) and unique (sickle cell) patient populations (Text Box 23.3).[7–9]

Despite their potential value, clinical guidelines are only as good as the evidence base and methods used to develop them. The production of a high-quality guideline requires a systematic review of empiric evidence relevant to a carefully specified question (while systematic reviews represent one step in

Determining When to Initiate or Continue Opioids for Chronic Pain

1. Nonpharmacologic therapy and non-opioid pharmacologic therapy are preferred for chronic pain. Clinicians should consider opioid therapy only if expected benefits for both pain and function are anticipated to outweigh risks to the patient. If opioids are used, they should be combined with nonpharmacologic therapy and non-opioid pharmacologic therapy, as appropriate.
2. Before starting opioid therapy for chronic pain, clinicians should establish treatment goals with all patients, including realistic goals for pain and function, and should consider how opioid therapy will be discontinued if benefits do not outweigh risks. Clinicians should continue opioid therapy only if there is clinically meaningful improvement in pain and function that outweighs risks to patient safety.
3. Before starting and periodically during opioid therapy, clinicians should discuss with patients known risks and realistic benefits of opioid therapy and patient and clinician responsibilities for managing therapy.

Opioid Selection, Dosage, Duration, Follow-Up, and Discontinuation

4. When starting opioid therapy for chronic pain, clinicians should prescribe immediate-release opioids instead of extended-release/long-acting (ER/LA) opioids.
5. When opioids are started, clinicians should prescribe the lowest effective dosage. Clinicians should use caution when prescribing opioids at any dosage, should carefully reassess evidence of individual benefits and risks when considering increasing dosage to ≥50 morphine milligram equivalents (MME)/day, and should avoid increasing dosage to ≥90 MME/day or carefully justify a decision to titrate dosage to ≥90 MME/day.
6. Long-term opioid use often begins with treatment of acute pain. When opioids are used for acute pain, clinicians should prescribe the lowest effective dose of immediate-release opioids and should prescribe no greater quantity than needed for the expected duration of pain severe enough to require opioids. Three days or less will often be sufficient; more than seven days will rarely be needed.
7. Clinicians should evaluate benefits and harms with patients within one to four weeks of starting opioid therapy for chronic pain or of dose escalation. Clinicians should evaluate benefits and harms of continued therapy with patients every three months or more frequently. If benefits do not outweigh harms of continued opioid therapy, clinicians should optimize other therapies and work with patients to taper opioids to lower dosages or to taper and discontinue opioids.

Assessing Risk and Addressing Harms of Opioid Use

8. Before starting and periodically during continuation of opioid therapy, clinicians should evaluate risk factors for opioid-related harms. Clinicians should incorporate into the management plan strategies to mitigate risk, including considering offering naloxone when factors that increase risk for opioid overdose, such as history of overdose, history of substance use disorder, higher opioid dosages (≥50 MME/day), or concurrent benzodiazepine use, are present.

9. Clinicians should review the patient's history of controlled substance prescriptions using state prescription drug monitoring program (PDMP) data to determine whether the patient is receiving opioid dosages or dangerous combinations that put him or her at high risk for overdose. Clinicians should review PDMP data when starting opioid therapy for chronic pain and periodically during opioid therapy for chronic pain, ranging from every prescription to every three months.

10. When prescribing opioids for chronic pain, clinicians should use urine drug testing before starting opioid therapy and consider urine drug testing at least annually to assess for prescribed medications as well as other controlled prescription drugs and illicit drugs.

11. Clinicians should avoid prescribing opioid pain medication and benzodiazepines concurrently whenever possible.

12. Clinicians should offer or arrange evidence-based treatment (usually medication-assisted treatment with buprenorphine or methadone in combination with behavioral therapies) for patients with opioid use disorder.

Source: *CDC Guideline for Prescribing Opioids for Chronic Pain—United States, 2016.*[1]

the guideline creation process, not all systematic reviews result in the creation of guidelines). Such reviews represent a prespecified, transparent, reproducible, highly structured approach to curating and critically appraising the totality of information required to address a topic of interest. These reviews are increasingly facilitated by a growing number of tools and techniques to search the published and unpublished literature. For example, checklists and collections of preferred reporting items exist to standardize the conduct and reporting of systematic reviews, including one of the most important elements of a review, the search strategy.[10] Once a search has identified a pool of potentially relevant studies, which may number in the thousands, guideline writers must sort and review each study to determine whether it merits inclusion in the guidelines and, if so, how the findings should shape recommendations. Tools to grade and evaluate evidence from studies such as randomized clinical trials

TEXT BOX 23.2 EXAMPLES OF PRESCRIBING GUIDELINES FROM SELECTED NATIONAL ORGANIZATIONS

Professional Group	Guideline Title	Link or Citation
American College of Emergency Physicians	Clinical Policy: Critical Issues in the Prescribing of Opioids for Adult Patients in the Emergency Department	https://www.acep.org/globalassets/new-pdfs/clinical-policies/opioids-2012.pdf *Ann Emerg Med.* 2012; 60:499–525
American College of Obstetricians and Gynecologists and American Society of Addiction Medicine	Opioid Use and Opioid Use Disorder in Pregnancy	https://www.ncsbn.org/2017_ACOG_Committee_Opinion.pdf
US Department of Veterans Affairs and US Department of Defense	Clinical Practice Guideline for Opioid Therapy for Chronic Pain	https://www.healthquality.va.gov/guidelines/Pain/cot/VADoDOTCPG022717.pdf
Federation of State Medical Boards	Guidelines for the Chronic Use of Opioid Analgesics	https://www.ncsbn.org/2017_FSMB_Guidelines.pdf

provide one way to standardize some parts of what is a complex process of synthesizing the evidence.

Guideline Challenges

One longstanding challenge of guideline development is a lack of transparency regarding how specific recommendations have been generated. In other words, while many steps of guideline development, such as conduct of searches of the peer-reviewed literature, can be heavily standardized, it is also vital that procedures regarding the development of recommendations are reported as transparently as possible. The absence of such transparency may lead to recommendations being called into question or even litigation, which occurred when the Infectious Disease Society of American released guidelines

TEXT BOX 23.3 SELECTED EXAMPLES OF STATE OPIOID AND/OR CONTROLLED SUBSTANCE PRESCRIBING GUIDELINES

State	Guideline Title(s)	Link
AZ	Arizona Opioid Prescribing Guidelines	https://azdhs.gov/audiences/clinicians/index.php#clinical-guidelines-and-references-rx-guidelines
CA	Guidelines for Prescribing Controlled Substances for Pain	http://www.mbc.ca.gov/licensees/prescribing/pain_guidelines.pdf
NM	New Mexico Clinical Guidelines on Prescribing Opioids for Treatment of Pain	https://nmhealth.org/publication/view/general/271/
OH	Opioid Prescribing Guidelines for: • Acute Pain Management • Chronic, Non-terminal pain • Emergency Care Settings	https://mha.ohio.gov/News/-GCOAT-Opiate-Action-Team/Opioid-Prescribing-Guidelines
OK	Oklahoma Opioid Prescribing Guidelines	https://www.ok.gov/health2/documents/Oklahoma_Opioid_Prescribing_Guidelines_2017.pdf
OR	Oregon Opioid Prescribing Guidelines	https://www.oregonpainguidance.org/oregon-health-authority/state-guidelines/
PA	Opioid Prescribing Guidelines for: • Treating Chronic Non-Cancer Pain • Opioids in Dental Practice • Geriatric Pain	https://www.health.pa.gov/topics/disease/Opioids/Pages/Prescribing-Guidelines.aspx
WA	Interagency Guidelines on Prescribing Opioids for Pain: Developed by the Washington State Agency Medical Directors' Group (AMDG)	http://agencymeddirectors.wa.gov/Files/2015AMDGOpioidGuideline.pdf

recommending against the use of antibiotics for treating chronic symptoms from Lyme disease in 2006.[11] A lack of transparency may also contribute to conflicting guidelines regarding a given topic, further challenging patients, clinicians, and others seeking a consistent approach to address a specific clinical question.

There will always be many clinical questions that guidelines fail to address.[12] For example, there is an overwhelming amount of evidence indicating that prescription opioids have an unfavorable risk/benefit balance among many patients in whom they have been used since the late 1990s, and the CDC Guideline provides many recommendations based on substantial evidence. However, the evidence base addressing some dimensions of opioid use remains relatively thin. For example, in 2013, at least 10 million Americans were using long-term opioids for chronic, non-cancer pain, and while guidelines support the avoidance of such use, there is relatively little information regarding optimal titration protocols for these patients.[13] Similarly, despite the more than 12 million Americans who reported nonmedical use of prescription opioids during the past month in 2015, there is relatively little evidence regarding the optimal clinical strategies to decrease the risk of overdose or progression to opioid use disorder among these individuals.[14]

While in some cases there may be an absolute paucity of evidence, other studies are threatened by confounding or bias.[15,16] The use of standard and transparent methods helps to reduce bias from the review process itself. For example, one of the most common types of bias that may be present is reporting bias, which may reflect publication bias (more difficulty publishing studies with negative findings), language bias (excluding studies not in English), or outcome reporting bias (selectively reporting only some outcomes). However, even the most robust methods cannot fully correct for bias inherent to studies used to shape recommendations. For guidelines on pharmaceutical products, financial conflicts of interest with drug manufacturers often exist and may directly shape how guidelines are developed. Companies and organizations with financial ties to drug manufacturers have criticized recommendations to limit or reduce therapies, as happened with the CDC Guideline when groups that had received funding from opioid manufacturers opposed recommended limits for opioid dosing and days' supply.[17]

Another challenge with guidelines is that within three to five years the recommendations in a majority of methodologically rigorous guidelines may become outdated and no longer represent the most up-to-date perspective.[18,19] Such a prospect is especially great in settings such as the opioid epidemic, where the scientific evidence base is rapidly growing.[19] This aging of the evidence argues for innovative methods of keeping guidelines dynamic and fresh, such as living systematic reviews, in which teams continuously update and incorporate new evidence into a systematic review.[20] Living guidelines based on this type of systematic review permits a seamless connection of evidence with practice, at the cost of additional time and money associated with searching for new evidence, screening studies, and incorporating new evidence into the existing recommendations.

Yet another challenge with the use of guidelines to improve practice is that there is no guarantee that once a guideline is developed it will actually be used. The reasons prescribers may fail to use guidelines in the course of the care they deliver have been well described and range from lack of knowledge of the guideline to the powerful influence that other drivers of prescriber behavior, such as insurers' coverage policies and pharmaceutical marketing and promotion, may play in ultimately determining who prescribers what for whom.[21] In addition, conflicting guidelines from different professional organizations, such as medical specialty societies, may sow confusion on the part of prescribers and diminish the credibility and standing of any one particular guideline, creating a "free-for-all" setting where heuristics and other drivers predominate over the evidence that is delivered in guidelines.[22]

A final concern with guidelines is that they may be applied with little concern to the needs of patients who have unique conditions or differ from those in the guidelines. Indeed, such concerns harken back to the enormous pushback that was generated against managed care in the late 1980s and early 1990s, grounded in the critique that it represented "cookbook medicine" and overlooked the needs of individuals in the interests of rigid guidelines and protocol-driven care.[23] More recently, appeals to personalized medicine and individualized care may be perceived as being at odds with clinical guidelines, despite the fact that guidelines apply to populations based on inclusion and exclusion criteria from clinical trials, and represent evidence aligned with populations broad enough to show a difference in outcomes. In their best form, guidelines represent guidance based on the best available evidence, not dictates that mandate a specific conduct of care.[24]

Despite these challenges, guidelines continue to serve an indispensable role in the delivery of evidence-based care, especially with opioid prescribing. The amount of available evidence is vast, and it is implausible to think that clinicians, patients, and other stakeholders can master the sheer volume of medical information on their own. This is not to suggest that there is no role for the careful analysis of individual studies, but rather to point out that there is an enormous value in careful, comprehensive, and well-articulated syntheses of the scientific literature relevant to highly relevant clinical questions. In the case of the opioid epidemic, where so many harms have been generated by the overuse of a prescription drug, such syntheses have been especially important in correcting misperceptions and providing evidence to clinicians.

Opioid Stewardship

Opioid stewardship is characterized by two important concepts. On the one hand, opioids have value in specific patient populations when used in accordance with the best evidence. On the other hand, opioids have been widely used beyond the evidence base, and thus in settings with an unfavorable risk/benefit balance. These concepts are particularly appropriate to consider in the context of identifying, implementing, and evaluating policies to optimize the role of opioids in clinical practice, just as antimicrobial stewardship seeks to do so with respect to the use of antimicrobials. A key concern that opioid stewardship must grapple with is the potential for unintended consequences from efforts to constrain opioid overuse. Some have argued that such efforts will invariably lead patients to physically suffer, while others have raised alarm that interventions targeting opioid overuse further stigmatize the millions of Americans living with chronic pain.[26] While there is no conflict between reducing opioid overuse and improving quality of care for those in pain, concerns about unintended consequences are important for public health officials, prescribers, and policymakers to consider as prescribing guidelines and other interventions are deployed to reverse opioid-related injuries and deaths.

Practical Steps for Implementing Guidelines

Health care systems play an indispensable role in improving opioid stewardship and implementing opioid prescribing guidelines. Consolidation among medical practices has diminished the role of lone prescribers as providers of health care, and the vast majority of clinicians provide care through one or more health care systems. The diversity of encounters within these organizations, ranging from primary care to specialty clinics, physical therapists to dentists, and acute care to long-term care settings, means that there is not a one-size-fits-all method to implement opioid guidelines. Rather, the information needs of patients and providers vary enormously depending on clinical circumstance, and this is especially true for large, complex health care organizations such as hospitals, physicians' groups, and integrated delivery networks. The implementation of opioid guidelines is best performed as part of a learning health care system,[27] which creates feedback cycles for learning and improvement by gathering data in real time and uses data to guide clinical care.

Many health care organizations fall under the auspices of accreditation groups such as the Joint Commission, which has issued and updated standards and regulations regarding the treatment of pain in response to negative reactions and unintended consequences of its policy.[28] In contrast to previous standards that focused on measuring pain ratings, in 2017 new standards from the Joint Commission recommended a broader and more holistic approach to pain management. The group also mandated that hospitals and other health care organizations collect and analyze data on safe opioid prescribing, though it stopped short of suggesting specific metrics to track. Whether stipulated by accreditation organizations or not, most organizations rely on a multidisciplinary teams to design, implement, and evaluate opioid prescribing guidelines. In addition to prescribers, the team should actively seek contributions from pharmacists, nurses, physician leadership, public health practitioners, and other leaders within the health care system.

Payer strategies to implement opioid prescribing guidelines may span utilization management and formulary controls, integration of pharmacologic and nonpharmacologic treatments for pain, and engagement with patients and prescribers, including surveillance for high-risk populations whose opioid utilization or prescribing suggests the need for more intensive intervention. Typical utilization management strategies include quantity limits, prior authorization, and step therapy. Quantity limits for the initial opioid prescription, in terms of either days' supply or pills dispensed, restrict the exposure of patients to opioids. Limiting the supply of new opioid prescriptions is particularly relevant given that the risk of inadvertent transition to long-term opioid use increases with every extra day of supply. Prior authorization, in which prescribers must obtain approval before the patient may receive a therapy, is typically reserved for less common settings where potential risks to patients from inappropriate treatments may be greater. For example, pharmacy benefits managers increasingly require prior authorization for long-term, extended-release/long-acting (ER/LR) opioids for the treatment of chronic, non-cancer pain. As a routine tool, prior authorization should be used judiciously given the increased burden it places on prescribers and the barriers to access it may pose to patients. Step therapy may be used to ensure prescribing practice aligns with guidelines. For example, patients should use non-opioid prescriptions and nonpharmacologic therapy prior to opioid therapy, and step therapy may be one tool to guide this desired behavior. Within a payer's system, opioid prescribing exists within the broader set of pain therapy. Examining the costs and coverage of nonpharmacologic and non-opioid pharmacologic therapies is also important to consider as a driver of opioid utilization, since ultimately opioids are part of a choice set that includes these other options.

Other approaches for payers to implement guidelines include directly engaging with patients and prescribers. Payers may engage with at-risk patients on high doses of opioids, and those with concerning utilization patterns may be subject to review and restriction programs, where they are "locked in" to receive opioid prescriptions from one prescriber and one pharmacy (Figure 23.1). While not routine, such programs may nudge these patients toward guideline-concordant care. For prescribers, payers may help correct information gaps for outlier prescribers who lack of awareness about contemporary evidence through a technique called academic detailing, which applies the face-to-face communication approach of pharmaceutical companies to disseminate best evidence. To avoid the cost of academic detailing, payers may use a range of outreach strategies that progress in a staged fashion, from mailing reports on how a prescriber's activity compares to peers, to calling prescribers to discuss their practices, to face-to-face meetings with prescribers whose activity raises sufficient concern.

WHAT YOU SHOULD KNOW ABOUT YOUR

OPIOID PAIN MEDICATIONS

TENNESSEE STATE LAW NOW LIMITS HOW MUCH YOUR
PRESCRIBER CAN WRITE FOR YOU

The Tennessee General Assembly has passed laws limiting how much
prescription pain medication you may be able to receive from your healthcare
provider unless an exemption applies. Effective July 1, 2018, state law restricts
initial supply of all opioids including but not limited to:

**Lortab • Vicodin • Oxycodone • Hydrocodone •
Percocet • Cough Syrups**

WHAT THIS MEANS FOR YOU:

- Your prescriber must consult with you and consider using alternative, non-opioid pain management medications and/or treatments.

- Your prescriber or a staff member must check the state's Controlled Substance Monitoring Database to ensure you are not receiving opioids from another prescriber.

- Your prescriber must require you to sign an Informed Consent form that includes warnings and education about the responsible use of opioids.

- Most patients who do receive opioids will be limited to a three-day supply.

- If you are prescribed up to a 10, 20 or 30-day prescription of opioids, your pharmacist can only fill half of your initial prescription per state law. You or someone on your behalf will be required to make a second visit to fill the remaining prescription, if needed.

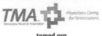

Physicians Caring for Tennesseans

tnmed.org

FIGURE 23.1. Example of a patient education card provided to physician offices for use with patients.

Source: Tennessee Medical Association (TMA). https://www.tnmed.org/TMA/Member_Resources/Opioid_Resource_Center

Federal and state municipalities implement opioid guidelines using a variety of methods, ranging from statute and regulation to decrees and informational items from the medical board and state department of health.[29] State laws and regulations represent one of the strictest approaches to implementing recommendations. By transforming a recommendation from a clinical guideline into a requirement backed by civil penalties, state laws leave little leeway in adapting guidelines to individual patients, although appeal processes generally remain available. Once legislation is enacted it may be difficult to change, despite the rapidly evolving evidence on opioid prescribing. As a result, state laws should address recommendations backed by broad consensus and robust evidence, leaving areas with less certainty to the oversight of state medical boards and departments of health. While some overlap exists in how states regulate opioid prescribing, differences in their approach create a patchwork of policies regulating opioid prescribing that make it difficult to understand the relative value of specific policies.

Summary

The opioid epidemic is a complex one that has developed over the course of two decades. Since a central driver of the epidemic has been the overuse of prescription opioids in clinical practice, prescribing guidelines and broader opioid stewardship are vital components of interventions to reduce opioid-related injuries and deaths, as well as to simultaneously improve the quality of care for the millions of Americans living with pain. There is a large and rapidly growing evidence base to support the continued development and re-finement of opioid guidelines, and a high demand for such information will remain for the foreseeable future. While guidelines may not always agree on every point, careful review of methods and process will often help to illuminate sources of disagreement when present; fortunately, there is growing consensus regarding many key principles that should govern opioid prescribing. Where concerns about the potential unintended consequence of guideline implementation may exist, opioid stewardship provides a helpful framework to ensure that the focus remains where it should be: maximizing the value of opioids in clinical practice by ensuring that they are used based on the best clinical evidence.

References

1. Dowell D, Haegerich TM, Chou R. CDC guideline for prescribing opioids for chronic pain—United States, 2016. *MMWR Morb Mortal Wkly Rep.* 2016; 65(1):1–49.
2. Shah A, Hayes CJ, Martin BC. Characteristics of initial prescription episodes and likelihood of long-term opioid use—United States, 2006–2015. *MMWR Morb Mortal Wkly Rep.* 2017; 66(10):265–269.
3. Barnett ML, Olenski AR, Jena AB. Opioid-prescribing patterns of emergency physicians and risk of long-term SSE. *N Engl J Med.* 2017; 376(7):663–673.
4. Bohnert ASB, Guy GP, Losby JL. Opioid prescribing in the United States before and after the Centers for Disease Control and Prevention's 2016 opioid guideline. *Ann Intern Med.* 2018; 169(6):367–375.
5. Cantrill S V, Brown MD, Carlisle RJ, et al. Clinical policy: Critical issues in the prescribing of opioids for adult patients in the emergency department. *Ann Emerg Med.* 2012; 60(4):499–525.

6. Rosenberg JM, Bilka BM, Wilson SM, Spevak C. Opioid therapy for chronic pain: Overview of the 2017 US Department of Veterans Affairs and US Department of Defense clinical practice guideline. *Pain Med*. 2018; 19(5):928–941.

7. Qaseem A, Wilt TJ, McLean RM, Forciea MA. Noninvasive treatments for acute, subacute, and chronic low back pain: A clinical practice guideline from the American College of Physicians. *Ann Intern Med*. 2017; 166(7):514–530.

8. Yawn BP, John-Sowah J. Management of sickle cell disease: Recommendations from the 2014 expert panel report. *Am Fam Physician*. 2015; 92(12):1069–1076.

9. Overton HN, Hanna MN, Bruhn WE, et al. Opioid-prescribing guidelines for common surgical procedures: An expert panel consensus. *J Am Coll Surg*. 2018; 227(4):411–418.

10. Moher D, Liberati A, Tetzlaff J, Altman DG, PRISMA Group. Preferred reporting items for systematic reviews and meta-analyses: The PRISMA statement. *Int J Surg*. 2010; 8(5):336–341.

11. Institute of Medicine. *Clinical Practice Guidelines We Can Trust*. Washington, DC: National Academies Press; 2011.

12. Del Fiol G, Workman TE, Gorman PN. Clinical questions raised by clinicians at the point of care: A systematic review. *JAMA Intern Med*. 2014; 174(5):710–718.

13. Sun EC, Jena AB. Distribution of prescription opioid use among privately insured adults without cancer: United States, 2001 to 2013. *Ann Intern Med*. 2017; 167(9):684–686.

14. Han B, Compton WM, Blanco C, et al. Prescription opioid use, misuse, and use disorders in U.S. adults: 2015 national survey on drug use and health. *Ann Intern Med*. 2017; 167(5):293.

15. Boutron I, Dutton S, Ravaud P, Altman DG. Reporting and interpretation of randomized controlled trials with statistically nonsignificant results for primary outcomes. *JAMA*. 2010; 303(20):2058–2064.

16. Porter J, Jick H. Addiction rare in patients treated with narcotics. *N Engl J Med*. 1980; 302(2):123.

17. Lin DH, Lucas E, Murimi IB, et al. Financial conflicts of interest and the Centers for Disease Control and Prevention's 2016 guideline for prescribing opioids for chronic pain. *JAMA Intern Med*. 2017; 177(3):427–428.

18. Shekelle PG, Ortiz E, Rhodes S, et al. Validity of the Agency for Healthcare Research and Quality clinical practice guidelines: How quickly do guidelines become outdated? *JAMA*. 2001; 286(12):1461–1467.

19. Shojania KG, Sampson M, Ansari MT, et al. How quickly do systematic reviews go out of date? A survival analysis. *Ann Intern Med*. 2007; 147(4):224–233.

20. Elliott JH, Synnot A, Turner T, et al. Living systematic review: 1. Introduction: The why, what, when, and how. *J Clin Epidemiol*. 2017; 91:23–30.

21. Cabana MD, Rand CS, Powe NR, et al. Why don't physicians follow clinical practice guidelines? A framework for improvement. *JAMA*. 1999; 282(15):1458–1465.

22. Greenfield S, Kaplan SH. When clinical practice guidelines collide: Finding a way forward. *Ann Intern Med*. 2017; 167(9):677–678.

23. Holoweiko M. What cookbook medicine will mean for you. *Med Econ*. 1989; 66(25):118–133.

24. Goldberger JJ, Buxton AE. Personalized medicine vs guideline-based medicine. *JAMA*. 2013; 309(24):2559–2560.
25. Moore PA, Hersh E V. Combining ibuprofen and acetaminophen for acute pain management after third-molar extractions. *J Am Dent Assoc*. 2013; 144(8):898–908.
26. Comerci G, Katzman J, Duhigg D. Controlling the swing of the opioid pendulum. *N Engl J Med*. 2018; 378(8):691–693.
27. Institute of Medicine. *The Learning Healthcare System*. Washington, DC: National Academies Press; 2007.
28. Baker DW. History of the Joint Commission's pain standards: Lessons for today's prescription opioid epidemic. *JAMA*. 2017; 317(11):1117–1118.
29. Soelberg CD, Brown RE, Du Vivier D, et al. The US opioid crisis: Current federal and state legal issues. *Anesth Analg*. 2017; 125(5):1675–1681.

24 | Developing a Culture of Opioid Stewardship

THE PENNSYLVANIA EXAMPLE

ALLISON MICHALOWSKI, SARAH BOATENG, MICHAEL R. FRASER, AND RACHEL L. LEVINE

THE COMMONWEALTH OF PENNSYLVANIA, along with other states in the Appalachian region, has been particularly hard hit by the opioid crisis. In January 2018, Pennsylvania Governor Tom Wolf declared the opioid epidemic a public health emergency to galvanize governmental efforts to respond to the crisis and use all means necessary to address it. With up to 15 Pennsylvanians dying each day from drug overdoses in 2017, "emergency" was the only suitable word to describe the severity of the situation.[1] As of 2016, the most recent year for which data are available nationwide, Pennsylvania ranked among the top five states in the country in drug-related overdose death rates.[2] Like several other states that have also declared opioid emergencies or disasters, Pennsylvania's declaration creates a unified response structure, reduces regulatory barriers to collaboration and partnership, bolsters efforts to increase access to treatment and recovery services, and expands availability to the overdose reversal medication naloxone.

Governor Wolf's emergency declaration was only part of Pennsylvania's comprehensive efforts to end the opioid misuse epidemic. In addition, the Pennsylvania Department of Health (PADOH) has led a collaboration of cross-sector partners across the Commonwealth to address opioid use disorder using public health's most powerful tool: prevention. This chapter examines the elements of Pennsylvania's efforts to prevent opioid use disorder by promoting a culture of opioid "stewardship" among providers, patients, and local and state policymakers. Similar to campaigns to promote the appropriate prescribing of antibiotic medications, such as the US Centers for Disease Control and Prevention (CDC)'s "Be Antibiotics Aware: Smart Use, Best Care" campaign, opioid stewardship focuses on activities to reduce inappropriate prescribing of opioid medication and to inform providers about best practices, to develop guidelines and standards, and to raise public awareness about the dangers of opioid misuse.[3]

The goal of opioid stewardship is to provide medical professionals with the education and tools they need to appropriately prescribe opioid medications to patients for whom an opioid is indicated and to reduce the overall supply of unused opioid medications that might be diverted and used by individuals other than the intended patient. Pennsylvania's experience illustrates that developing a statewide culture of opioid stewardship is a process requiring the active involvement of health care professionals, provider and patient groups, law enforcement agencies, academic institutions and large health systems, state policymakers and politicians, and the general public (Figure 24.1). PADOH has played a lead role in initiating the state's opioid stewardship efforts and supporting its development through research, partnerships, innovation, overall strategy, and tactical implementation. By describing Pennsylvania's experience of building a culture of opioid stewardship, we hope that other states can learn how to foster opioid stewardship among their state's health care provider communities and evolve the concept to ensure its effective spread within states and across the nation.

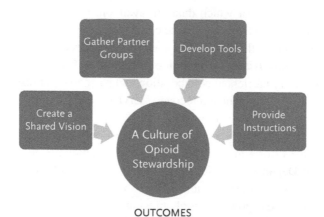

OUTCOMES
Comprehensive Evidence-Based Prescriber Education
Judicious Prescription of Opioids that Follows Established Guidelines
Increased Use of Non-Opioid Alternative Treatments for Pain
Compassionate Care for Patients that Reduces Risk of Addiction
A Healthier Pennsylvania

FIGURE 24.1. Pennsylvania's approach to developing a culture of opioid stewardship.
Source: PADOH.

Developing the Vision for a Culture of Opioid Stewardship

From first-year medical students to veteran health care professionals, establishing opioid stewardship requires changing the way prescribers think about opioid medications and their use by developing a vision that encourages judicious prescribing of opioids and promotes alternative treatments for pain. This new vision is necessary because of the way opioids were originally presented to practitioners soon after their development and introduction to the health care market. Throughout the 1990s, pharmaceutical companies that produced opioid medications promoted their widespread use to treat chronic pain.[4] These companies' provider marketing and educational materials cast their novel medications as rarely, if ever, addictive and as the most effective way to relieve a patient's pain.[4] The few studies that were used to support these claims involved small sample sizes and were often not generalizable to the broader population.[4] Nonetheless, the calls for increased prescribing of opioids for chronic pain spread.

From the Joint Commission to the American Pain Society, many professional organizations and patient advocacy groups emphasized the importance of pain relief.[5] The movement to include pain as the "fifth vital sign" swept through hospitals and doctors' offices throughout the nation. Facilities and providers were rated by patients as to how well their pain was treated, and satisfaction scores were used in part to determine a facility's quality scores and to compensate health care providers. Patient attitudes toward pain relief also shifted from viewing pain as a natural part of the healing process that could be managed but not eliminated to expectations that health care providers could make pain disappear altogether.

The combination of industry promotion of opioids and the emphasis on pain relief was reflected in providers' prescribing habits: Prescriptions for opioids rose quickly throughout the late 1990s and the 2000s.[5] In 2015, opioids were prescribed three times more than they were in 1999.[6] Throughout the 1990s and 2000s, the prescribing of opioids became standard medical practice for many types of pain, including both acute and chronic. Furthermore, this approach to pain management began to be taught in American medical schools. Opioid prescribing habits were reinforced through practice among experienced practitioners and learned through schooling and observation by newly trained providers.

With this history in mind, contemporary policymakers, public health professionals, and professional organizations saw two clear objectives in the current push to change prescribing habits that included liberal use of opioids:

1. Medical professionals in training needed to be taught comprehensive opioid education and non-opioid alternatives to evidence-based

pain management. This included a comprehensive understanding of the appropriate uses of opioids and the dangers of addiction, training in methods and medicines for treating pain that did not include opioid medications, judicious opioid prescribing using clinical guidelines and recommendations, and comprehensive pain management approaches.

2. Practicing providers needed to be informed on current practice guidelines and updated clinical recommendations, and retrained on the risks and benefits of prescribing opioids for chronic pain management.

All of this needed to include the compassionate treatment of pain, realizing that opioids are an appropriate medication for some patients, including those in palliative or hospice care and those for whom other medicines were not effective, and efforts to reduce opioid availability could have an adverse impact on this small but significant group of patients.

Gathering Partners Around the Table

With a mission to "promote healthy lifestyles, prevent injury and disease, and to assure the safe delivery of quality health care for all Commonwealth citizens," the PADOH took the lead in promoting statewide opioid stewardship efforts.[7] However, to effectively change the medical and dental prescribing cultures with buy-in from practitioners, many perspectives had to be included in the PADOH's activities. Several key partners were involved in the development and implementation of opioid stewardship–related policies, programs, and publications. These included other Pennsylvania state agencies such as the Department of Human Services, which oversees the state's Medicaid program and the state's substance misuse and addiction programs; the Department of Drug and Alcohol Programs (DDAP); and the Department of State, which licenses and sanctions health care providers through various boards. Nongovernmental organizations were also involved, including representatives from the Pennsylvania Medical Society (PAMED), the Hospital Association of Pennsylvania, the Pennsylvania State Nurses Association, the Pennsylvania Society of Physician Assistants, the Pennsylvania Coalition of Nurse Practitioners, the Pennsylvania Pharmacists Association, the Pennsylvania Dental Association, leaders from the state's medical colleges, and representatives from addiction medicine specialty groups.

Though the name and classification of organizations and departments may vary from state to state, it is important for any state working to foster opioid stewardship to identify and work with partners that fill certain roles. Working with other relevant departments within a state is crucial. Beyond offering research and experience, different departments may have the authority to support different programmatic and policy aspects of opioid stewardship. For example, the Department of Drug and Alcohol Program's expertise helped in the creation of the prescribing guidelines and the state's prescription drug monitoring program (PDMP), and the Department of State, through legislation, was able to require opioid-specific continuing education for annual licensure of medical practitioners.

Specialists in addiction medicine are important partners because they bring specific training and the experience of their practice to the table. Those whose whole work is dedicated to treating addiction have extensive knowledge about origins and triggers of addiction. Opioid stewardship is not solely about limiting the number of opioids prescribed. When necessary, it also includes prescribing in a way that limits the risk of addiction, whether through short duration, careful monitoring, or otherwise. Thus, the knowledge and experience that addiction specialists possess is critical to developing thorough and clinically feasible opioid prescribing guidelines. In Pennsylvania, which is home to 10 medical schools, addiction medicine specialists in academic medical centers served as equal partners with physicians in solo practice in the development of guidelines such that recommendations were based in the best science available at the time and grounded in the reality of implementing such measures at the practice level.

Medical educators represented another important partnership. Since medical school faculty teach the next generation of medical practitioners, they provide an excellent opportunity to advance opioid stewardship and make it a part of the work of doctoring. Working with educators and their institutions has many advantages, but medical schools are also often requested to add various content to their training curricula, creating pressure to add hours to an already years-long training program. Many schools partner with top health care systems that have addiction and pain management specialists, and these practitioners have expertise that can help in the development of curricula, core competencies, and guidelines development that are essential elements of opioid stewardship.

A state's health care professional associations and societies have considerable expertise and influence that make them essential partners in the work of opioid stewardship. Ultimately, the goal of professional organizations, including PAMED, the Pennsylvania Osteopathic Medical Association, the Pennsylvania Coalition of Nurse Practitioners, and the Pennsylvania Society of Physician Assistants, is to bring health care practitioners together to practice good medicine for the sake of their patients. Often, medical societies facilitate trainings and conduct continuing education seminars. They regularly communicate with their membership about new regulations and requirements, which was critical in informing providers about new continuing education requirements for state licensure related to opioid stewardship. State medical societies maintain up-to-date listings of all physicians in their state, so they are excellent resources for outreach and education efforts for physicians. Professional associations comprise clinically knowledgeable, respected medical professionals, many of whom have significant sway in the medical community and ties to the state political system.

Working with PAMED, the state health department developed practical, science-based opioid guidelines to guide opioid stewardship efforts. Because guideline development was collaborative, the PADOH gained professional support to establish statewide recommendations for prescribing opioids without having to go through the long and often contentious legislative process to require them. This led to quicker adoption and adherence to guidelines for proper prescribing of opioids. Furthermore, PAMED worked with other state health associations, such as the Pennsylvania State Nurses Association and the Pennsylvania Dental Association, to develop continuing education for opioid stewardship (including materials on opioid prescribing and the PDMP), which it offered free of charge for all physicians on its website. This partnership helped the PADOH reach doctors and other medical professionals across the state. PAMED had led several prior efforts to educate physicians about appropriate opioid prescribing, including the "Pills for Ills, Not Thrills" and "Be Smart. Be Safe. Be Sure." (Figures 24.2 and 24.3) educational campaigns and actively supporting physician training in the area of addiction and the creation of a skills assessment and training program for physicians identified as needing additional competence in opioid prescribing.

Pennsylvania's partnership activities and collaborative approach demonstrated that with the right set of partners working together, a state can change how medical practitioners approach opioid prescribing and pain management. Casting a "wide net" and engaging all those who had a role in opioid stewardship in the state, the PADOH managed to bring attention to the problem while also stressing the importance of preventing overdose death, appropriate prescribing of opioids, and the broader approach to preventing addiction in the first place. As a result, Pennsylvania has been frequently identified as a leader in making progress toward ending the opioid epidemic nationwide, and PADOH staff frequently work with other states and national public health leaders to share strategies and evolve the state's approach.

Developing State-Specific Opioid Stewardship Tools

The PADOH and its partners worked together to develop two complementary tools that formed the foundation of the state's opioid stewardship effort. The first of these tools, Pennsylvania Prescribing Guidelines, provided medical

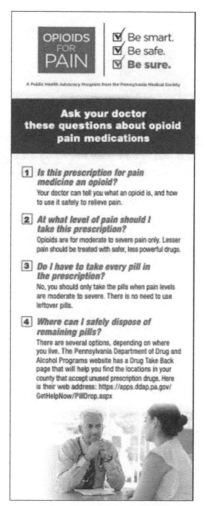

FIGURE 24.2. PAMED's "Be Smart. Be Safe. Be Sure." patient education card for use in health care providers' offices.

providers with facility-specific or physician specialty–specific information to guide prescribing practices using evidence-based prescribing options and recommendations. The other tool, Pennsylvania's PDMP, provides medical professionals with technical resources that improve their ability to practice judicious prescribing (Text Box 24.1).

In partnership with DDAP, members of PAMED, addiction specialists, and other stakeholders, the PADOH published a series of guidelines pertaining to opioid prescribing in a variety of health care settings. By working with these partners to adopt them, the PADOH was able to publish helpful, respected, and influential guidelines without having to resort to the lengthy process of

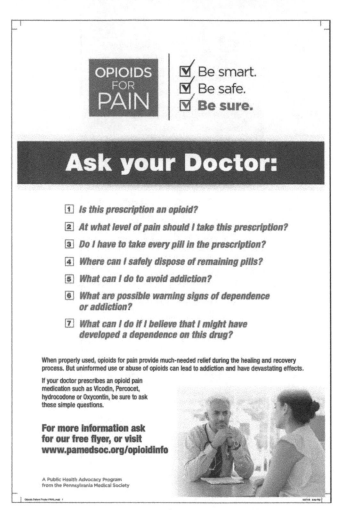

FIGURE 24.3. PAMED's "Be Smart. Be Safe. Be Sure." patient education poster for use in examination rooms and other clinical settings.

establishing their use through legislation. Each set of guidelines provides specific advice in a concise, easy-to-use document that gives providers easy access to "state of the art" clinical practice. The guidelines range from the more general "Treating Chronic Non-Cancer Pain" to the more specific, such as "The Safe Prescribing of Opioids in Orthopedics and Sports Medicine." As of August 2018, Pennsylvania had published 11 sets of prescribing guidelines. The most recent of these, "Safe Prescribing for Workers' Compensation," was published in July 2018, while the first guideline was published in 2014. These efforts also complement the work of national medical specialties that have published national guidelines and the CDC's Guideline for Prescribing Opioids for Chronic Pain.

**TEXT BOX 24.1 PENNSYLVANIA'S OPIOID STEWARDSHIP
ONLINE RESOURCES**

Pennsylvania Opioid Prescribing Guidelines:
https://www.health.pa.gov/topics/disease/Opioids/Pages/Prescribing-Guidelines.aspx
  • Treating Chronic Non-Cancer Pain
  • Emergency Department Pain Treatment Guidelines
  • Opioids in Dental Practice
  • Opioid Dispensing Guidelines
  • Obstetrics & Gynecology Opioid Prescribing Guidelines
  • Geriatric Pain
  • Use of Addiction Treatment Medications in Treatment of Pregnant
    Patients with OUD
  • Safe Prescribing of Benzodiazepines for Acute Treatment of Anxiety &
    Insomnia
  • Safe Prescribing of Opioids in Orthopedics and Sports Medicine
  • Safe Prescribing of Opioids in Pediatric and Adolescent Populations
  • Safe Prescribing for Workers' Compensation
Pennsylvania PDMP: https://www.health.pa.gov/topics/programs/PDMP/
    Pages/PDMP.aspx
Evidence-Based Prescribing Tools: https://www.health.pa.gov/topics/
    programs/PDMP/Pages/Education.aspx
LifeGuard® Program: https://www.foundationpamedsoc.org/lifeguard/
    LifeGuard-services
Pennsylvania State Core Competencies for Education on Opioids and
    Addiction: https://www.ncbi.nlm.nih.gov/pubmed/28339890
Searching for Patients Across State Lines: https://www.health.pa.gov/topics/
    programs/PDMP/Pages/Interstate.aspx
PDMP Tutorials and Policies: https://www.health.pa.gov/topics/programs/
    PDMP/Pages/Tutorial.aspx
Clinical Resources: https://www.health.pa.gov/topics/programs/PDMP/Pages/
    Clinical.aspx
Pennsylvania Medical Society Opioid-Related CMEs: https://www.pamedsoc.
    org/detail/article/Opioid-Crisis-CME
Pennsylvania State Board of Medicine: https://www.dos.pa.gov/
    ProfessionalLicensing/BoardsCommissions/Medicine/Pages/default.aspx

---

There are several characteristics that make the Pennsylvania guidelines
practical and useful to practitioners, and each of these characteristics can
be incorporated in the development or revision of guidelines in other states.
In contrast with the CDC's single Guideline document, Pennsylvania's
guidelines are specific to facilities or specialties. Each of these targets specific
fields of medicine that may need different prescribing advice because they

have different current practices, treat different types of conditions, work with various at-risk populations, or any of a variety of other reasons that influence prescribing perspectives. The variety and specificity of these guidelines make them more practical for a greater number of medical professionals because they address specific situations that practitioners can encounter. For example, specific guidelines are available for pharmacists and dentists, who require very different recommendations from physicians prescribing to chronic pain populations. To ensure these guidelines were specific, practical, and applicable to the specific medical fields for which they were designed, the PADOH worked with experts in each specific guideline setting or specialty. The guidelines are also routinely updated to make sure they include best practices in accordance with the most recent evidence available.

While designing specialty- and facility-specific guidelines is important, effective guidelines need content that is thorough and applicable as well. Effective guidelines include more than just recommended dosages and pre-scription durations. Rather, they address the whole of the opioid prescribing process, including whether to prescribe opioids in the first place. Guidelines also include how to evaluate a patient for opioid prescribing. This process includes warning practitioners of addiction risk factors, raising awareness of alternative treatments for pain, and recommending tools for addiction screening. Alternative treatments are especially important because they pro-vide practitioners with effective options that allow patients to avoid opioids altogether.

The prescribing process does not end after the initial prescription is pro-vided but rather lasts until a patient has been tapered off opioids. As such, guidelines need to provide practitioners with advice for care throughout opioid therapy so that they can monitor patients for signs of addiction, refer patients appropriately for addiction treatment, and instruct them on how to change doses. Finally, guidelines also address when and how to discontinue opioid therapy. There are many components to opioid discontinuation, in-cluding when to discontinue, the speed at which to taper, and resources to assist with drug tapering for individuals showing signs of addiction. While es-sential information should be presented concisely in the guidelines, it is also helpful to refer practitioners to other resources for additional information. For example, Pennsylvania's opioid stewardship guidelines refer providers to the CDC's *Pocket Guide for Tapering Opioids* as another respected source of information.[8]

The state's PDMP complements the prescribing guidelines by helping practitioners monitor the opioid history of patients as well as their own prescribing behaviors as providers. Pennsylvania's PDMP contains records of prescribing and dispensing of controlled drugs. This means that when-ever a controlled substance is dispensed to a patient, it is recorded in the PDMP. Beyond recording their own prescribing history, the PDMP gives health care providers access to a patient's full history of controlled substance prescriptions. Pennsylvania law requires prescribers to conduct a PDMP query in three situations:[9]

1. The first time the patient is prescribed a controlled substance by the prescriber for purposes of establishing a baseline and a thorough medical record
2. When a prescriber believes or has reason to believe, using sound clinical judgment, that a patient may be abusing or diverting drugs
3. Every time a patient is prescribed an opioid drug product or benzodiazepine by the prescriber.

According to a nationwide study involving 24 states, statewide use of a PDMP is associated with a 30% decrease in opioid prescriptions.[10] In 2016, the first year that Pennsylvania's PDMP was operational, the number of opioids dispensed decreased by 12.6%. Pennsylvania also saw a decrease in "doctor shopping" for opioid prescriptions, with the number of patients visiting five or more doctors or pharmacists for Schedule II drugs like opioids decreasing drastically.[11] Likewise, the number of patients visiting 10 or more doctors or pharmacists for such purposes decreased as well. Pennsylvania's experience shows that PDMP use is associated with more judicious prescribing practices for the reasons described below.

When providers query the PDMP, they receive a patient's controlled substance prescription history to assist with clinical decision making. When evaluating a patient prior to initiating and throughout opioid therapy, the prescribing data help providers screen patients for opioid use disorder. These data can be used to evaluate the risk of a patient developing substance use disorder should the doctor initiate therapy, or the data may show that a patient currently taking opioids is demonstrating signs of substance use disorder. Additionally, the PDMP discourages doctors from overprescribing by establishing a concrete record of their opioid prescribing activity. Regulatory authorities, including the Pennsylvania's Board of Medicine, have access to this information and can use it to identify potential overprescribing. The agencies can then contact prescribers to learn more about their practices, communicate concerns about opioid prescribing, and provide access to opioid stewardship training. In addition, practitioners are aware that data in the PDMP can be used as evidence in legal actions against them if they continuously prescribe opioids negligently or maliciously.

Providing the Instructions, Not Just the Tools

Having access to a PDMP and prescribing guidelines is necessary but not sufficient to developing a culture of opioid stewardship. In addition to these two tools, prescribers often have to change their practice of medicine, and this requires clear instructions. Education is the cornerstone of complex, dynamic fields such as medicine and health care. Practitioners enter the field knowing that they will spend their whole careers learning, and continuing education is a well-known aspect of medical practice. While many practitioners are ready to learn, they are also very busy and need access to high-quality, evidence-based education that fits the demands of busy clinical practice. Easy-to-access guides and "instruction manuals" are valued by busy trainees and practitioners seeking to add new information about opioid stewardship to their already full training and practice schedules.

As mentioned above, medical educators are key to preparing the next generation of prescribers to better understand the opioid crisis and practice opioid stewardship. Pennsylvania has the fifth highest number of total residents and fellows enrolled in primary care accredited programs in the United States, and 60% of active physicians in Pennsylvania completed their graduate medical education in the state.[12] With that in mind, Pennsylvania established several opioid-related core competencies that must be taught at every medical school in Pennsylvania. The PADOH and PAMED worked with deans from each medical school in the state to develop these core competencies.[13] The six core competencies focusing on judicious prescribing are:

1. Proper patient assessment when treating pain
2. Proper use of multimodal treatment options when treating acute pain
3. Proper use of opioids for the treatment of acute pain (after consideration of alternatives)
4. The role of opioids in the treatment of chronic non-cancer pain
5. Patient risk assessment related to the use of opioids to treat chronic non-cancer pain, including the assessment for substance use disorder or increased risk for aberrant drug- related behavior
6. The process for patient education, initiation of treatment, patient monitoring, and discontinuation of therapy when using opioids to treat chronic non-cancer pain.

Each of these topics allows for significant variability in what is taught in different schools and can be tailored depending on that school's approach. This allows schools to make the curriculum their own while still ensuring that students graduate from Pennsylvania medical schools with a thorough understanding of opioid stewardship. With this education, these graduates will enter the medical field prepared to establish a culture of opioid stewardship in their practice of medicine.

Training the next generation of prescribers is incredibly important, but with 48,549 physicians practicing in Pennsylvania as of March 2018, educating current practitioners was a priority as well. In many states, including Pennsylvania, medical licensing boards require a specific number of continuing education units to renew practice licenses. This provides the regulatory means necessary to require that every practitioner in Pennsylvania receives at least foundational knowledge in the area of opioid stewardship. While practitioners often have many potential continuing education topics to choose from, the Pennsylvania General Assembly passed, and the governor signed, legislation requiring all prescribers to complete approved opioid-related continuing education training for license renewal starting in the 2017–2018 license renewal period.[14]

In addition to the state's legislature, several other partners were essential for establishing the continuing education requirements as an effective way to increase opioid stewardship among prescribers. The Pennsylvania Board of Medicine requires documentation verifying that approved opioid education has been completed, and the Pennsylvania Department of State enforces the continuing education requirements for license renewal. Furthermore, PAMED established approved opioid stewardship trainings that are free for prescribers and can be used to meet the licensure requirement. In addition to being free, these trainings are easily accessible, as they are promoted on the websites of both PADOH and PAMED. These comprehensive trainings blend judicious prescribing practices and alternative treatments and instruct prescribers how to use the PDMP. In partnership with the University of Pittsburgh School of Medicine and the PADOH's PDMP office, PADOH worked to develop trainings in evidence-based prescribing practices. Available free on the PADOH's website, these trainings address a variety of topics, including use of the PDMP, overviews of the Commonwealth's various opioid prescribing guidelines, substance abuse risk identification, and many other crucial topics.

The topics covered in the trainings are only one part of what makes them successful; the way the content is presented makes the trainings particularly effective and relevant. These trainings focus on clinical integration and practical application in a clinical setting. Learning information is necessary, but once practice habits are established it can be difficult to change existing ways of thinking and practicing. For example, incorporating a new tool like the PDMP into patient visits means changing the workflow for a provider who may have been practicing for years. Training is needed to address best practices on how to incorporate the PDMP into patient visits and how to integrate the PDMP with electronic medical records. In addition to addressing clinically relevant subjects, these trainings also provide resources that can be used routinely during practice to reinforce the training such as checklists, pocket cards, and flowcharts that can each be used to guide clinical practice on a daily basis. To further make this information clinically relevant, Pennsylvania offers onsite training for those who request it.

In addition to preventing overprescribing, it is important to provide education specifically designed for those who are identified as not following guidelines and/or who are overprescribing opioids. Many of these prescribers are not operating "pill mills" or engaged in criminal activity; rather, they are practitioners who need help managing the patient volume and demand for opioids or have become the physician of "last resort" when a practice closes or a health system "cracks down" on opioid prescribing. The PAMED Foundation led the development of the LifeGuard program to address this population of physicians.[15] The program offers a multi-day in-person training with experienced professionals to support physicians in implementing best practices in their clinics. The in-person, interactive format allows for one-on-one training and opportunities for learners to ask questions and share insights about their practice situation. Furthermore, the program offers monitoring after the completion of the training to measure physicians' compliance with the guidelines and make sure they learned and are implementing the necessary practice changes in prescribing behaviors.

Part of opioid stewardship is identifying why prescribers may not be following guidelines and helping to inform and educate them rather than rush to judgment about aberrant prescribing behavior. With these instructional resources, prescribers are better able to use the tools provided by the PADOH and its partners to build a culture of opioid stewardship. These trainings approach judicious opioid prescribing from multiple perspectives, and together, they provide practitioners with the knowledge they need to do their part in curbing the opioid epidemic.

Summary

This chapter details Pennsylvania's experience of confronting the opioid epidemic by developing the overall concept of "opioid stewardship." While the examples are state specific, the strategies described can be applied in jurisdictions nationwide. Prevention is the cornerstone of public health. To prevent opioid addiction, opioids need to be prescribed more judiciously and efforts to retrain prescribers are needed. To build a culture of opioid stewardship, state public health agencies need to provide useful tools and instructions that address each facet of prescribing behavior and patient care related to opioid misuse and addiction. Pennsylvania's experience demonstrates that partnerships form the foundation on which a culture of opioid stewardship can be built. It is our hope that the approach used, lessons learned, and insights gleaned in Pennsylvania inform and motivate other states and territories to take similar action, adopt novel approaches, and iterate and expand the concept of opioid stewardship for their own contexts.

Disclaimer

Michael R. Fraser was the executive vice president of PAMED from 2013 to 2016. The views expressed in this chapter do not necessarily represent the views of PAMED or its members.

References

1. US Drug Enforcement Agency. DEA announces 5,456 drug-related overdose deaths in Pennsylvania in 2017. https://www.dea.gov/press-releases/2018/08/21/dea-announces-5456-drug-related-overdose-deaths-pennsylvania-2017-0. Accessed September 28, 2018.
2. US Centers for Disease Control and Prevention. Drug overdose mortality by state. https://www.cdc.gov/nchs/pressroom/sosmap/drug_poisoning_mortality/drug_poisoning.htm. Accessed September 28, 2018.
3. US Centers for Disease Control and Prevention. Be antibiotics aware: Smart use, best care. https://www.cdc.gov/features/antibioticuse/index.html. Accessed September 28, 2018.
4. Zee AV. The promotion and marketing of OxyContin: Commercial triumph, public health tragedy. *Am J Public Health*. 2009; 99(2):221–227.
5. Kolodny A, Courtwright DT, Hwang CS, et al. The prescription opioid and heroin crisis: A public health approach to an epidemic of addiction. *Ann Rev Public Health*. 2015; 36:559–574.
6. US Centers for Disease Control and Prevention. Opioid prescribing. https://www.cdc.gov/vitalsigns/opioids/infographic.html. Accessed September 28, 2018.
7. Pennsylvania Department of Health. About the Department of Health. https://www.health.pa.gov/About/Pages/About.aspx. Accessed September 28, 2018.
8. US Centers for Disease Control and Prevention. Pocket guide: Tapering opioids for chronic pain. https://www.cdc.gov/drugoverdose/pdf/clinical_pocket_guide_tapering-a.pdf. Accessed September 28, 2018.
9. Pennsylvania General Assembly. 2015 Act 191—Achieving Better Care by Monitoring All Prescriptions Program (ABC-MAP) Act. http://www.legis.state.pa.us/cfdocs/legis/li/uconsCheck.cfm?yr=2014&sessInd=0&act=191. Accessed September 28, 2018.
10. Bao Y, Pan Y, Taylor A, et al. Prescription drug monitoring programs are associated with sustained reductions in opioid prescribing by physicians. *Health Aff*. 2016; 35(6):1045–1051.
11. Pennsylvania Department of Health. Interactive data report. https://www.health.pa.gov/topics/programs/PDMP/Pages/Data.aspx. Accessed September 28, 2018.
12. Association of American Medical Colleges. Pennsylvania physician workforce profile. https://www.aamc.org/download/484584/data/pennsylvaniaprofile.pdf. Accessed March 3, 2019.
13. Ashburn MA, Levine RL. Pennsylvania state core competencies for education on opioids and addiction. *Pain Med*. 2017; 18(10):1890–1894.

14. Pennsylvania Medical Society. Answers to FAQs on new opioids continuing education requirements. https://www.pamedsoc.org/detail/article/faqs-new-opioids-CME-requirements. Accessed September 28, 2018.

15. The Foundation of the Pennsylvania Medical Society. LifeGuard services. https://www.foundationpamedsoc.org/lifeguard/LifeGuard-services. Accessed September 28, 2018.

AFTERWORD

Our Collaborative Journey

My awareness (Michael R. Fraser) of the US opioid crisis grew significantly in 2013 when I became the executive vice president of the Pennsylvania Medical Society. While I had been introduced to the issue of neonatal abstinence syndrome several years earlier when serving as chief executive officer of the Association of Maternal and Child Health Programs, my experience in Pennsylvania made the extent of the crisis clear in a state hard hit by opioid misuse and addiction. Physician leaders were not only concerned about overdose deaths and effectively treating patients with substance misuse and addiction, they were also concerned about being seen as contributing to the crisis due to perceived lax prescribing practices, the many barriers to screening for and treating addiction in the primary care setting (including stigma), and concerns that patients who legitimately needed opioids for chronic pain would be made to jump through hoops to get them.

Many physician leaders were also concerned about the impact of public health and law enforcement actions on their ability to practice to medicine in the ways they deemed most appropriate. Pennsylvania was the second-to-last state to implement a modern prescription drug program (PDMP) by replacing a paper system run by the state's Attorney General's office. When the new system was introduced, many prescribers asked for it to be voluntary for fear that mandatory use would interrupt their clinical workflow. Efforts to require mandated continuing medical education (CME) in opioid prescribing as a condition of physician licensure were resisted by some physicians who wanted to choose their own CME courses, did not prescribe opioids, or believed there were already enough requirements to licensure as it was. Statewide opioid prescribing guidelines,[1] as well as the Center for Disease Control and Prevention (CDC)'s opioid prescribing guideline,[2] were initially seen by some as a move to limit the "art" of medicine and could serve as unapproved standards instead of clinical suggestions to health care providers. What I learned during those three years at the Pennsylvania Medical Society was that the scope of the crisis was growing at an alarming rate, my peers leading other medical and health professional societies at the state and national level were equally concerned about the crisis, and the solutions to the crisis would not come from a clinical focus but rather an approach that stressed community-wide solutions that addressed root causes of addiction versus treating patients individually.

While my orientation to the crisis was as an association executive working on the issue with physician leaders and state policymakers, my co-author (Jay C. Butler)'s experience as a frontline infectious disease physician working with individuals using injection drugs in a clinical setting, and then as Alaska's state health officer working to address the crisis at the community level, led to many different learnings from Alaska and public health and health care agencies across the country.

My (Butler) interest in addiction was piqued by clinical work I was doing before my appointment as state health official. A number of my patients were infected with hepatitis C virus acquired through self-injection drug use, and with the release of highly effective antiviral agents, cure was finally within reach. As a clinician, this was incredibly satisfying, bringing back memories of two decades earlier when speaking with AIDS patients about new drugs that we believed could suppress HIV. But in the case of hepatitis C, we were discussing high likelihood of *cure*. However, a few of my patients troubled me; some returned to using self-injected drugs. Another patient with hepatitis C said that she had entered into treatment for opioid addiction only after a friend had asked to use her needle and syringe. Her friend told her that impending withdrawal would make her too sick to care for her family and get to work on time, so she did not care if she became infected by sharing gear with someone with documented hepatitis C. She and I pondered why an intelligent and caring person with much to live for would do something so apparently irrational. It got me thinking: As an infectious diseases physician, I realized that my life was full of patients who had lost control of their lives to addiction, and I had to question my past assumptions about what addiction really is. Addiction is more than a series of bad decisions or a lack of will.

As Alaska's state health official, I was able to continue the conversations with people in recovery. I realized that these people were mostly invisible to my clinical colleagues and me because many people do recover but are hesitant to share their past experience with health care providers because of stigma. Some were willing to share their experiences with opioids. One person described the sensation of injecting heroin as "like Jesus came and gave me a big, warm hug." This insight and the knowledge of how the reward centers of the brain function and are altered by addiction changed my view of persons with addiction. Who would not want to feel unconditional love and forgiveness? It helped me to understand why someone would use, to see that no one is totally immune to addiction, and that persons who have experienced trauma can be particularly vulnerable. The shared experiences provided the insight I needed into how the emerging epidemiologic data and our understanding of the neurobiology of addiction can translate into policy to address the opioid crisis. The long-lasting changes in brain function that occur in addiction convinced me that public health approaches to the opioid crisis should be founded on the concept of addiction as a chronic health condition involving the brain. This was reinforced by colleagues in law enforcement who were making similar observations. One drug enforcement officer told me, "I spent years undercover and have lived with these people— none of them would ever have chosen to be where they ended up," any more than someone would "choose" to develop lung cancer as a result of nicotine addiction.

As awareness of the crisis grew, I was not surprised when the first agenda item for a one-hour health briefing with Alaska Governor Bill Walker was the opioid crisis. In preparing for the brief, I cleaned up a graphic of an opioid prevention pyramid (see Chapter 3) that I had initially doodled while my mind wondered during a long finance committee hearing during the prior legislative session. The pyramid features three levels of public health activities: those that prevent life-threatening complications of addiction (tertiary prevention), those that remove barriers and increase access to treatment and long-term recovery (secondary prevention), and those that prevent addiction from developing in the first place by addressing the supply and demand drivers of the crisis (primary prevention). The governor was engaged and supportive, and we never got past the first item on our agenda. Leaving the meeting, I knew that I had my marching orders for the rest of my time as state health official and the theme for the Association of State and Territorial Health Officials (ASTHO) President's Challenge for the coming year.

Past Perspectives of Addiction: Partners in Recovery

In 2016, our paths crossed when Fraser became the ASTHO's CEO and Butler assumed the office of ASTHO president. Butler's President's Challenge to peer state and territorial public health leaders was to take a public health approach to the opioid crisis and lead efforts within states and territories that address prevention of substance misuse and addiction. Fraser's second day as ASTHO's chief executive was spent with Butler in a room full of representatives from over 60 different groups working on various aspects of the opioid crisis. The

2017 ASTHO President's Challenge developed out of that convening and catalyzed ASTHO's efforts to promote a public health approach to ending the crisis and increased federal investment for states to move upstream and fund primary prevention programs that addressed the root causes of addiction, not just opioid misuse but also alcohol, tobacco, and other substances. ASTHO's work continues to be informed by Jay's challenge and was reaffirmed by Dr. John Wiesman, Secretary of Health for Washington State, when he became ASTHO's president in 2017 and continued the effort for an additional year. Dr. Nicole Alexander-Scott, Director of the Rhode Island Department of Health, moves the issue even farther with the 2019 ASTHO President's Challenge by focusing on building healthy and resilient communities.

The idea for a public health *Guide* to ending the opioid crisis is rooted in our individual and shared journeys. From the vantage point of a medical society executive looking at how to best support state efforts to prevent opioid use disorder, Fraser should not have been surprised by the lack of attention to the primary prevention of addiction but was surprised at how little was being implemented at the local and state levels when it came to preventing opioid use disorder at the community versus individual patient level. Butler's journey as a physician and state health officer included insights that a broader focus on addiction was needed. As others have pointed out, there are more deaths due to alcohol than opioid overdoses, and that was indeed true in Alaska. What made the opioid and overdose response so critical, however, was the rapid increase in deaths in both Alaska and nationwide, which urgently raised the need for rapid public health action.

Our shared journey at ASTHO underscored the need for national attention to the opioid crisis from the vantage point of public health. While numerous efforts were being undertaken to respond to the crisis in states and territories in 2016, the role of public health was still varied in states and federal investments focused mostly on overdose prevention and surveillance. New or rekindled partnerships were being developed among public health; existing substance abuse, drug, and alcohol programs; and health care provider organizations and professional societies. However, public health was also forging new collaborative ground with law enforcement, housing, education, and employment agencies by taking a "health in all policies" approach with a specific focus on opioid use disorder and addiction.

As is typical with emerging issues, states were experimenting with different approaches to addiction prevention, leading to a variety of lessons about what works and what does not when it comes to prevention of substance misuse and addiction. Some of those innovations and experiments are described in this volume with an eye toward replication and/or customization at the local and state levels. However, there was a clear need for a synthesis of emerging approaches to prevention as well as review of the fundamentals of a public health approach to the opioid crisis.

Two events reaffirmed our observation that more was needed to describe the role that public health practitioners could play in ending the opioid epidemic. The first was the passage of the 21st Century Cures/CARES Act in December 2016. That Act primarily funded treatment and recovery services, as well as US National Institutes of Health (NIH) research on addiction, but not broader work around primary prevention of addiction. Second, the declaration of the opioid overdose crisis as a public health emergency by the Trump administration in October 2017 demonstrated to us the urgent need for both overdose prevention and a commensurate focus on the primary prevention of addiction in communities nationwide. These events led to advocacy by ASTHO and its partners for funds specifically addressing the primary prevention of substance use disorder and addiction that resulted in $350 million to CDC in FY2019.

Core to this *Guide* is the simple, yet also extremely complex, insight that a public health approach brings to ending the opioid crisis: that the best way to end the crisis is to prevent substance misuse and addiction in the first place. Over the past several years, public health leaders working on ending the crisis have recognized that we will not treat or arrest our way out of the current situation; instead, we must focus on preventing it. This is not to minimize the lifesaving work of overdose reversal or to diminish the role of important tools such as PDMPs, public health surveillance efforts in tandem with law enforcement interdiction activities, prescribing guidelines, and education and awareness raising. Rather, it is taking a core public health principle (preventing disease in the first place is the best way to treat it) and applying it to the opioid crisis.

Experience with our nation's other drug crises, including methamphetamines and crack cocaine, illustrates that while opioid misuse is on the radar screen now, as efforts to reduce the supply of opioids are successful, the demand will shift to another substance unless we do not treat and prevent addiction in the first place. The "war on drugs" is seen by some as a failure not because it failed to cut off the supply of drugs to the United States but because it only focused on the supply side and did little to effectively address demand.

Numerous academic studies, papers, and reports and several practical guides have been written to describe the public health and health care impact of the crisis and guide efforts to end it. Stories of addiction have illustrated the deep personal effect that opioid misuse and addiction have had on the lives of so many of our family members, friends, and neighbors. The successful journeys of so many individuals in recovery have inspired us and helped us see hope in what is often portrayed as hopeless. This *Guide* is meant to inspire and inform the work of public health practitioners, students, and others with an interest in practical approaches to preventing opioid misuse and the address the root causes of addiction.

References

1. Pennsylvania Department of Health. Opioid Prescribing Guidelines. https://www.health.pa.gov/topics/disease/Opioids/Pages/Prescribing-Guidelines.aspx. Accessed February 13, 2019.
2. US Centers for Disease Control and Prevention. CDC Guideline for Prescribing Opioids for Chronic Pain. https://www.cdc.gov/drugoverdose/prescribing/guideline.html. Accessed February 12, 2019.

ABOUT THE AUTHORS

Caleb Alexander, MD, MS
Dr. Alexander is an associate professor of epidemiology and medicine at the Johns Hopkins Bloomberg School of Public Health, where he serves as founding co-director of the Center for Drug Safety and Effectiveness and principal investigator of the Johns Hopkins–FDA Center of Excellence in Regulatory Science and Innovation. Dr. Alexander is a practicing general internist and pharmacoepidemiologist and is internationally recognized for his research examining prescription drug utilization, safety, and effectiveness.

Nicole Alexander-Scott, MD, MPH
Dr. Alexander-Scott serves as the director of the Rhode Island Department of Health. Dr. Alexander-Scott is the 2018–2019 president of the Association of State and Territorial Health Officials (ASTHO), the national organization for state and territorial health directors. Dr. Alexander-Scott is board certified in pediatrics, internal medicine, pediatric infectious diseases, and adult infectious diseases.

Leigh Alderman, JD, MPH
Leigh Alderman serves as the senior advisor to the director of the Georgia Health Policy Center. Leigh's focus is in partnering with the community stakeholders to address identifying the health determinants using the skills from strategy planning, systems, health policy and design, and facilitation. Alderman helps to support the Robert Wood Johnson Foundation–sponsored *Bridging for Health: Improving Community Health through Innovations in Financing*, the Legislative Healthy Policy Certificate Program, and a statewide strategic planning initiative to address the opioid crisis.

Samantha Arsenault, MACD

Samantha Arsenault is the director of National Treatment Quality Initiatives for Shatterproof. In this role, Sam manages the Substance Use Treatment Task Force and provides strategic guidance and support to critical stakeholders across sectors to improve the quality of substance use disorder treatment nationally. Prior to joining Shatterproof, Sam worked on the Substance Use Prevention and Treatment Initiative at the Pew Charitable Trusts. In this role, Sam worked to advance programs and policies that improve access to and the quality of substance use disorder treatment at the state and federal levels, with a focus on medication-assisted treatment for opioid use disorder, and changes to infrastructure and payment systems.

John Auerbach, MBA

John Auerbach is the president and CEO of the Trust for America's Health, a nonprofit, nonpartisan organization dedicated to saving lives by protecting the health of every community and working to make disease prevention a national priority. Formerly he served as the associate director for policy and the acting director of the Office for State, Tribal, Local, and Territorial Support at the US Centers for Disease Control and Prevention. From 2012 to 2014, Auerbach was a professor of practice in health sciences and the director of the Institute on Urban Health Research and Practice at Northeastern University.

Sarah Bacon, PhD

Dr. Bacon leads two of the US Centers for Disease Control and Prevention (CDC)'s opioid overdose prevention initiatives: Prevention for States and the Data-Driven Prevention Initiative. Dr. Bacon began her time at CDC in 2010 in the National Center for Injury Prevention and Control's Division of Violence Prevention, where she was the lead scientist for the National Centers of Excellence in Youth Violence Prevention, a strategic initiative for implementing and evaluating violence prevention strategies in high-burden communities. While much of her work focuses on evaluation, Sarah is also fully immersed in implementation science and has significant hands-on experience with the implementation realities that often challenge our scientific agendas. Sarah moved to the Division of Unintentional Injury Prevention in 2015, where she leads the division's efforts to prevent prescription drug overdose.

Grant Baldwin, PhD, MPH

Since 2008, Grant Baldwin has served as the director of the Division of Unintentional Injury Prevention at the National Center for Injury Prevention and Control in the Centers for Disease Control and Prevention (CDC). Dr. Baldwin has been with the CDC since 1996 and in 2006 joined the CDC Injury Center, where he served as deputy director. With nearly a decade of leadership at the Injury Center, he has assisted in improving motor vehicle injury prevention and has aided in the response to the prescription drug overdose epidemic. He has also enhanced efforts of older adult fall prevention and CDC's prevention of traumatic brain injury.

Colleen L. Barry, PhD, MPP

Dr. Barry is the Fred and Julie Soper Professor and Chair of the Department of Health Policy and Management at the John Hopkins Bloomberg School of Public Health. She has a joint appointment in the Department of Mental Health. Professor Barry's research focuses on how health and social policies can affect a range of outcomes for individuals with mental illness and substance use disorders, including access to medical care and social services, care quality, health care spending, financial protection, and mortality.

Mark Bicket, MD

Since 2015, Dr. Bicket has been a part of the Johns Hopkins Department of Anesthesiology/Critical Care Medicine. He takes care of patients at the Blaustein Pain Treatment Center in Baltimore, Maryland, and dedicates his time to research. Dr. Bicket specializes in the treatment of chronic and neuropathologic pain. He performs fluoroscopically guided or ultrasound-guided interventions, and he focuses on applications of ultrasound in chronic pain. He is currently leading research on treatments for lower back pain and their evidence base. Dr. Bicket is also working toward a master's degree in health sciences in the Johns Hopkins Bloomberg School of Public Health.

Sarah Boateng

Sarah Boateng is the executive deputy secretary at the Pennsylvania Department of Health, where she focuses on the state's response to the opioid crisis. She led the development of the state's evidence-based, specialty-specific prescribing guidelines. Boateng also contributed to the development of the PacMAT treatment model and Pennsylvania's warm-handoff protocol. She previously served as the special assistant to the physician general at the Pennsylvania Department of Health and the director of public affairs at Planned Parenthood Keystone.

Michael Botticelli, M.Ed.

Michael serves as the executive director of the Grayken Center for Addiction Medicine at the Boston Medical Center. He previously served as the director of the White House Office of National Drug Control under President Obama. He was also the director of the Bureau of Substance Abuse Services at the Massachusetts Department of Public Health.

Jane Branscomb, MPH

For over a decade, Jane has delivered research, technical assistance, and evaluation for local and national clients of Georgia Health Policy Center. She utilizes systems thinking and tools to aid stakeholders collaborate and share strategies. She helped initiate the creation of 2010 Minimum Elements and Practice and

Standards for Health Impact Assessment and the creation of SOPHIA, an international professional association focused on advancing excellence in the practice of health impact assessment.

Jay C. Butler, MD
Dr. Butler is the former director of the Public Health Division and chief medical officer for the Alaska Department of Health & Social Services (DHSS). Prior to his DHSS appointments in December 2014, he was senior director for community health services and also the medical director for infection control and employee health at the Alaska Native Tribal Health Consortium. He worked for DHSS between 2005 and 2009 as the chief medical officer and the state epidemiologist. Dr. Butler completed over 23 years of service as a US Public Health Service medical officer, during which he served as the director of the US Centers for Disease Control and Prevention (CDC)'s Arctic Investigations Program in Anchorage, Alaska, and as a medical epidemiologist in the CDC's National Center for Infectious Diseases in Atlanta, Georgia.

Ruben Cantu
Ruben Cantu is a program manager for community trauma, mental health, and violence prevention. He has more than 20 years of nonprofit experience in public health, equity, program and organizational management, and technical assistance and capacity building. Most recently Associate Director at the California Pan-Ethnic Health Network (CPEHN), Ruben managed development, outreach, and communications initiatives to inform, mobilize, and advocate for the constituents of the state's largest multicultural health policy organization. Before his nine years at CPEHN, Ruben was Senior Specialist and Project Director at Mosaica: The Center for Nonprofit Development and Pluralism in Washington, DC, where he led activities funded by the U.S. Department of Health and Human Services, Office of HIV/AIDS Policy and provided technical assistance to small and large community organizations across the country. He has held positions at the National Minority AIDS Council and Human Rights Campaign, also in Washington, D.C. A native Texan and graduate of the University of Houston, he serves on Regional Asthma Management and Prevention's advisory committee and several state mental health advisory committees. He has worked extensively with organizations and community members fighting to advance health equity for the underserved.

Alexis Captanian
Alexis Captanian is a Masters Candidate at the NYU Robert F. Wagner Graduate School of Public Service. She was previously a Program Coordinator at Prevention Institute where she played a central role in the Institute's projects to advance mental health and wellbeing. The Institute combines a passion for equity and community change with expertise in developing strategies, best

practices, writing, and training in the fields of health system transformation, injury and violence prevention, chronic disease prevention, healthy eating and physical activity, and mental health and wellbeing. She holds a BA in Public Health from the University of California at Berkeley.

Jennifer J. Carroll, PhD, MPH

Dr. Carroll is a medical anthropologist, research scientist, and subject matter expert on substance use and public health. She is currently an assistant professor of anthropology at Elon University, North Carolina, and an adjunct assistant professor of medicine at the Alpert Medical School at Brown University, Rhode Island. Dr. Carroll's first book, *Narkomania: The Addiction Imaginary at Peace and at War*, is forthcoming from Cornell University Press. Based on her dissertation work, *Narkomania* is an ethnographic study of internationally funded treatment programs for opioid use disorder in Ukraine and the impact of drug use and drug users on the ongoing geopolitical conflict in this region.

Jac A. Charlier, MPA

Jac Charlier is the executive director for Treatment Alternatives for Safe Communities (TASC)'s Center for Health and Justice. A national expert in crime reduction and pre-arrest diversion, he specializes in practical solutions that bring together justice system partners, behavioral health service providers, and community leaders in common aims of creating safer, healthier communities. Since 2011, he has led the growth and evolution of TASC's Center for Health and Justice, which provides national and international consulting, training, public policy strategy, and research dissemination to help create more just justice systems. As the co-founder in 2017 of the national Police, Treatment and Community Collaborative and a leader in justice system strategies to fight the national opioid epidemic, Jac led the development of a framework for preventing and reducing opioid overdose and death among justice populations, as well as community-based post-overdose response strategies for law enforcement.

Sana Chehimi

Sana Chehimi joined Prevention Institute in 2003. Sana leads Prevention Institute's federal engagement and partnership outreach efforts by directing the organization's policy and advocacy portfolio, aimed at supporting upstream prevention policies and investments to advance health, safety, wellbeing, and health equity. She provides core staffing to the Convergence Partnership, a collaboration of seven leading foundation and healthcare institutions working to foster healthier and more equitable environments for all children and families. Sana provides training and technical assistance to philanthropies, government agencies, coalitions, and community-based organizations on cutting-edge prevention practices and strategy development to address underlying community determinants of health and improve community health and equity. She co-edited one of the first academic texts on primary prevention, Prevention Is Primary: Strategies for Community Wellbeing (jointly published by Jossey-Bass/Wiley and the American Public Health Association in 2007 and 2010), with PI Founder Larry Cohen and Dr. Vivian Chavez of San Francisco State University. She is lead writer of and contributor to numerous articles and publications on community wellbeing and comprehensive primary prevention strategies to advance social justice and promote healthy communities. Before joining Prevention Institute, Sana worked in the HIV field as an outreach and education associate. She leveraged her background in biology and research to support the development of California's first statewide certificate program for HIV Education, and conducted local, state, and national HIV health education trainings for health and human service providers. She holds a master's degree in Public Health from the University of California, Berkeley and a BA from Columbia University.

Jennifer G. Clarke, MD, MPH, FACP

Dr. Clarke is the medical programs director at the Rhode Island Department of Corrections. She is also an associate professor of medicine at the Warren Alpert Medical School of Brown University. She has been the principal investigator on several grants funded by the National Institute of Health and has over 100 peer-reviewed publications. She is a national leader in expanding access to medications for addiction treatment for people in corrections.

Jeffery P. Engel, MD

Dr. Engel is the executive director of the Council of State and Territorial Epidemiologists (CSTE), an organization that involves members of states and territories that represent state and local government epidemiologists. From 2002 to 2009 Dr. Engel served as North Carolina's health director, in which he directed various public health achievements. He led the state's response and increased prevention services during the H1N1 pandemic, initiated a statewide ban on smoking in restaurants and bars, helped to significantly decrease the incidence rates of HIV infection rate, and helped to reduce infant mortality rates to an all-time low.

Dana Fields-Johnson, MPA

Dana Fields-Johnson joined the Prevention Institute staff in September 2016 and works in the Health Equity and Violence Prevention focus areas. Dana has more than 20 years of professional experience and has worked in public health to address maternal and child well-being, chronic disease and obesity prevention, healthy eating, and active living with an emphasis on policy, systems and environmental change, community safety, and violence prevention. Most recently, Dana was director of programs for the Health Education Council in West Sacramento, California, where she provided leadership to the agency's regional prevention programs and was responsible for implementing the overall agency strategy and approach to improving the health and quality of life for low-income families and communities of color.

Elizabeth M. Finkelman, MPP

Elizabeth Finkelman is a program officer in the Office of the President at the National Academy of Medicine (NAM), where she manages special projects and initiatives, including the Action Collaborative on Countering the US Opioid Epidemic, Healthy Longevity Grand Challenge, and the Vital Directions for Health and Health Care initiative. She completed her undergraduate degree at McGill University, double-majoring in cell and molecular biology and political science, and has a Master of Public Policy degree with a concentration in health policy from the George Washington University.

Anthony Folland, BA

Tony Folland serves as the clinical services manager and state opioid treatment authority for the Vermont Department of Health, Division of Alcohol and Drug Abuse Programs, and has been in state service since 2010. In the Vermont system of care, Tony has regulatory oversight of both the hub and spoke parts of the provider system. Prior to state government, he served for nearly 20 years as a clinician, program director, and clinical director in various mental health/substance abuse organizations, both in rural and urban settings, and for several years was the clinical director of Vermont's initial buprenorphine induction hub.

Derek C. Ford, PhD

Dr. Ford is a fellow on the Morbidity & Behavioral Surveillance Team within the Surveillance Branch in the Division of Violence Prevention at the National Center for Injury Prevention and Control at the US Centers for Disease Control and Prevention. Much of his current work is focused on examining risk and protective factors for adverse childhood experiences and their impact on subsequent mental and physical health outcomes throughout the life course. Dr. Ford participates in several cross-cutting projects and partnerships related to his work on the Adverse Childhood Experiences Study in the Division of Violence Prevention.

Michael R. Fraser, PhD, MS, CAE

Dr. Fraser is the chief executive officer of the Association of State and Territorial Health Officials (ASTHO). Previously, he served as the executive vice president and CEO of the Pennsylvania Medical Society in Harrisburg. In addition to nationally recognized work at the Pennsylvania Medical Society to address the state's opioid misuse and drug abuse crisis, Dr. Fraser has been a distinguished leader in public health for almost 20 years. He served as CEO of the Association of Maternal and Child Health Programs from 2007 to 2013 and as Deputy Director of the National Association of County and City Health

Officials, and worked in various roles at the US Department of Health and Human Services. He is affiliated faculty at George Mason University College of Health and Human Services' Department of Community Health and an adjunct professorial lecturer at the Milken Institute School of Public Health at George Washington University.

Brett P. Giroir, MD

Dr. Giroir serves as assistant secretary for health at the US Department of Health and Human Services (HHS). Dr. Giroir is a physician, scientist, and innovator. He is a former medical school executive and biotech startup CEO and has served in several leadership positions in the federal government as well as academia. He also serves as senior advisor to the secretary for opioid policy. In this capacity, he is responsible for coordinating HHS's efforts across the Trump administration to fight America's opioid crisis.

Valerie N. Goodson, MPA

Valerie Goodson is an associate research analyst for the Council of State and Territorial Epidemiologists (CSTE). She is tasked with building capacity for substance abuse and mental health surveillance within local jurisdictions, states, tribal centers, and territories.

Nicholas E. Hagemeier, PharmD, PhD

Dr. Hagemeier serves as associate professor at the Gatton College of Pharmacy, East Tennessee State University (ETSU). He is the co-investigator of the $2.2 million Diversity-Promoting Institutions Drug Abuse Research Program at ETSU, funded by the National Institute of Health, and is principal investigator on one of the core projects focused on prescription drug abuse interprofessional communication. Dr. Hagemeier is also the Research Director of ETSU's Center for Prescription Drug Abuse Prevention and Treatment. He also serves as director of the College of Pharmacy's Community Pharmacy Practice Research Fellowship.

Debra E. Houry, MD, MPH

Dr. Houry is the director of the National Center for Injury Prevention and Control at the US Centers for Disease Control and Prevention (CDC). Dr. Houry serves as a leader in key research and science-based programs to prevent injury and violence and decrease their consequences. She has helped to increase support for programs that aid states in preventing prescription drug overdose and improve reporting of violent death rates. Prior to joining the CDC, she served as vice-chair and associate professor in the Department of Emergency Medicine at Emory University School of Medicine and associate professor in the Departments of Behavioral Science and Health Education and in Environmental Health at the Rollins School of Public Health.

Rachel Katonak, PhD, RN

Dr. Katonak is a public health analyst for Dr. Vanila Singh, chief medical officer in the Office of the Assistant Secretary for Health, US Department of Health and Human Services, and an officer with the US Public Health Service. Since 2009, LCDR Katonak worked with the Indian Health Service as a nurse case manager. She dedicated her graduate education to building her expertise in chronic pain and health disparity issues with the completion of her PhD in nursing at the University of Arizona.

Karmen Kurtz

Karmen Kurtz is the Open Homes Causes Coordinator at Airbnb. Previously she was a Program Assistant with Prevention Institute where she provided core programmatic support to several of the Institute's topical teams. She holds a BA in International Relations and Affairs with a minor in Africana Studies from University of North Carolina at Asheville.

Michael Landen, MD, MPH

Dr. Landen is the state epidemiologist with the New Mexico Department of Health. Dr. Landen served as a family physician and clinical director for the Indian Health Service in Arizona and New Mexico, and as a volunteer physician in Belize. In 1995, he worked as an Epidemic Intelligence Service officer assigned to the Alaska Department of Health and Social Services.

Mark Levine, MD

Dr. Levine is the commissioner of the Vermont Department of Health. He was previously a professor of medicine at the University of Vermont (UVM), associate dean for graduate medical education, and institutional officer at the College of Medicine and UVM Medical Center. He has served on the American College of Physicians Board of Regents and was elected vice president and president-elect of the Vermont Medical Society.

Rachel L. Levine, MD

Dr. Levine is the secretary of health and physician general for the Commonwealth of Pennsylvania and professor of pediatrics and psychiatry at the Penn State College of Medicine. Dr. Levine has made substantial efforts combating the opioid epidemic by helping to establish opioid prescribing guidelines and establishing opioid prescribing education for medical students. She was previously vice-chair for clinical affairs for the Department of Pediatrics and chief of the Division of Adolescent Medicine and Eating Disorders at Penn State Hershey Children's Hospital/Milton S. Hershey Medical Center.

Kumiko Lippold, PhD

Dr. Lippold is an ORISE fellow in the Office of the Assistant Secretary for Health (OASH) in the Department of Health and Human Services. As a fellow, she provides scientific support on a broad range of health topics, including drug overdose, kidney disease, sickle cell disease, and others. Her primary research in OASH focuses on the intersection of race/ethnicity and urbanicity in opioid-involved overdoses. Prior to joining HHS, she received her PhD in Pharmacology and Toxicology in 2018 from the Virginia Commonwealth University. Her doctoral dissertation work focused on the preclinical development of opioid-sparing adjunctive therapies for the treatment of acute pain. She received her bachelors of Science degree from Virginia Tech in 2014. She is also currently studying at the George Washington University for her Masters of Public Health Degree and will complete it in 2019.

Jan L. Losby, PhD, MSW

Dr. Losby is a behavioral scientist who serves as the team lead for the Opioid Overdose Health Systems Team, Division of Unintentional Injury Prevention, at the US Centers for Disease Control and Prevention (CDC). Dr. Losby is responsible for evaluating and advancing the implementation of CDC's Guideline for Prescribing Opioids for Chronic Pain; conducting applied health systems research; and building scientific evidence to support state, community, and tribal efforts to address the opioid overdose epidemic. Prior to working with CDC, Dr. Losby managed the evaluation arm of a nonprofit organization where she designed and conducted evaluations of social service and public health programs in welfare reform, asset development, refugee services, mental health, substance abuse, and employment.

Mark Lysyshyn, MD, MPH

Dr. Lysyshyn serves as a medical health officer with Vancouver Coastal Health, where he leads the health authority's response to the opioid overdose emergency. He specializes in public health and preventive medicine and internal medicine. In the past, he practiced addiction medicine at St. Paul's Hospital in Vancouver. Dr. Lysyshyn is currently a clinical assistant professor at the University of British Columbia School of Population and Public Health.

Brigitte Manteuffel, PhD, MA

Dr. Manteuffel is a senior research associate at the Georgia Health Policy Center, where she leads efforts to address the opioid epidemic through policy, practice, and research. Her interests focus on improving the infrastructure for addressing the opioid epidemic, as well as the evidence-based prevention and treatment of behavioral health disorders. Manteuffel is an expert in mixed-methods evaluation of children's mental health systems of care (including mental health, child welfare, juvenile justice, education, and primary care) and has special expertise in youth substance use and substance use disorder treatment.

Rosemarie A. Martin, PhD

Dr. Martin is an assistant professor at the Center for Alcohol and Addiction Studies, Department of Behavioral and Social Sciences at Brown University School of Public Health, and is the program evaluation director for the medication-assisted treatment program at the Rhode Island Department of Corrections. Dr. Martin co-directs the New England Addiction Technology Transfer Center and the New England State Targeted Response Technical Assistance Center. These two centers, funded by the US Substance Abuse and Mental Health Services Administration, provide training and technical assistance to address substance use and opioid use disorder prevention, treatment, and recovery.

Kenneth J. Martz, PsyD, CAS

Dr. Martz is a licensed psychologist and the special assistant to the secretary in the Commonwealth of Pennsylvania. He has worked in substance use disorder treatment and management of special populations including criminal justice clients in community corrections and in prison settings for the past 20 years. Dr. Martz has also worked in a variety of settings, including outpatient and residential and therapeutic communities, providing treatment of addictions, including gambling.

Melissa T. Merrick, PhD
President & CEO

Dr. Merrick is a behavioral scientist with the Surveillance Branch in the Division of Violence Prevention at the US Center for Disease Control and Prevention's National Center for Injury Prevention and Control. Dr. Merrick's key work involves studying safe and nurturing relationships and environments, as they relate to child maltreatment prevention, and examining the effects of adverse childhood experiences, particularly maltreatment, throughout the lifespan. She also serves as the Science Lead for the Adverse Childhood Experiences (ACE) Study. Dr. Merrick leads other projects, including the Division of Violence Prevention's surveillance of safe, stable, nurturing relationships in collaboration with the US Department of Justice, Office of Juvenile Justice and Delinquency Prevention, and the National Survey of Children's Exposure to Violence.

J. Michael McGinnis, MD, MA, MPP

Dr. McGinnis is the senior scholar and executive director of the National Academy of Medicine. He was the founder of multiple programs, such as Healthy People, the HHS/USDA Dietary Guidelines for Americans, the US Preventative Task Force, and Ten Essential Services for Public Health. He received his bachelor's degree at Berkeley, his master's and medical degrees at UCLA, and his master of public policy degree at Harvard's Kennedy School of Government.

Jamie Mells, PhD

Dr. Mells has a diverse background in nutritional biochemistry and biology, having completed a master's degree in biology from Austin Peay State University and recently a PhD in nutrition and health sciences from Emory University. He joined the US Public Health Service in 2013 and began his work at the US Centers for Disease Control and Prevention in 2014 as a quarantine public health officer in the Division of Global Migration and Quarantine. Stationed at Hartsfield Jackson Airport, he was an integral part of the Ebola response at the airport, providing technical assistance and training to federal partner and city stakeholders. Previously he served as the director of minority affairs at Tennessee Technological University.

Benjamin F. Miller, PsyD

Benjamin Miller is the chief strategy officer of the Well Being Trust. At the Department of Family Medicine at the University of Colorado School of Medicine, he was the founding director of the Eugene S. Farley, Jr. Health Policy Center, where he remains a senior advisor. Ben has been a principal investigator on many federal and foundation grants as well as state contracts related to health and health care integration. Ben is a technical expert panelist for the US Centers for Medicare & Medicaid Services on quality measure development for Medicaid beneficiaries as well as for the Medicaid Innovation Accelerator Program.

Allison Michalowski

Allison Michalowski is an Eugene DuPont Distinguished Scholar at the University of Delaware, pursuing her bachelor's degrees in psychology and liberal studies of public health. During her internship with Dr. Rachel Levine, Pennsylvania's secretary of health and physician general, Allison researched best practices, developed new policies, and led a group of highly qualified individuals and created a strategic model for the group to sustain a robust Institutional Review Board. At the University of Delaware, Allison has developed local policy tools through the Complete Communities group at the Institute for Public Administration and conducts food access research with the Center for Research in Education and Social Policy.

Karen Minyard, PhD, MN

Dr. Minyard has been director of the Georgia Health Policy Center since 2001 and is also a research professor with the Department of Public Management and Policy. Minyard connects the research, policy, and programmatic work of the center across issue areas including population health, health philanthropy, public and private health coverage, and the uninsured. Minyard has experience with the state Medicaid program, both with the design of program reforms and external evaluation.

Rita K. Noonan, PhD

Dr. Noonan is the leader of the Health Systems and Trauma Branch in the Division of Unintentional Injury, National Center for Injury Prevention and Control, at the US Centers for Disease Control and Prevention (CDC), where both drug overdose and traumatic brain injury prevention activities reside. Before joining the CDC, Dr. Noonan taught sociology and women's studies as a professor at the University of Iowa. She led research in Latin America on global debt crisis, gender, social movements, and health outcomes.

Alexandra Nowalk, MPH, CPH, CHES

Alexandra is the screening, brief intervention, and referral to treatment (SBIRT) program director at the University of Pittsburgh, School of Pharmacy, for the Program Evaluation and Research Unit. Her background includes mental health research and work in the nonprofit sector to address health disparities in minority populations. She earned her master's degree in public health with a certificate in global health from the University of Pittsburgh, specializing in behavioral and community health sciences.

Janice Pringle, PhD

Dr. Pringle is an epidemiologist by training with extensive experience in health services research. Her areas of focus include addiction services research, especially involving the application of screening, brief intervention, and referral to treatment (SBIRT) within various health care settings. She served as director of Pennsylvania's SBIRT Initiative's Data Coordinating Center and is one of the principal investigators funded by the Substance Abuse Mental Health Services Association to develop and implement an SBIRT curriculum for medical residencies throughout Pennsylvania. Dr. Pringle is also leading the evaluation of a Pharmacy Quality Alliance–funded initiative within Pennsylvania that has involved the application of SBI techniques with community pharmacists for improving medication adherence.

Wesley M. Sargent, Jr., EdD

Dr. Sargent is a health scientist on the Prescription Drug Overdose Health Systems Team in the US Centers for Disease Control and Prevention (CDC)'s Division of Unintentional Injury Prevention (DUIP). He joined DUIP in 2014 as an evaluation fellow, working on multiple prescription drug overdose projects, which included the CDC Guideline for Prescribing Opioids for Chronic Pain and the evaluation of the Substance Abuse and Mental Health Administration's Prescription Drug Monitoring Program (PDMP)'s Electronic Health Records Integration and Interoperability Expansion Program. Sargent's current responsibilities include working with CDC-funded states to enhance PDMPs, implement community or insurer/health system interventions, evaluate policy/ legislative initiatives, and provide scientific and technical assistance.

Sheila Savannah, MA

Sheila Savannah is the director of the Prevention Institute, where her work has focused on building local assets for multi-sector systems transformation. Sheila serves on the FRIENDS National Advisory Council on Community-Based Child Abuse Prevention and previously served as an expert advisor for several bodies, including the Center for Health Care Strategies Committee on Consumer Advancement, the Harris County Regional Advisory Council on Medicaid Managed Care, and the Texas Commission on Alcohol and Drug Abuse Multicultural Advisory Committee. In 2009, she was a children's mental health panelist for Vice President Al Gore's Conference on Families and Health, and in 2014 she was a US Centers for Disease Control and Prevention Grand Rounds Panelist on Preventing Youth Violence.

Vanila M. Singh, MD

Dr. Singh serves as the chief medical officer for the Office of the Assistant Secretary for Health at the US Department of Health and Human Services (HHS). Her main role is to serve as the primary medical advisor to the assistant secretary for health on the development and implementation of HHS-wide public health policy recommendations. Dr. Singh has been a clinical associate professor of anesthesiology and perioperative and pain medicine at Stanford University School of Medicine. Board-certified in both anesthesiology and pain medicine, she treats patients with complex chronic pain.

Gary Tennis, JD

Gary Tennis serves as president and CEO of the National Alliance for Model State Drug Laws. He is a specialist in drafting and developing treatment, intervention, and prevention model laws, policies, guidelines and strategies. Tennis was a prosecutor in the Philadelphia District Attorney's Office from 1980 to 2006. In 2012, he became the first secretary of Pennsylvania's Department of Drug and Alcohol Programs, during which he served as an officer on the National Association of Substance Abuse Drug and Alcohol Directors (NASADAD) Board. Tennis was awarded the NASADAD Award for Exceptional Leadership and Support of Substance Abuse Prevention and Treatment in 2014 and the National Ramstad-Kennedy award in 2015.

Megan Toe, MSW

Megan Toe is a senior research analyst at the Council of State and Territorial Epidemiologists (CSTE), where she focuses on behavioral health. She previously worked for the Mental Health Liberia Initiative at the Carter Center, where she managed activities in partnership with the Liberian government to help strengthen the national mental health system through training, policy, and advocacy.

Philicia Tucker, MPH
Philicia Tucker is the research assistant for the Association of State and Territorial Health Officials (ASTHO). She received her master's degree in public health with a concentration in global health from the George Mason University Department of Health and Human Services.

Mark Tyndall, MD, ScD
Dr. Tyndall is the executive medical director of British Columbia's Center for Disease Control. He is the deputy provincial health officer, the director of the University of British Columbia (UBC) Centre for Disease Control Research Institute, and a professor at the UBC School of Population and Public Health. Previously, Dr. Tyndall was the chief of the Division of Infectious Diseases at the University of Ottawa and a senior scientist at the Ottawa Hospital Research Institute. He lived in Kenya for four years as part of the World Health Organization's collaborative research group on HIV. Dr. Tyndall was also the program director for epidemiology at the British Columbia Center for Excellence in HIV/AIDS and was a co-lead investigator on the evaluation of Insite, North America's first supervised injection site.

Anne Van Donsel
Anne Van Donsel is the director of performance management and evaluation for the Division of Alcohol and Drug Abuse Programs at the Vermont Department of Health, where she has worked for over 20 years. Her work identifies areas of opportunity for change, supports new and existing programming, and monitors the effectiveness of the activities undertaken by the division.

Meena Vythilingam, MD
CDR (USPHS) Meena Vythilingam is a board certified psychiatrist and the Deputy Director of Psychological Health for the US Marine Corp. She attended Yale University School of Medicine for her residency training in psychiatry in addition to training at the National Institute of Mental Health and Neurosciences (NIMHANS), Bangalore, India. After her post-doctoral fellowship at Yale University, she served on the faculty as an Assistant Professor. She then led clinical research for 8.5 years at the Mood and Anxiety Disorders Program at the National Institute of Mental Health (NIMH), Bethesda, MD. Over the course of her time at Yale, NIMHANS and the NIMH, CDR Vythilingam published more 75 peer-reviewed articles on posttraumatic stress disorder, depression and psychological resilience. She joined the Department of Defense (DoD) in 2009 as the Deputy Director of Psychological Health (PH) Strategic Operations at Force Health Protection & Readiness, in the Office of the Assistant Secretary of Defense (Health Affairs) where she led policies

on deployment mental health assessment and combat operational stress. She also served in leadership positions in the Defense Centers of Excellence for Psychological Health and Traumatic Brain Injury (DCoE) where she led numerous DoD PH efforts including program evaluation. She has received numerous awards to include the DoD and USPHS Meritorious Service Medals, Commendation Medals, Applied Public Health Physician of the Year, and an Army Achievement Medal.

Joseph Wendelken
Joseph Wendelken is the public information officer for the Rhode Island Department of Health. He previously worked in the fields of print journalism and translation. He is a graduate of Providence College.

Greg Williams, MA
Greg Williams is a filmmaker and recovery leader. He made the award-winning documentary *The Anonymous People*, which follows the history and struggles of over 23 million individuals living in recovery. He was also the co-founder of Facing Addiction, a national nonprofit organization dedicated to discovering solutions to the addiction crisis by unifying the voice of over 45 million Americans and their families directly impacted by addiction. Greg served as the campaign director and one of the executive producers of the historic Unite to Face Addiction Rally on the National Mall in Washington, DC, on October 4, 2015.

Jessica Wolff, MPH
Jessica Wolff has six years of program evaluation and project management experience in a variety of public health fields, including global HIV/AIDS prevention, youth suicide prevention, and children's mental health services. She is project manager for the Heroin Response Strategy, a 20-state collaborative between public health (Centers for Disease Control and Prevention) and public safety (High Intensity Drug Trafficking Areas) to address the opioid epidemic. Prior to her work with the Heroin Response Strategy, Jessica was a senior research associate at a public health consulting firm, providing evaluation training and technical assistance to federally funded grantees.

INDEX

Tables, figures, and boxes are indicated by *t*, *f*, and *b* following the page number

For the benefit of digital users, indexed terms that span two pages (e.g., 52–53) may, on occasion, appear on only one of those pages.

economic mobility, and comprehensive approach to opioid crisis, 174, 178
economic security, and systems-based prevention strategies, 216
education
 core competencies of judicious prescribing, 318
 and developing a culture of opioid stewardship, 317–320
 of health professionals in addiction, 14–15, 37–38
 patient counseling and education, community pharmacies and, 67
 patient education card, 303*f*, 313*f*
 patient education poster, 314*f*
 pharmacy accreditation standards, 65–66
educators, public health agency collaboration with, 152–153
electronic health information, and integration of care, 15
"Emergence of an Epidemic, The," 7–18
emergency medical services (EMS), public health agency collaboration with, 148–149
EMPOWER Center for Health, Blair County, Pennsylvania, 83*b*
Engel, Jeffrey P., "Public Health Surveillance and the Opioid Crisis," 253–264
Enhanced State Opioid Overdose Surveillance, 256
epidemic, emergence of opioid, 7–8
 drivers of epidemic, 10–16
 evolution of opioid use in United States, 8–10
 implications for controlling the epidemic, 16–17
epidemiologists, workforce needs and public health surveillance, 261
equity, promoting in broad terms, 192
Essentials for Childhood: Assuring Safe, Stable, Nurturing Relationships and Environments for All Children, 217, 218*b*, 219
exercise therapy, and nonpharmacologic pain management, 58

Facing Addiction in America, 14
faith communities, public health agency collaboration with, 151
families
 parental substance misuse, impacts of, 214–215
 strengthening economic security of, 216
 and "upstream" approach to preventing addiction, 188–189, 189*b*
federal drug-control spending, priorities, 36*f*
Feedback-Listening-Options brief intervention model, 85–86
fentanyl
 drug checking for, 25
 early warning program in Ohio, 245–246, 246*f*
 EMS personnel safety and, 148–149
Fentanyl Overdose Reduction Checking Analysis Study (FORECAST), 25
Fields-Johnson, Dana, "Addressing Community Trauma and Building Community Resilience to Prevent Opioid Misuse and Addiction," 199–209
financing disincentives, and integration of care, 16
Finkelman, Elizabeth M., "The Emergence of an Epidemic," 7–18
first responders
 collaboration with public health agencies, 148–149
 overdose prevention and, 26–27
Folland, Anthony, "Expanding Access to Treatment and Recovery Services Using a Hub-and-Spoke Model of Care," 95–105
Fraser, Michael R.
 "A Comprehensive Approach to Addressing the Opioid Crisis," 171–179
 "Developing a Culture of Opioid Stewardship: The Pennsylvania Example," 307–321

"The Role of Public Health Agencies in Convening Partnerships and Collaborations to Respond to the Opioid Crisis," 137–157

"Why a Public Health Guide to Ending the Opioid Crisis?", 3–6

Georgia, systems thinking and opioid epidemic in, 159–160, 168–169
  application of systems thinking, 160, 161*f*, 162
  describing misuse, treatment, and recovery, 162–167
  leveraging change, 167–168
  misuse and overuse strategic map, 163*f*
  Opioid Systems Map, 161*f*, 162–167
Giroir, Brett P., "Countering the Opioid Epidemic," xv–xx
Goodson, Valerie N., "Public Health Surveillance and the Opioid Crisis," 253–264
"Guideline for Prescribing Opioids for Chronic Pain," 294, 295*b*

Hagemeier, Nicholas E., "The Role of Community Pharmacy in Addressing and Preventing Opioid Use Disorder," 65–76
harm reduction, 29
  definition of, 23
  drug checking and alerting, 25–26
  hydromorphone distribution, 28
  injectable therapies, 27
  peer engagement and, 28–29
  public health approaches to, 23–31
  supervised consumption, 24–25
  "take-home" naloxone, 26–27
Harrison Narcotic Act of 1914, 8
health, biopsychosocial model of, 56
Health and Human Services, U.S. Department of
  five-point strategy to combat opioids crisis, xvi*f*
  opioid crisis response priorities, 173*t*
Healthcare Cost and Utilization Project (HCUP), 258

healthcare facilities, public health agency collaboration with, 145
healthcare professionals
  building workforce capacity among, 14–15
  burnout among, 144
  education in addiction, 14–15
  public health agency collaboration with, 143–145
health insurance coverage, substance use disorders and, 37, 107–109, 119
  adequacy of plan network, 113–114
  alternative payment models, 115–116
  carve-outs and fragmentation, 112–113
  cost sharing, 111–112
  covered services, 109, 111
  data sharing, 117
  high out-of-network utilization, 113–114
  payment timeliness, 114
  prior-authorization policies, 118
  reimbursement rates, 114
  utilization management, 118–119
  value-based payment models, 115–116
Health Insurance Portability and Accountability Act (HIPAA) of 1996, 243–244
health insurers, public health agency collaboration with, 153
health system, as driver of opioid epidemic, 14–16
Helping to End Addiction Long Term, xviii
heroin
  development and medicinal use of, 8
  and injectable therapies, 27
  and return of veterans from Vietnam War, 225, 227
  1960s rates of illegal use, 11
heroin addiction, and former use of prescription opioids, 13
"high-impact" chronic pain, prevalence of, 55
High Intensity Drug Trafficking Areas (HIDTAs), 241–242, 242*f*

mood-altering effects, use of opiates for, 9
morbidity and mortality, opioid misuse
   community pharmacies, role in
      preventing, 66–70
   opioid addiction, xv, 7
   primary prevention of, 67–70
   secondary prevention of, 71–73
   tertiary prevention of, 73–74
mortality surveillance, 260
muscle relaxants, and non-opioid pain
   management, 61

naloxone
   improving access to, xvi*f*,
      xvii–xviii, 19–20
   and public health agency collaborations
      with EMS, 148
   "take-home" naloxone, 26–27
   and tertiary prevention of morbidity
      and mortality, 73–74
National Association of Drug Court
   Professionals, 232
National Center for Injury Prevention and
   Control (NCIPC), 259
National Council on Alcoholism and Drug
   Dependence (NCADD), xii–xiii
National Hospital Care Survey (NHCS), 258
National Institutes of Health, xviii
National Resilience Strategy, "upstream"
   prevention efforts and, 182, 183*b*
National Survey on Drug Use and Health
   (NSDUH), 255, 257–258
National Syndromic Surveillance Program
   (NSSP), 259–260
Nationwide Emergency Department
   Sample (NEDS), 258
needle service programs, 19
negative affect stage of addiction, 47–48
neonatal abstinence syndrome (NAS)
   prevention, 70
neuropathic pain, non-opioid
   management of, 61
neuroscience of addiction, 45, 51
   and evidence base to destigmatize
      opioid addiction, 49–50
   neurologic function, 45–47, 46*f*

and public health practice and
   policy, 48–50
stages of addiction, 47–48
tolerance, development of, 47
New Mexico, Project ECHO in, 144
news media, public health agency
   collaboration with, 147–148,
   147*f*, 149*f*
New York
   overdose response in Erie County,
      247–248
   RxStat initiative in New York City,
      246–247
NMDA-receptor antagonists, and non-
   opioid pain management, 61
nonsteroidal anti-inflammatory drugs, and
   non-opioid pain management, 60–61
Noonan, Rita K., "Building Effective
   Public Health and Public Safety
   Collaborations to Prevent Opioid
   Overdose at the Local, State, and
   Federal Levels," 241–251
North American Opiate Medication
   Initiative (NAOMI), 27
Nowalk, Alexandra, "Screening, Brief
   Intervention, and Referral to
   Treatment (SBIRT) as a Public
   Health and Prevention Strategy to
   Address Substance Misuse and
   Addiction," 77–94

Ohio
   prescription-drug monitoring program
      (PDMP), 285
   promoting community-level solutions
      in, 205*b*
   public health and safety collaboration
      in, 245–246, 246*f*
opioid abuse, increase in rates of, 13
opioid addiction
   access to treatment, xvi, 14–16
   increase in rates of, 13
   increase in 1960s, 9
   morbidity and mortality, xv, 7
   prevalence of, xv
   primary prevention of, 50, 67–70